SECOND EDITION

Essential Medical Statistics

Betty R. Kirkwood

MA MSc DIC, Hon MFPHM, FMedSci
Professor of Epidemiology and International Health
London School of Hygiene and Tropical Medicine
University of London

Jonathan A.C. Sterne

MA MSc PhD
Reader in Medical Statistics and Epidemiology
Department of Social Medicine
University of Bristol

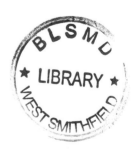

Blackwell
Science

© 1988, 2003 by Blackwell Science Ltd
a Blackwell Publishing company
Blackwell Science, Inc., 350 Main Street,
  Malden, Massachusetts 02148–5020, USA
Blackwell Publishing Ltd, 9600 Garsington Road, Oxford
  OX4 2DQ, UK
Blackwell Science Asia Pty Ltd, 550 Swanston Street,
  Carlton, Victoria 3053, Australia

First published 1988
Second edition 2003
Reprinted 2003, 2004, 2005

Library of Congress Cataloging-in-Publication Data
Kirkwood, Betty R.
  Essential medical statistics/Betty R. Kirkwood,
  Jonathan A.C. Sterne.—2nd ed.
    p. ; cm.
Rev. ed. of: Essentials of medical statistics/Betty R. Kirkwood. 1988.
Includes bibliographical references and index.
  ISBN 0–86542–871–9

  1. Medicine–Research–Statistical methods. 2. Medical statistics.
    [DNLM: 1. Statistics. 2. Biometry. WA 950 K59e 2003]
      I. Sterne, Jonathan A. C. II. Kirkwood, Betty R. Essential
      medical statistics. III. Title.

  R853.S7 K497 2003
  610′. 7′27—dc21
                                                    2002015537
ISBN 0–86542–871–9

A catalogue record for this title is available from the British Library

Set in 10/13pt Times by Kolam Information Services Pvt. Ltd, Pondicherry, India
Printed and bound in United Kingdom by MPG Books Ltd, Bodmin, Cornwall

Commissioning Editor: Fiona Goodgame
Editorial Assistant: Vicky Pinder
Production Editor: Karen Moore
Production Controller: Kate Charman
For further information on Blackwell Publishing, visit our website:
www.blackwellpublishing.com

Contents

Preface to the second edition

The practice of medical statistics has changed considerably since the first edition was written. At that time the age of the personal computer was just beginning, and serious statistical analyses were conducted by specialist statisticians using mainframe computers. Now, there is ready access to statistical computing—even the most sophisticated statistical analyses can be done using a personal computer. This has been accompanied by the growth of the evidence-based medicine movement and a commitment of medical journals to improve the statistical rigour of papers they publish.

These changes mean that the boundary between what used to be considered 'basic' or 'essential' statistics and more advanced methods has been blurred. A statistical analysis presented in a leading general medical journal is more likely to use logistic regression (formerly considered a specialist technique) than to present results from χ^2 tests. In this second edition we describe the most commonly used regression models—multiple linear regression, logistic regression, Poisson regression and Cox regression—and explain how these include many basic methods as special cases. By including chapters on general issues in regression modelling, interpretation of analyses and likelihood, we aim to present a unified view of medical statistics and statistical inference, and to reflect the shift in emphasis in modern medical statistics from hypothesis testing to estimation. Other new chapters introduce methods, some relatively new, that allow common problems in statistical analysis to be addressed; these include meta-analysis, bootstrapping, robust standard errors, and analysis of clustered data.

Our aim throughout has been to retain the strengths of the first edition, by keeping the emphasis on enabling the reader to know which method to apply when. We have therefore structured the book into parts relating to the analysis of different types of outcome variable, and included new chapters on linking analysis to study design, measures of association and impact, and general strategies for analysis.

A number of the larger datasets used in the chapters on regression modelling are available for downloading from the book's website (www.blackwellpublishing. com/essentialmedstats), to allow readers to reproduce the analyses presented or try out further analyses for themselves. Readers are also invited to visit the website to check for corrections and updates and to give feedback, which we welcome.

In writing this second edition, we have benefited from advice and support from many colleagues, students and friends. In particular, we would like to thank the many readers who gave feedback on the first edition and inspired us to embark on this, Cesar Victora, Kate Tilling and Simon Cousens for so willingly commenting on early drafts in detail, David Clayton and Michael Hills for generous advice and unstinting help on many occasions, George Davey Smith for helpful comments on a number of draft chapters and the late Paul Arthur for his enduring encouragement and advice. We would like to express our appreciation to Christopher Baum, James Carpenter, Matthias Egger, Stephen Frankel, David Gunnell, Richard Hayes, Sharon Huttly, Mike Kenward, Peter McCarron, Roger Newson, Steven Oliver, Andrew Polmear, Bianca de Stavola, and Lesley Wood for helpful discussions and for sharing their insights into statistical issues. We are grateful to James Carpenter, Erik Christensen, Shah Ebrahim, Alison Elliot, Richard Hayes, David Kessler, Carl-Johan Lamm, Debbie Lawlor, Steven Oliver, Mary Penny, Seif Shaheen and Bianca de Stavola, who generously provided datasets for use as examples. We would also like to thank Maggie Rae and Alan Haworth, whose generous hospitality facilitated much writing, and last but not least Harriet Aston, Emily, Kitty and Max Sterne, Alex Khot, and Sam and Daisy Kirkwood, for their support and the difference they make in our lives.

Betty Kirkwood
Jonathan Sterne

Preface to the first edition

The aim in writing this book has been to put the multitude of statistical methods applicable to medical research into their practical context, and in doing this I hope I have combined simplicity with depth. I have adopted a somewhat different ordering of topics than found in most books, based on a logical progression of practical concepts, rather than a formal mathematical development. Statistical ideas are introduced as and when needed, and all methods are described in the context of relevant examples drawn from real situations. There is extensive cross-referencing to link and contrast the alternative approaches which may apply in similar situations. In this way the reader is led more quickly to the analysis of practical problems and should find it easier to learn which procedures are applicable and when.

This book is suitable for self-instruction, as a companion to lecture courses on medical statistics, and as a reference text. It covers all topics which a medical research worker or student is likely to encounter. Some advanced (or uncommon) methods are described only briefly, and the reader referred to more specialist books. It is hoped, however, that it will be a rare event to look for a topic in the index, and not to find even a mention. All formulae are clearly highlighted for easy reference, and there is a useful summary of methods on the inside front and back covers.

The book is a concise and straightforward introduction to the basic methods and ideas of medical statistics. It does not, however, stop here. It is intended also to be a reasonably comprehensive guide to the subject. For anyone seriously involved in statistical applications, it is not sufficient just to be able to carry out, for example, a t test. It is also important to appreciate the limitations of the simple methods, and to know when and how they should be extended. For this reason, chapters have been included on, for example, analysis of variance and multiple regression. When dealing with these more advanced methods the treatment concentrates on the principles involved and the interpretation of results, since with the wide availability of computing facilities it is no longer necessary to acquire familiarity with the details of the calculations. The more advanced sections may be omitted at a first reading, as indicated at the relevant points in the text. It is recommended, however, that the introductions of all chapters are read, as these put the different methods into context.

The reader will also find such topics as trend tests for contingency tables, methods of standardization, use of transformations, survival analysis and case–control studies. The last quarter of the book is devoted to issues involved in the design and conduct of investigations. These sections are not divorced in any way from the sections on methods of analysis and reflect the importance of an awareness of statistics throughout the execution of a study. There is a detailed summary of how to decide on an appropriate sample size, and an introduction to the use of computers, with much of the common jargon explained.

This book has been compiled from several years' experience both of teaching statistics to a variety of medical personnel and of collaborative research. I hope that the approach I have adopted will appeal to anyone working in or associated with the field of medical research, and will please medical workers and statisticians alike. In particular, I hope the result will answer the expressed need of many that the problem in carrying out statistical work is not so much learning the mechanics of a particular test, but rather knowing which method to apply when.

I would like to express my gratitude to the many colleagues, students, and friends who have assisted me in this task. In particular, I would like to thank David Ross and Cesar Victora for willingly reading early drafts and commenting in great detail, Richard Hayes for many discussions on teaching over the years, Laura Rodrigues for sharing her insight into epidemiological methodology with me, Peter Smith for comments and general support, Helen Edwards for patient and skilled help with the typing, and Jacqui Wright for assistance in compiling the appendix tables. I would also like to thank my husband Tom Kirkwood not only for comments on many drafts, endless discussions and practical help, but also for providing unfailing support and encouragement throughout. It is to him this book is dedicated. Finally, I would like to mention Daisy and Sam Kirkwood, whose birth, although delaying the finalization of an almost complete manuscript, provided me with an opportunity to take a fresh look at what I had written and make a number of major improvements.

Betty Kirkwood

PART A

BASICS

Statistics is the science of collecting, summarizing, presenting and interpreting data, and of using them to estimate the magnitude of associations and test hypotheses. It has a central role in medical investigations. Not only does it provide a way of organizing information on a wider and more formal basis than relying on the exchange of anecdotes and personal experience, it takes into account the intrinsic variation inherent in most biological processes. For example, not only does blood pressure differ from person to person, but in the same person it also varies from day to day and from hour to hour. It is the interpretation of data in the presence of such variability that lies at the heart of statistics. Thus, in investigating morbidity associated with a particular stressful occupation, statistical methods would be needed to assess whether an observed average blood pressure above that of the general population could simply be due to chance variations or whether it represents a real indication of an occupational health risk.

Variability can also arise *unpredictably* (randomly) within a population. Individuals do not all react in the same way to a given stimulus. Thus, although smoking and heavy drinking are in general bad for the health, we may hear of a heavy smoker and drinker living to healthy old age, whereas a non-smoking teetotaller may die young. As another example, consider the evaluation of a new vaccine. Individuals vary both in their responsiveness to vaccines and in their susceptibility and exposure to disease. Not only will some people who are unvaccinated escape infection, but also a number of those who are vaccinated may contract the disease. What can be concluded if the proportion of people free from the disease is greater among the vaccinated group than among the unvaccinated? How effective is the vaccine? Could the apparent effect just be due to chance? Or, was there some bias in the way people were selected for vaccination, for example were they of different ages or social class, such that their baseline risk of contracting the disease was already lower than those selected into the non-vaccinated group? The methods of statistical analysis are used to address the first two of these questions, while the choice of an appropriate design should exclude the third. This example illustrates that the usefulness of statistics is not confined to the analysis of results. It also has a role to play in the design and conduct of a study.

In this first part of the book we cover the basics needed to understand data and commence formal statistical analysis. In Chapter 1 we describe how to use the book to locate the statistical methods needed in different situations, and to progress from basic techniques and concepts to more sophisticated analyses.

Before commencing an analysis it is essential to gain an understanding of the data. Therefore, in Chapter 2 we focus on defining the data, explaining the concepts of populations and samples, the structure of a dataset and the different types of variables that it may contain, while in Chapter 3 we outline techniques for displaying and tabulating data.

CHAPTER 1

Using this book

1.1 INTRODUCTION

People usually pick up a statistics book when they have data to analyse, or when they are doing a course. This has determined the structure of this book. The ordering of topics is based on a logical progression of both methods and practical concepts, rather than a formal mathematical development. Because different statistical methods are needed for different types of data, we start by describing how to define and explore a dataset (rest of Part A). The next three parts (B, C and D) then outline the standard statistical approaches for the three main types of outcome variables (see Section 1.3). Statistical ideas are introduced as needed, methods are described in the context of relevant examples drawn from real situations, and the data we have used are available for you to reproduce the examples and try further analyses (see Section 1.6). In Part E, we introduce a collection of more advanced topics, which build on common themes in Parts B to D. These are beyond the scope of most introductory texts. The final part of the book (Part F) is devoted to issues involved in the design and conduct of a study, and how to develop an analysis strategy to get the best out of the data collected.

This book is intended to appeal to a wide audience, and to meet several needs. It is a concise and straightforward introduction to the basic methods and ideas of medical statistics, and as such is suitable for self-instruction, or as a companion to lecture courses. It does not require a mathematical background. However, it is not just an introductory text. It extends well beyond this and aims to be a comprehensive reference text for anyone seriously involved in statistical analysis. Thus it covers the major topics a medical research worker, epidemiologist or medical statistician is likely to encounter when analysing data, or when reading a scientific paper. When dealing with the more advanced methods, the focus is on the principles involved, the context in which they are required and the interpretation of computer outputs and results, rather than on the statistical theory behind them.

1.2 GETTING STARTED (PART A)

The other chapters in Part A deal with the basics of getting to know your data. In Chapter 2 ('Defining the data') we explain the link between populations and samples, and describe the different types of variables, while in Chapter 3 we outline simple techniques for tabulating and displaying them.

In particular, we introduce the distinction between **exposure variables** or **risk factors** (that is variables which influence disease outcomes, including medical treatments) and **outcome variables** (the variables whose variation or occurrence we are seeking to understand). Assessing the size and strength of the influence of one or more exposure variables on the outcome variable of interest is the core issue that runs throughout this book, and is at the heart of the majority of statistical investigations.

1.3 FINDING THE RIGHT STATISTICAL METHOD (PARTS B–D)

The appropriate statistical methods to use depend on the nature of the outcome variable of interest. Types of outcome variables are described in detail in Chapter 2; they may be essentially one of three types:

1 Numerical outcomes, such as birthweight or cholesterol level.
2 Binary outcomes, summarized as proportions, risks or odds, such as the proportion of children diagnosed with asthma, the proportion of patients in each treatment group who are no longer hypertensive, or the risk of dying in the first year of life.
3 Rates of mortality, morbidity or survival measured longitudinally over time, such as the survival rates following different treatments for breast cancer, or the number of episodes of diarrhoea per person per year among AIDS patients.

Parts B, C and D comprehensively cover the full range of standard methods for these three types of outcome respectively, and will be sufficient for the majority of analysis requirements. The emphasis throughout is on how to choose the right method for the required analysis, how to execute the method and how to interpret the results from the computer output. A quick guide to the appropriate statistical methods for the analysis of the different types of outcome variable is included on the inside covers.

The key concepts underlying statistical methods are all introduced in Part B in the context of analysing numerical outcomes, but they apply equally to all the statistical methods in the book. Statistics is used to evaluate the association between an exposure variable and the outcome of interest. More specifically, it is used to measure this association in the data collected from the particular sample of individuals in our study and to make inferences about its likely size and strength in the population from which the sample was derived. In Chapter 6, we introduce the use of a **confidence interval**, to give a range of values within which the size of the association in the population is likely to lie, taking into account **sampling variation** and **standard error**, which reflect the inherent variation between individuals.

Hypothesis tests (also known as **significance tests**) and **P-values**, introduced in Chapter 7, are used to assess the strength of the evidence against the **null hypothesis** that there is no true association in the population from which the sample was drawn.

The methods in these three core parts of the book range from simple techniques such as *t*-tests or chi-squared tests for comparing two exposure groups, to the use of regression models for examining the effect of several exposure variables. Throughout we aim to show how these **regression models** arise as natural extensions to the simpler methods. These more sophisticated analyses are no longer the preserve of the trained statistician. They are widely available in statistical software packages and can be used by anyone with a desktop or notebook/laptop computer, and a moderate level of computer expertise. *The more advanced sections can be omitted at a first reading, as indicated at the relevant points in the text.* It is recommended, however, that the introductions of all chapters be read, as these put the different methods into context.

1.4 GOING FURTHER (PART E)

Parts B, C and D comprehensively cover the full range of standard methods for the three types of outcome variables. This range of methods will be sufficient for the majority of analysis requirements. Part E is for those who wish to go further, and to understand general issues in statistical modelling. It can be omitted until needed.

In Part E we explain the idea of **likelihood**, upon which most statistical methods are based, discuss generic issues in regression modelling, so that skills learned in applying one type of regression model can be applied directly to the others, and describe methods that allow us to relax the assumptions made in standard statistical methods. We also include chapters for two specialised areas of analysis. The first is the analysis of **clustered data**, which arise, for example, in cluster-randomized trials where communities, rather than individuals, are randomized to receive the intervention or to act as control. The second is on **systematic reviews** and **meta-analyses**, which synthesize findings from several independent studies. Finally, we include a brief overview of the **Bayesian approach** to statistical inference.

In these more advanced chapters our emphasis is on a practical approach, focussing on what the reader needs to know to conduct such analyses, and what is needed to critically appraise their reporting in scientific papers. However, we recommend that only the introductions of the chapters be attempted at first reading. The detail can be omitted and used only when the necessity arises, and/ or the reader has acquired experience of basic regression modelling.

1.5 UNDERSTANDING THE LINKS BETWEEN STUDY DESIGN, ANALYSIS AND INTERPRETATION (PART F)

The results of a study are only as good as the data on which they are based. Part F addresses the links between study design, analysis and interpretation. It starts by explaining how to choose the right analysis for each of the main types of study

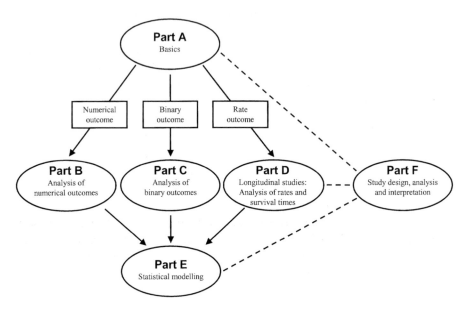

Fig. 1.1 Organization of this book.

design. It then describes how to choose an appropriate sample size, the effects of measurement error and misclassification, and the different ways in which associations can be measured and interpreted.

Finally, it is essential to plan and conduct statistical analyses in a way that maximizes the quality and interpretability of the findings. In a typical study, data are collected on a large number of variables, and it can be difficult to decide which methods to use and in what order. In Part F we aim to navigate you through this, by describing how to plan and conduct an analysis. Time invested here before you start pays off. Millions of trees must have been sacrificed to unplanned data analyses, where the data were looked at in every way imaginable. Equally often, gaps in analyses are discovered when the analyst tries to present the results. In fact it is not uncommon for people to find themselves going back to the drawing board at this stage. Careful planning of analyses should avoid these frustrations.

Of course, the issues discussed in Part F will affect all stages of the analysis of a study. This is illustrated in Figure 1.1, which shows how this book is organized.

1.6 TRYING OUT OUR EXAMPLES

Almost all statistical analyses are now done using computers, and all but very large datasets (those with measurements made on hundreds of thousands of individuals) can now be analysed using standard (desktop or laptop) office or home computers. Although simple analyses can be done with a hand-held calculator, even for these the use of a computer is recommended because results will be produced more quickly and be more accurate. For more complex analyses it is essential to use computers. Computers also allow production of high quality graphical displays.

For these reasons, we have conducted all analyses in this book using a computer. We have done these using the statistical package Stata (Stata Corporation, College Station, TX, USA; see www.stata.com). For simple analyses, we have included raw data where possible to enable readers to try out our examples for themselves. Most regression analyses presented in this book are based on datasets that are available for downloading from the book's web site, at www.blackwellpublishing.com/ EssentialMedStats. Readers may wish to use these datasets either to check that they can reproduce the analyses presented in the book, or to practice further analyses.

In general, hand-held calculators do not provide facilities to perform a large enough range of statistical analyses for most purposes. In particular, they do not allow the storage of data or analysis commands that are needed to make sure that an analysis can be reproduced (see Chapter 38). However, calculators are useful for quick calculations and checking of results (both one's own and those in scientific papers). The minimum requirements are keys for scientific functions (such as square root and logarithm) and at least one memory. The new generation of handheld computers and personal organizers is blurring the distinction between calculators and computers, and it is likely that statistical software for such devices will become available in the future.

1.7 THIS BOOK AND EVIDENCE-BASED MEDICINE

As discussed above, statistics is the science of collecting, summarizing, presenting and interpreting data, and of using them to estimate the size and strengths of associations between variables. The core issue in medical statistics is how to assess the size and strength of the influence of one or more exposure variables (risk factors or treatments) on the outcome variable of interest (such as occurrence of disease or survival). In particular it aims to make inferences about this influence by studying a selected sample of individuals and using the results to make more general inferences about the wider population from which the sample was drawn.

The approach of evidence-based medicine is like a mirror to this. Inferences are made the other way around; by appraising the evidence based on the average effect of a treatment (or exposure) assessed on a large number of people, and judging its relevance to the management of a particular patient. More specifically, practitioners need to ask themselves what to consider before they can assume that the general finding will apply to a particular patient. For example, does the patient share the same characteristics as the group from which the evidence was gathered, such as age, sex, ethnic group, social class and the profile of related risk factors, such as smoking or obesity?

The evidence that the practitioner needs to appraise may come from a single study or, increasingly, from a systematic review of many. There has been an explosion in research evidence in recent decades: over two million articles are published annually in the biomedical literature and it is common for important issues to be addressed in several studies. Indeed, we might be reluctant to introduce a new treatment based on the result of one trial alone. A **systematic review**, or

overview, of the literature is a 'systematic assembly, critical appraisal and synthesis of all relevant studies on a specific topic'. The statistical methods for combining the results of a number of studies are known as **meta-analysis**. It should be emphasized that not all systematic reviews will contain a meta-analysis: this depends on the systematic review having located studies which are sufficiently similar that it is reasonable to consider combining their results. The increase in interest in meta-analysis is illustrated by the fact that while in 1987 there were 25 MEDLINE citations using the term 'meta-analysis'; this had increased to around 380 by 1991 and around 580 by 2001.

The majority of practitioners are concerned with using and appraising this evidence base, whereas the main focus of this book is on how to conduct the statistical analyses of studies that contribute to the evidence base. There are several excellent specialized evidence-based medicine books that lay out the issues in critically appraising a scientific paper or systematic review. We have therefore decided to refer the reader to these, rather than including a detailed discussion of critical appraisal in this book. We recommend Crombie (1996), Clarke and Croft (1998), Silagy and Haines (1998), Greenhalgh (2000) and Sackett *et al.* (2000).

The parts of this book that are particularly relevant to those practising evidence-based medicine are Chapters 32, 34 and 37. Thus in Chapter 32 on 'Systematic reviews and meta-analysis', we include a discussion of the sources of bias in meta-analysis and how these may be detected. In Chapter 34 we briefly review the most important aspects of the quality of randomized controlled trials. In Chapter 37 we describe the various different 'Measures of association and impact' and how to interpret them. These include numbers needed to treat or harm as well as risk ratios, odds ratios, attributable risks and absolute risk reductions. In addition, this book will be a useful companion for any practitioner who, as well as appraising the quality and relevance of the evidence base, wishes to understand more about the statistics behind the evidence generated.

CHAPTER 2

Defining the data

2.1 POPULATIONS AND SAMPLES

Except when a full census is taken, we collect data on a **sample** from a much larger group called the **population**. The sample is of interest not in its own right, but for what it tells the investigator about the population. Statistics allows us to use the sample to make inferences about the population from which it was derived, as illustrated in Figure 2.1. Because of chance, different samples from the population will give different results and this must be taken into account when using a sample to make inferences about the population. This phenomenon, called **sampling variation**, lies at the heart of statistics. It is described in detail in Chapter 4.

The word 'population' is used in statistics in a wider sense than usual. It is not limited to a population of people but can refer to any collection of objects. For

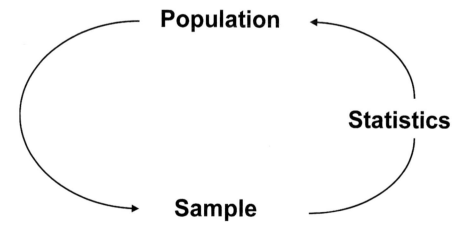

Fig. 2.1 Diagram to show the role of statistics in using information from a sample to make inferences about the population from which the sample was derived.

example, the data may relate to a sample of 20 hospitals from the population of all hospitals in the country. In such a case it is easy to imagine that the entire population can be listed and the sample selected directly from it. In many instances, however, the population and its boundaries are less precisely specified, and care must be taken to ensure that the sample truly represents the population about which information is required. This population is sometimes referred to as the **target population**. For example, consider a vaccine trial carried out using student volunteers. If it is reasonable to assume that in their response to the vaccine and exposure to disease students are typical of the community at large, the results will have general applicability. If, on the other hand, students differ in any respect which may materially affect their response to the vaccine or exposure to disease, the conclusions from the trial are restricted to the population of students and do not have general applicability. Deciding whether or not 'students are typical' is not a statistical issue, but depends on an informed judgement taking into account relevant biological and epidemiological knowledge.

Note that the target population often includes not only all persons living at present but also those that may be alive at some time in the future. This is the case in this last example evaluating the efficacy of the vaccine. It is obvious that the complete enumeration of such a population is not possible.

2.2 TYPES OF VARIABLE

The raw data of an investigation consist of **observations** made on individuals. In many situations the individuals are people, but they need not be. For instance, they might be red blood cells, urine specimens, rats, or hospitals. The number of individuals is called the **sample size**. Any aspect of an individual that is measured, like blood pressure, or recorded, like age or sex, is called a **variable**. There may be only one variable in a study or there may be many. For example, Table 2.1 shows the first six lines of data recorded in a study of outcome of treatment in tuberculosis patients treated in three hospitals. Each row of the table shows the data collected on a particular individual, while the columns of the table show the different variables which have been collected.

Table 2.1 First six lines of data from a study of outcome after diagnosis of tuberculosis.

Id	Hospital	Date of birth	Sex	Date of diagnosis	Weight (kg)	Smear result	Culture result	Skin test diameter (mm)	Alive after 6 months?
001	1	03/12/1929	M	23/08/1998	56.3	Positive	Negative	18	Y
002	1	13/04/1936	M	12/09/1998	73.5	Positive	Negative	15	Y
003	1	31/10/1931	F	17/06/1999	57.6	Positive	Positive	21	N
004	2	11/11/1922	F	05/07/1999	65.6	Uncertain	Positive	28	Y
005	2	01/05/1946	M	20/08/1999	81.1	Negative	Positive	6	Y
006	3	18/02/1954	M	17/09/1999	56.8	Positive	Negative	12	Y

A first step in choosing how best to display and analyse data is to classify the variables into their different types, as different methods pertain to each. The main division is between numerical (or quantitative) variables, categorical (or qualitative) variables and rates.

Numerical variables

A **numerical** variable is either **continuous** or **discrete**. A continuous variable, as the name implies, is a measurement on a continuous scale. In Table 2.1, weight is a continuous variable. In contrast, a discrete variable can only take a limited number of discrete values, which are usually whole numbers, such as the number of episodes of diarrhoea a child has had in a year.

Binary and other categorical variables

A **categorical** variable is non-numerical, for instance place of birth, ethnic group, or type of drug. A particularly common sort is a **binary variable** (also known as a **dichotomous** variable), which has only two possible values. For example, sex is male or female, or the patient may survive or die. We should also distinguish **ordered categorical** variables, whose categories, although non-numerical, can be considered to have a natural ordering. A common example of an ordered categorical variable is social class, which has a natural ordering from most deprived to most affluent. Table 2.2 shows the possible categories and sub-types of variable for each of the categorical variables in the data displayed in Table 2.1. Note that it could be debated whether smear result should be classified as ordered categorical or simply as categorical, depending on whether we can assume that "uncertain" is intermediate between 'negative' and 'positive'.

Rates

Rates of disease are measured in follow-up studies, and are the fundamental measure of the frequency of occurrence of disease over time. Their analysis forms the basis for Part D, and their exact definition can be found there. Examples include the survival rates following different treatments for breast cancer, or the number of episodes of diarrhoea/person/year among AIDS patients.

Table 2.2 Categorical (qualitative) variables recorded in the study of outcome after diagnosis of tuberculosis.

Variable	Categories	Type of variable
Hospital	1, 2, 3	Categorical
Sex	Male, female	Binary
Smear result	Negative, uncertain, positive	Ordered categorical
Culture result	Negative, positive	Binary
Alive at 6 months?	No, yes	Binary

2.3 DERIVED VARIABLES

Often, the variables included in a statistical analysis will be **derived** from those originally recorded. This may occur in a variety of different ways, and for a variety of reasons.

Calculated or categorized from recorded variables

We commonly derive a patient's *age* at diagnosis (in years) by calculating the number of days between their date of birth and date of diagnosis, and dividing this by 365.25 (the average number of days in a year, including leap years). We will often proceed to categorize age into *age groups*, for example we might define ten-year age groups as 30 to 39, 40 to 49, and so on. Age group is then an ordered categorical variable.

Another example is where the range of values observed for average monthly income is used to divide the sample into five equally-sized income groups (quintiles, see Section 3.3), and a new variable 'income group' created with '1' corresponding to the least affluent group in the population and '5' to the most affluent group.

Similarly, body mass index (BMI), which is calculated by dividing a person's weight (in kg) by the square of their height (in m), may be categorized into a 5-point scale going from $< 16 \, \text{kg/m}^2$ being malnourished to $\geq 30 \, \text{kg/m}^2$ defining obese. In contrast to the income group variable where the categorization is specific to the particular set of data, the categorization of the BMI scale has been carried out using conventionally agreed cut-off points to define the different groups. This type of variable, where the categorizing is based on pre-defined threshold values, is described in the next paragraph.

Variables based on threshold values

A particular group of derived variables are those based on **threshold values** of a measured variable. Two examples are given in Table 2.3. LBW is a binary variable for low birthweight ('yes' if the baby's birthweight was below 2500 g, and 'no' if

Table 2.3 Examples of derived variables based on threshold values.

Derived variable	Original variable
LBW (Low birthweight):	Birthweight:
Yes	$< 2500 \, \text{g}$
No	$\geq 2500 \, \text{g}$
Vitamin A status:	Serum retinol level:
Severe deficiency	$< 0.35 \, \mu\text{mol/l}$
Mild/moderate deficiency	$0.35–0.69 \, \mu\text{mol/l}$
Normal	$\geq 0.70 \, \mu\text{mol/l}$

the birthweight was 2500 g or above). Vitamin A status is an ordered categorical variable, derived from the serum retinol level.

Variables derived from reference curves, based on standard population values

A more refined comparison is based on comparing the value of a variable for the individual with **reference curves** based on the average and range of values for the whole population. For example, a child's growth can be monitored by plotting his/her weight (and height) against standard **growth curves**. This allows not only an assessment of where the child's weight (or height) lays compared to the average child at this age, but also allows growth faltering to be detected, if their growth curve appears to be dropping below what is usually expected for a child with their birthweight. How to calculate variables derived from a comparison with reference curves is postponed until Chapter 13 ('Transformations') at the end of Part B, since it requires an understanding of means, the normal distribution and z-scores, all of which are covered in Part B.

Transformed variables

In some cases it may be necessary to *transform* a numerical variable onto another scale in order to make it satisfy the assumptions needed for the relevant statistical methods. The **logarithmic transformation**, in which the value of the variable is replaced by its logarithm, is by far the most frequently applied. Its use is appropriate for a great variety of variables including incubation periods, parasite counts, titres, dose levels, concentrations of substances, and ratios. The reasons why a variable should be transformed, the different types of transformation, and how to choose between them are covered in detail in Chapter 13 at the end of part B.

2.4 DISTINGUISHING BETWEEN OUTCOME AND EXPOSURE VARIABLES

In order to choose appropriate data displays and statistical methods, it is very important to distinguish between *outcome* and *exposure* variables, in addition to identifying the types of each of the variables in the data set. The **outcome** variable is the variable that is the focus of our attention, whose variation or occurrence we are seeking to understand. In particular we are interested in identifying factors, or **exposures**, that may influence the size or the occurrence of the outcome variable. Some examples are given in Table 2.4. The purpose of a statistical analysis is to quantify the magnitude of the association between one or more exposure variables and the outcome variable.

A number of different terms are used to describe exposure and outcome variables, depending on the context. These are listed in Table 2.5. In particular, in a

Table 2.4 Examples of outcome and exposure variables.

Outcome variable	Exposure variable
Baby born with low birth weight (yes, no)	Mother smoked during pregnancy (yes, no)
Anthropometric status at 1 year of age (weight-for-age z-score)	Duration of exclusive breastfeeding (weeks)
Number of diarrhoea episodes experienced in a year	Access to clean water supply (yes, no)
Child develops leukaemia (yes, no)	Proximity to nuclear power station (miles)
Survival time (months) following diagnosis of lung cancer	Socio-economic status (6 groups)

Table 2.5 Commonly used alternatives for describing exposure and outcome variables.

Outcome variable	Exposure variable
Response variable	Explanatory variable
Dependent variable	Independent variable
y-variable	x-variable
Case–control group	Risk factor
	Treatment group

clinical trial (see Chapter 34) the exposure is the **treatment** group, and in a **case–control study**, the outcome is the case–control status, and the exposure variables are often called **risk factors**.

The type of outcome variable is particularly important in determining the most appropriate statistical method. Part B of this book describes statistical methods for numerical outcome variables. Part C describes methods for binary outcome variables, with a brief description (Section 20.5) of methods for categorical outcomes with more than two types of response. Part D describes methods to be used for rates, arising in studies with binary outcomes in which individuals are followed over time.

CHAPTER 3

Displaying the data

3.1 INTRODUCTION

With ready access to statistical software, there is a temptation to jump straight into complex analyses. This should be avoided. An essential first step of an analysis is to summarize and display the data. The familiarity with the data gained through doing this is invaluable in developing an appropriate analysis plan (see Chapter 38). These initial displays are also valuable in identifying **outliers** (unusual values of a variable) and revealing possible errors in the data, which should be checked and, if necessary, corrected.

This chapter describes simple tabular and graphical techniques for displaying the distribution of values taken by a single variable, and for displaying the association between the values of two variables. Diagrams and tables should always be clearly labelled and self-explanatory; it should not be necessary to refer to the text to understand them. At the same time they should not be cluttered with too much detail, and they must not be misleading.

3.2 FREQUENCIES, FREQUENCY DISTRIBUTIONS AND HISTOGRAMS

Frequencies (categorical variables)

Summarizing categorical variables is straightforward, the main task being to count the number of observations in each category. These counts are called **frequencies**. They are often also presented as **relative frequencies**; that is as proportions or percentages of the total number of individuals. For example, Table 3.1 summarizes the method of delivery recorded for 600 births in a hospital. The

Table 3.1 Method of delivery of 600 babies born in a hospital.

Method of delivery	No. of births	Percentage
Normal	478	79.7
Forceps	65	10.8
Caesarean section	57	9.5
Total	600	100.0

variable of interest is the method of delivery, a categorical variable with three categories: normal delivery, forceps delivery, and caesarean section.

Frequencies and relative frequencies are commonly illustrated by a **bar chart** (also known as a **bar diagram**) or by a **pie chart**. In a bar chart the lengths of the bars are drawn proportional to the frequencies, as shown in Figure 3.1. Alternatively the bars may be drawn proportional to the percentages in each category; the shape is not changed, only the labelling of the scale. In either case, for ease of reading it is helpful to write the actual frequency and/or percentage to the right of the bar. In a pie chart (see Figure 3.2), the circle is divided so that the areas of the sectors are proportional to the frequencies, or equivalently to the percentages.

Frequency distributions (numerical variables)

If there are more than about 20 observations, a useful first step in summarizing a numerical (quantitative) variable is to form a **frequency distribution**. This is a table showing the number of observations at different values or within certain ranges. For a discrete variable the frequencies may be tabulated either for each value of the variable or for groups of values. With continuous variables, groups have to be formed. An example is given in Table 3.2, where haemoglobin has been measured

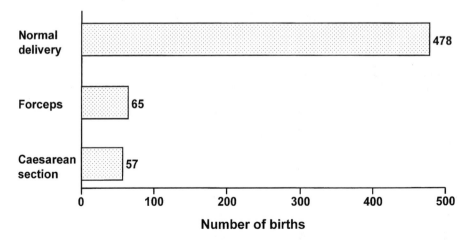

Fig. 3.1 Bar chart showing method of delivery of 600 babies born in a hospital.

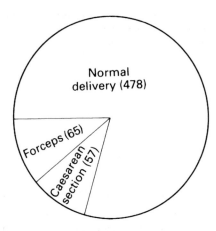

Fig. 3.2 Pie chart showing method of delivery of 600 babies born in a hospital.

to the nearest 0.1 g/100 ml and the group 11–, for example, contains all measurements between 11.0 and 11.9 g/100 ml inclusive.

When forming a frequency distribution, the first things to do are to count the number of observations and to identify the lowest and highest values. Then decide

Table 3.2 Haemoglobin levels in g/100 ml for 70 women.

(a) Raw data with the highest and lowest values underlined.

10.2	13.7	10.4	14.9	11.5	12.0	11.0
13.3	12.9	12.1	9.4	13.2	10.8	11.7
10.6	10.5	13.7	11.8	14.1	10.3	13.6
12.1	12.9	11.4	12.7	10.6	11.4	11.9
9.3	13.5	14.6	11.2	11.7	10.9	10.4
12.0	12.9	11.1	8.8	10.2	11.6	12.5
13.4	12.1	10.9	11.3	14.7	10.8	13.3
11.9	11.4	12.5	13.0	11.6	13.1	9.7
11.2	15.1	10.7	12.9	13.4	12.3	11.0
14.6	11.1	13.5	10.9	13.1	11.8	12.2

(b) Frequency distribution.

Haemoglobin (g/100 ml)	No. of women	Percentage
8–	1	1.4
9–	3	4.3
10–	14	20.0
11–	19	27.1
12–	14	20.0
13–	13	18.6
14–	5	7.1
15–15.9	1	1.4
Total	70	100.0

whether the data should be grouped and, if so, what grouping interval should be used. As a rough guide one should aim for 5–20 groups, depending on the number of observations. If the interval chosen for grouping the data is too wide, too much detail will be lost, while if it is too narrow the table will be unwieldy. The starting points of the groups should be round numbers and, whenever possible, all the intervals should be of the same width. There should be no gaps between groups. The table should be labelled so that it is clear what happens to observations that fall on the boundaries.

For example, in Table 3.2 there are 70 haemoglobin measurements. The lowest value is 8.8 and the highest 15.1 g/100 ml. Intervals of width 1 g/100 ml were chosen, leading to eight groups in the frequency distribution. Labelling the groups 8–, 9–, ... is clear. An acceptable alternative would have been 8.0–8.9, 9.0–9.9 and so on. Note that labelling them 8–9, 9–10 and so on would have been confusing, since it would not then be clear to which group a measurement of 9.0 g/100 ml, for example, belonged.

Once the format of the table is decided, the numbers of observations in each group are counted. If this is done by hand, mistakes are most easily avoided by going through the data in order. For each value, a mark is put against the appropriate group. To facilitate the counting, these marks are arranged in groups of five by putting each fifth mark horizontally through the previous four (卌); these groups are called **five-bar gates**. The process is called **tally-ing**.

As well as the number of women, it is useful to show the percentage of women in each of the groups.

Histograms

Frequency distributions are usually illustrated by **histograms**, as shown in Figure 3.3 for the haemoglobin data. Either the frequencies or the percentages may be used; the shape of the histogram will be the same.

The construction of a histogram is straightforward when the grouping intervals of the frequency distribution are all equal, as is the case in Figure 3.3. If the intervals are of different widths, it is important to take this into account when drawing the histogram, otherwise a distorted picture will be obtained. For example, suppose the two highest haemoglobin groups had been combined in compiling Table 3.2(b). The frequency for this combined group (14.0–15.9 g/100 ml) would be six, but clearly it would be misleading to draw a rectangle of height six from 14 to 16 g/100 ml. Since this interval would be twice the width of all the others, the correct height of the line would be three, half the total frequency for this group. This is illustrated by the dotted line in Figure 3.3. The general rule for drawing a histogram when the intervals are not all the same width is to make the heights of the rectangles proportional to the frequencies divided by the widths, that is to make the areas of the histogram bars proportional to the frequencies.

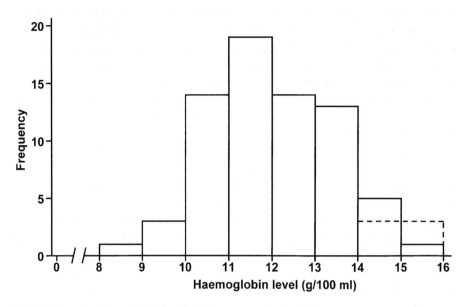

Fig. 3.3 Histogram of haemoglobin levels of 70 women.

Frequency polygon

An alternative but less common way of illustrating a frequency distribution is a **frequency polygon**, as shown in Figure 3.4. This is particularly useful when comparing two or more frequency distributions by drawing them on the same diagram. The polygon is drawn by imagining (or lightly pencilling) the histogram and joining

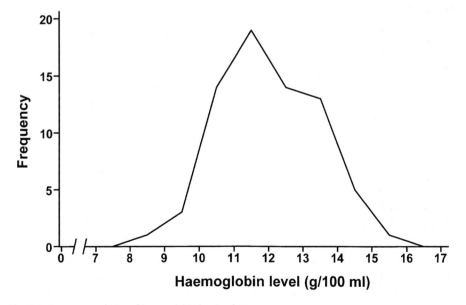

Fig. 3.4 Frequency polygon of haemoglobin levels of 70 women.

the midpoints of the tops of its rectangles. The endpoints of the resulting line are then joined to the horizontal axis at the midpoints of the groups immediately below and above the lowest and highest non-zero frequencies respectively. For the haemoglobin data, these are the groups 7.0–7.9 and 16.0–16.9 g/100 ml. The frequency polygon in Figure 3.4 is therefore joined to the axis at 7.5 and 16.5 g/100 ml.

Frequency distribution of the population

Figures 3.3 and 3.4 illustrate the frequency distribution of the haemoglobin levels of a sample of 70 women. We use these data to give us information about the distribution of haemoglobin levels among women in general. For example, it seems uncommon for a woman to have a level below 9.0 g/100 ml or above 15.0 g/100 ml. Our confidence in drawing general conclusions from the data depends on how many individuals were measured. The larger the sample, the finer the grouping interval that can be chosen, so that the histogram (or frequency polygon) becomes smoother and more closely resembles the distribution of the total population. At the limit, if it were possible to ascertain the haemoglobin levels of the whole population of women, the resulting diagram would be a smooth curve.

Shapes of frequency distributions

Figure 3.5 shows three of the most common shapes of frequency distributions. They all have high frequencies in the centre of the distribution and low frequencies at the two extremes, which are called the **upper** and **lower tails** of the distribution. The distribution in Figure 3.5(a) is also **symmetrical** about the centre; this shape of curve is often described as 'bell-shaped'. The two other distributions are asymmetrical or **skewed**. The upper tail of the distribution in Figure 3.5(b) is longer than the lower tail; this is called **positively skewed** or skewed to the right. The distribution in Figure 3.5(c) is **negatively skewed** or skewed to the left.

All three distributions in Figure 3.5 are **unimodal**, that is they have just one peak. Figure 3.6(a) shows a **bimodal** frequency distribution, that is a distribution with two peaks. This is occasionally seen and usually indicates that the data are a mixture of

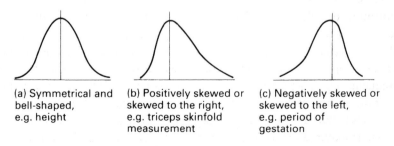

(a) Symmetrical and bell-shaped, e.g. height

(b) Positively skewed or skewed to the right, e.g. triceps skinfold measurement

(c) Negatively skewed or skewed to the left, e.g. period of gestation

Fig. 3.5 Three common shapes of frequency distributions with an example of each.

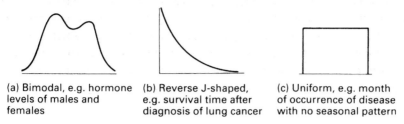

(a) Bimodal, e.g. hormone levels of males and females

(b) Reverse J-shaped, e.g. survival time after diagnosis of lung cancer

(c) Uniform, e.g. month of occurrence of disease with no seasonal pattern

Fig. 3.6 Three less-common shapes of frequency distributions with an example of each.

two separate distributions. Also shown in Figure 3.6 are two other distributions that are sometimes found, the **reverse J-shaped** and the **uniform** distributions.

3.3 CUMULATIVE FREQUENCY DISTRIBUTIONS, QUANTILES AND PERCENTILES

Cumulative frequency distributions

Frequency distributions (and histograms) indicate the way data are distributed over a range of values, by showing the number or percentage of individuals within each group of values. **Cumulative distributions** start from the lowest value and show how the number and percentage of individuals accumulate as the values increase. For example, the cumulative frequency distribution for the first five observations of haemoglobin levels is shown in Table 3.3. There were 70 observations, so each represents $100/70 = 1.43\%$ of the total distribution. Rounding to one decimal place, the first observation ($8.8\,g/100\,ml$) corresponds to 1.4% of the distribution, the first and second observations to 2.9% of the distribution, and so on. Table 3.3 shows the values of these **cumulative percentages**, for different observations in the range of observed haemoglobin levels in the 70 women. A total of four women (5.7%) had levels below $10\,g/100\,ml$. Similarly, 18 women (25.7%) had haemoglobin levels below $11\,g/100\,ml$.

The **cumulative frequency distribution** is illustrated in Figure 3.7. This is drawn as a **step function**: the vertical jumps correspond to the increases in the cumulative percentages at each observed haemoglobin level. (Another example of plots that use step functions is **Kaplan–Meier** plots of cumulative survival probabilities over time; see Section 26.3.) Cumulative frequency curves are steep where there is a concentration of values, and shallow where values are sparse. In this example, where the majority of haemoglobin values are concentrated in the centre of the distribution, the curve is steep in the centre, and shallow at low and high values. If the haemoglobin levels were evenly distributed across the range, then the cumulative frequency curve would increase at a constant rate; all the steps would be the same width as well as the same height. An advantage of cumulative frequency distributions is that they display the shape of the distribution without the need for grouping, as required in plotting histograms (see Section 3.2). However the shape of a distribution is usually more clearly seen in a histogram.

Table 3.3 Cumulative percentages for different ranges of haemoglobin levels of 70 women.

Observation	Cumulative percentage	Haemoglobin level (g/100 ml)		Quartile
1	1.4	8.8	Minimum = 8.8	1
2	2.9	9.3		1
3	4.3	9.4		1
4	5.7	9.7		1
5	7.1	10.2		
⋮	⋮	⋮		
15	21.4	10.8		1
16	22.9	10.9		1
17	24.3	10.9	Lower quartile = 10.9	1
18	25.7	10.9		1
19	27.1	11.0		2
20	28.6	11.0		2
⋮	⋮	⋮		
33	47.1	11.7		2
34	48.6	11.8		2
35	50.0	11.8	Median = 11.85	2
36	51.4	11.9		3
37	52.9	11.9		3
38	54.3	12.0		3
⋮	⋮	⋮		
50	71.4	12.9		3
51	72.9	12.9		3
52	74.3	13.0		3
53	75.7	13.1	Upper quartile = 13.1	4
54	77.1	13.1		4
55	78.6	13.2		4
⋮	⋮	⋮		
66	94.3	14.6		4
67	95.7	14.6		4
68	97.1	14.7		4
69	98.6	14.9		4
70	100	15.1	Maximum = 15.1	4

Median and quartiles

Cumulative frequency distributions are useful in recoding a numerical variable into a categorical variable. The **median** is the midway value; half of the distribution lies below the median and half above it.

$$\text{Median} = \frac{(n+1)\text{th}}{2} \text{ value of the ordered observations}$$
$$(n = \text{number of observations})$$

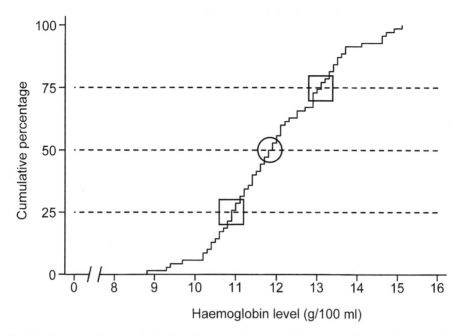

Fig. 3.7 Cumulative frequency distribution of haemoglobin levels of 70 women, with the median marked by a circle, and lower and upper quartiles marked by squares.

For the haemoglobin data, the median is the $71/2 = 35.5$th observation and so we take the average of the 35th and 36th observations. Thus the median is $(11.8+11.9)/2 = 11.85$, as shown in Table 3.3. Calculation of the median is also described in Section 4.2. When the sample size is reasonably large, the median can be estimated from the cumulative frequency distribution; it is the haemoglobin value corresponding to the point where the 50% line crosses the curve, as shown in Figure 3.7.

Also marked on Figure 3.7 are the two points where the 25% and 75% lines cross the curve. These are called the **lower** and **upper quartiles** of the distribution, respectively, and together with the median they divide the distribution into four equally-sized groups.

$$\text{Lower quartile} = \frac{(n+1)\text{th}}{4} \text{ value of the ordered observations}$$

$$\text{Upper quartile} = \frac{3 \times (n+1)\text{th}}{4} \text{ value of the ordered observations}$$

In the haemoglobin data, the lower quartile is the $71/4 = 17.75$th observation. This is calculated by taking three quarters of the difference between the 17th and 18th observations and adding it to the 17th observation. Since both the 17th and 18th observations equal 10.9 g/100 ml, so does the lower quartile, as shown in Table 3.3. Similarly, $3 \times 71/4 = 53.25$, and since both the 53rd and 54th observations equal 13.1 g/100 ml, so does the upper quartile.

The **range** of the distribution is the difference between the minimum and maximum values. From Table 3.3, the minimum and maximum values for the haemoglobin data are 8.8 and 15.1 g/100 ml, so the range is $15.1 - 8.8 = 6.3$ g/ 100 ml. The difference between the lower and upper quartiles of the haemoglobin data is 2.2 g/100 ml. This is known as the **interquartile range**.

> Range = highest value − lowest value
>
> Interquartile range = upper quartile − lower quartile

A useful plot, based on these values, is a **box and whiskers plot**, as shown in Figure 3.8. The box is drawn from the lower quartile to the upper quartile; its length gives the interquartile range. The horizontal line in the middle of the box represents the median. Just as a cat's whiskers mark the full width of its body, the 'whiskers' in this plot mark the full extent of the data. They are drawn on either end of the box to the minimum and maximum values.

The right hand column of Table 3.3 shows how the median and lower and upper quartiles may be used to divide the data into equally sized groups called **quartiles**.

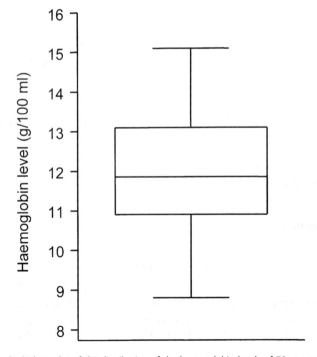

Fig. 3.8 Box and whiskers plot of the distribution of the haemoglobin levels of 70 women.

Values between 8.8 and 10.9 g/100 ml are in the first quartile, those between 11 and 11.8 g/100 ml are in the second quartile and so on. Note that equal values should always be placed in the same group, even if the groups are then of slightly different sizes.

Quantiles and percentiles

Equal-sized divisions of a distribution are called **quantiles**. For example, we may define **tertiles**, which divide the data into three equally-sized groups, and **quintiles**, which divide them into five. An example was described in Section 2.3, where the range of values observed for average monthly income was used to divide the sample into five equally-sized income groups, and a new variable 'income group' created with '1' corresponding to the least affluent group in the population and '5' to the most affluent group. Quintiles are estimated from the intersections with the cumulative frequency curve of lines at 20%, 40%, 60% and 80%. Divisions into ten equally sized groups are called **deciles**.

More generally, the kth **percentile** (or **centile** as it is also called) is the point below which k% of the values of the distribution lie. For a distribution with n observations, it is defined as:

$$k\text{th percentile} = \frac{k \times (n+1)\text{th}}{100} \text{ value of ordered observations}$$

It can also be estimated from the cumulative frequency curve; it is the x value corresponding to the point where a line drawn at k% intersects the curve. For example, the 5% point of the haemoglobin values is estimated to be 9.6 g/100 ml.

3.4 DISPLAYING THE ASSOCIATION BETWEEN TWO VARIABLES

Having examined the distribution of a single variable, we will often wish to display the way in which the distribution of one variable relates to the distribution of another. Appropriate methods to do this will depend on the type of the two variables.

Cross tabulations

When both variables are categorical, we can examine their relationship informally by cross-tabulating them in a **contingency table**. A useful convention is for the rows of the table to correspond to the exposure values and the columns to the outcomes. For example, Table 3.4 shows the results from a survey to compare the principal water sources in 150 households in three villages in West Africa. In this example, it would be natural to ask whether the household's village affects their likely water source, so that water source is the *outcome* and village is the *exposure*.

Table 3.4 Comparison of principal sources of water used by household in three villages in West Africa.

	Water source		
Village	River	Pond	Spring
A	20	18	12
B	32	20	8
C	18	12	10

The interpretability of contingency tables can be improved by including **marginal totals** and **percentages**:
- The marginal row totals show the total number of households in each village, and the marginal columns show the total numbers using each water source.
- Percentages (or proportions) can be calculated with respect to the row variable, the column variable, or the total number of individuals. A useful guide is that the percentages should correspond to the *exposure* variable. If the exposure is the row variable, as here, then row percentages should be presented, whereas if it is the column variable then column percentages should be presented.

In Table 3.4, the exposure variable, village, is the row variable, and Table 3.5 therefore shows row percentages together with marginal (row and column) totals. We can now see that, for example, the proportion of households mainly using a river was highest in Village B, while village A had the highest proportion of households mainly using a pond. By examining the column totals we can see that overall, rivers were the principal water source for 70 (47%) of the 150 households.

Table 3.5 Comparison of principal sources of water used by households in three villages in West Africa, including marginal totals and row percentages.

	Water source			
Village	River	Pond	Spring	Total
A	20 (40%)	18 (36%)	12 (24%)	50 (100%)
B	32 (53%)	20 (33%)	8 (13%)	60 (100%)
C	18 (45%)	12 (30%)	10 (25%)	40 (100%)
Total	70 (47%)	50 (33%)	30 (20%)	150 (100%)

Scatter plots

When we wish to examine the relationship between two numerical variables, we should start by drawing a scatter plot. This is a simple graph where each pair of values is represented by a symbol whose horizontal position is determined by the value of the first variable and vertical position is determined by the value of the second variable. By convention, the outcome variable determines vertical position and the exposure variable determines horizontal position.

For example, Figure 3.9 shows data from a study of lung function among 636 children aged 7 to 10 years living in a deprived suburb of Lima, Peru. The maximum volume of air which the children could breath out in 1 second (Forced Expiratory Volume in 1 second, denoted as FEV_1) was measured using a spirometer. We are interested in how FEV_1 changes with age, so that age is the exposure variable (horizontal axis) and FEV_1 is the outcome variable (vertical axis). The plot gives the clear impression that FEV_1 increases in an approximately linear manner with age.

Scatter plots may also be used to display the relationship between a categorical variable and a continuous variable. For example, in the study of lung function we are also interested in the relationship between FEV_1 and respiratory symptoms experienced by the child over the previous 12 months. Figure 3.10 shows a scatter plot that displays this relationship.

This figure is difficult to interpret, because many of the points overlap, particularly in the group of children who did not report respiratory symptoms. One solution to this is to scatter the points randomly along the horizontal axis, a process known as '**jittering**'. This produces a clearer picture, as shown in Figure 3.11. We can now see that FEV_1 tended to be higher in children who did not report respiratory symptoms in the previous 12 months than in those who did.

An alternative way to display the relationship between a numerical variable and a discrete variable is to draw **box and whiskers plots**, as described in Section 3.3. Table 3.6 shows the data needed to do this for the two groups of children: those who did and those who did not report respiratory symptoms. All the statistics displayed are

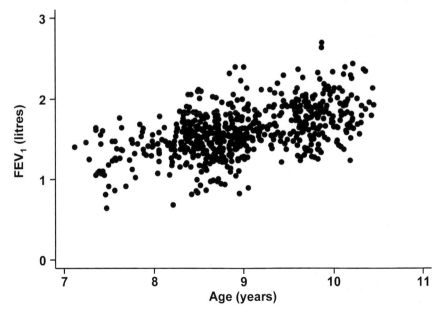

Fig. 3.9 Scatter plot showing the relationship between FEV_1 and age in 636 children living in a deprived suburb of Lima, Peru.

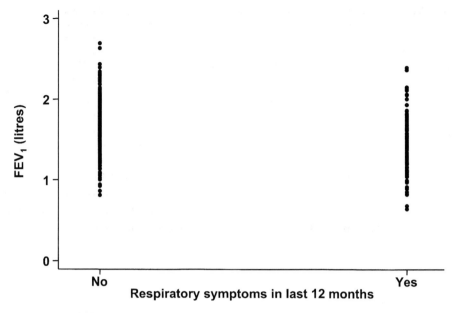

Fig. 3.10 Scatter plot showing the relationship between FEV$_1$ and respiratory symptoms in 636 children living in a deprived suburb of Lima, Peru.

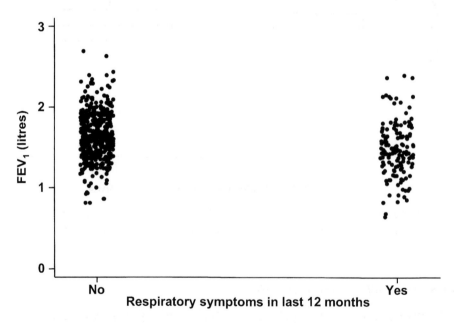

Fig. 3.11 Scatter plot showing the relationship between FEV$_1$ and respiratory symptoms in 636 children living in a deprived suburb of Lima, Peru. The position of the points on the horizontal axis was moved randomly ('jittered') in order to separate them.

Table 3.6 Median, interquartile range, and range of FEV$_1$ measurements on 636 children living in a deprived suburb of Lima, Peru, according to whether the child reported respiratory symptoms in the previous 12 months.

Respiratory symptoms in the previous 12 months	n	Lowest FEV$_1$ value	Lower quartile (25th centile)	Median	Upper quartile (75th centile)	Highest FEV$_1$ value
No	491	0.81	1.44	1.61	1.82	2.69
Yes	145	0.64	1.28	1.46	1.65	2.39
Totals	636	0.64	1.40	1.58	1.79	2.69

lower in children who reported symptoms. This is reflected in Figure 3.12, where all the points in the box and whiskers plot of FEV$_1$ values for children who reported respiratory symptoms are lower than the corresponding points in the box and whiskers plot for children who did not report symptoms.

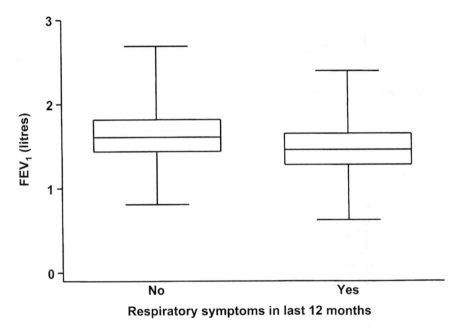

Fig. 3.12 Box and whiskers plots of the distribution of FEV$_1$ in 636 children living in a deprived suburb of Lima, Peru, according to whether they reported respiratory symptoms in the previous 12 months.

3.5 DISPLAYING TIME TRENDS

Graphs are also useful for displaying trends over time, such as the declines in child mortality rates that have taken place in all regions of the world in the latter half of the twentieth century, as shown in Figure 3.13. The graph also indicates the enormous differentials between regions that still remain. Note that the graph shows absolute changes in mortality rates over time. An alternative would be to

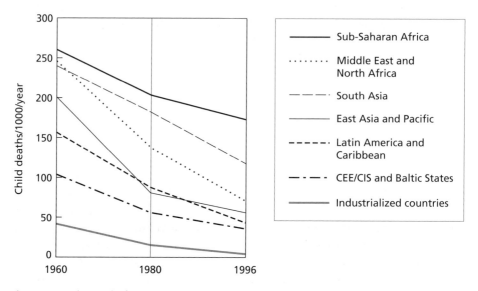

Fig. 3.13 Trends in under-five mortality rates by region of the world.

plot the logarithms of the death rates (see Chapter 13). The slopes of the lines would then show proportional declines, enabling rates of progress between regions to be readily compared.

Breaks and discontinuities in the scale(s) should be clearly marked, and avoided whenever possible. Figure 3.14(a) shows a common form of misrepresentation due to an inappropriate use of scale. The decline in infant mortality rate (IMR) has been made to look dramatic by expanding the vertical scale, while in reality the decrease over the 10 years displayed is only slight (from 22.7 to 22.1 deaths/1000 live births/year). A more realistic representation is shown in Figure 3.14(b), with the vertical scale starting at zero.

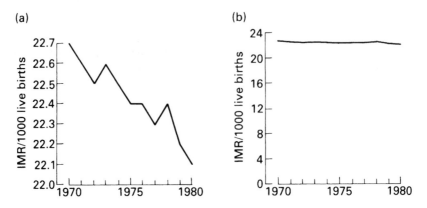

Fig. 3.14 Decline in infant mortality rate (IMR) between 1970 and 1980. (a) Inappropriate choice of scale has misleadingly exaggerated the decline. (b) Correct use of scale.

PART B

ANALYSIS OF NUMERICAL OUTCOMES

In this part of the book we describe methods for the analysis of studies where the outcome variable is **numerical**. Examples of such variables include blood pressure, antibody levels, birth weight and so on. We begin, in Chapter 4, by describing how to summarize characteristics of the distribution of a numerical variable; having defined the **mean** and **standard deviation** of a distribution, we introduce the important concept of **sampling error**. Chapter 5 describes the **normal distribution**, which occupies a central role in statistical analysis. We explain that the normal distribution is important not only because it is a good empirical description of the distribution of many variables, but also because the **sampling distribution** of a mean is normal, even when the individual observations are not normally distributed. We build on this in the next three chapters, introducing the two fundamental ways of reporting the results of a statistical analysis, **confidence intervals** (Chapters 6 and 7) and *P*-values (Chapters 7 and 8).

Chapter 6 deals with the analysis of a single variable. The remainder of this part of the book deals with ways of analysing the relationship between a numerical outcome (response) variable and one or more exposure (explanatory) variables. We describe how to compare means between two exposure groups (Chapters 7 and 8), and extend these methods to comparison of means in several groups using **analysis of variance** (Chapter 9) and the use of **linear regression** to examine the association between numerical outcome and exposure variables (Chapter 10). All these methods are shown to be special cases of **multiple regression**, which is described in Chapter 11.

We conclude by describing how we can examine the assumptions underlying these methods (Chapter 12), and the use of **transformations** of continuous variables to facilitate data analysis when these assumptions are violated (Chapter 13).

CHAPTER 4

Means, standard deviations and standard errors

4.1 INTRODUCTION

A frequency distribution (see Section 3.2) gives a general picture of the distribution of a variable. It is often convenient, however, to summarize a numerical variable still further by giving just two measurements, one indicating the average value and the other the spread of the values.

4.2 MEAN, MEDIAN AND MODE

The average value is usually represented by the arithmetic mean, customarily just called the **mean**. This is simply the sum of the values divided by the number of values.

$$\text{Mean, } \bar{x} = \frac{\Sigma x}{n}$$

where x denotes the values of the variable, Σ (the Greek capital letter sigma) means 'the sum of' and n is the number of observations. The mean is denoted by $\bar{x}$ (spoken 'x bar').

Other measures of the average value are the **median** and the **mode**. The median was defined in Section 3.3 as the value that divides the distribution in half. If the observations are arranged in increasing order, the median is the middle observation.

$$\text{Median} = \frac{(n+1)}{2} \text{th value of ordered observations}$$

If there is an even number of observations, there is no middle one and the average of the two 'middle' ones is taken. The **mode** is the value which occurs most often.

Example 4.1
The following are the plasma volumes of eight healthy adult males:

$$2.75, 2.86, 3.37, 2.76, 2.62, 3.49, 3.05, 3.12 \text{ litres}$$

(a) $n = 8$
  $\Sigma x = 2.75 + 2.86 + 3.37 + 2.76 + 2.62 + 3.49 + 3.05 + 3.12 = 24.02 \text{ litres}$
  Mean, $\bar{x} = \Sigma x / n = 24.02/8 = 3.00 \text{ litres}$

(b) Rearranging the measurements in increasing order gives:
  $$2.62, 2.75, 2.76, 2.86, 3.05, 3.12, 3.37, 3.49 \text{ litres}$$
  Median $= (n + 1)/2 = 9/2 = 4\frac{1}{2}$th value
    $=$ average of 4th and 5th values
    $= (2.86 + 3.05)/2 = 2.96 \text{ litres}$

(c) There is no estimate of the mode, since all the values are different.

The mean is usually the preferred measure since it takes into account each individual observation and is most amenable to statistical analysis. The median is a useful descriptive measure if there are one or two extremely high or low values, which would make the mean unrepresentative of the majority of the data. The mode is seldom used. If the sample is small, either it may not be possible to estimate the mode (as in Example 4.1c), or the estimate obtained may be misleading. The mean, median and mode are, *on average*, equal when the distribution is symmetrical and unimodal. When the distribution is positively skewed, a **geometric mean** may be more appropriate than the arithmetic mean. This is discussed in Chapter 13.

4.3 MEASURES OF VARIATION

Range and interquartile range

Two measures of the amount of variation in a data set, the range and the interquartile range, were introduced in Section 3.3. The **range** is the simplest measure, and is the difference between the largest and smallest values. Its disadvantage is that it is based on only two of the observations and gives no idea of how the other observations are arranged between these two. Also, it tends to be larger, the larger the size of the sample. The **interquartile range** indicates the spread of the middle 50% of the distribution, and together with the median is a useful adjunct to the range. It is less sensitive to the size of the sample, providing that this is not too small; the lower and upper quartiles tend to be more stable than the extreme values that determine the range. These two ranges form the basis of the **box and whiskers plot**, described in Sections 3.3 and 3.4.

> Range = highest value − lowest value
>
> Interquartile range = upper quartile − lower quartile

Variance

For most statistical analyses the preferred measure of variation is the **variance** (or the **standard deviation**, which is derived from the variance, see below). This uses all the observations, and is defined in terms of the *deviations* $(x-\bar{x})$ of the observations from the mean, since the variation is small if the observations are bunched closely about their mean, and large if they are scattered over considerable distances. It is not possible simply to average the deviations, as this average will always be zero; the positive deviations corresponding to values above the mean will balance out the negative deviations from values below the mean. An obvious way of overcoming this difficulty would be simply to average the sizes of the deviations, ignoring their sign. However, this measure is not mathematically very tractable, and so instead we average the *squares* of the deviations, since the square of a number is always positive.

$$\text{Variance, } s^2 = \frac{\Sigma(x - \bar{x})^2}{(n - 1)}$$

Degrees of freedom

Note that the sum of squared deviations is divided by $(n - 1)$ rather than n, because it can be shown mathematically that this gives a better estimate of the variance of the underlying population. The denominator $(n - 1)$ is called the number of **degrees of freedom** of the variance. This number is $(n - 1)$ rather than n, since only $(n - 1)$ of the deviations $(x - \bar{x})$ are independent from each other. The last one can always be calculated from the others because all n of them must add up to zero.

Standard deviation

A disadvantage of the variance is that it is measured in the square of the units used for the observations. For example, if the observations are weights in grams, the variance is in grams squared. For many purposes it is more convenient to express the variation in the original units by taking the *square root* of the variance. This is called the **standard deviation** (s.d.).

$$\text{s.d., } s = \sqrt{\frac{\Sigma(x - \bar{x})^2}{(n - 1)}}$$

or equivalently

$$s = \sqrt{\frac{\Sigma x^2 - (\Sigma x)^2/n}{(n - 1)}}$$

When using a calculator, the second formula is more convenient for calculation, since the mean does not have to be calculated first and then subtracted from each of the observations. The equivalence of the two formulae is demonstrated in Example 4.2. (Note: Many calculators have built-in functions for the mean and standard deviation. The keys are commonly labelled $\bar{x}$ and σ_{n-1}, respectively, where σ is the lower case Greek letter sigma.)

Example 4.2
Table 4.1 shows the steps for the calculation of the standard deviation of the eight plasma volume measurements of Example 4.1.

$$\Sigma x^2 - (\Sigma x)^2/n = 72.7980 - (24.02)^2/8 = 0.6780$$

gives the same answer as $\Sigma(x - \bar{x})^2$, and

$$s = \sqrt{(0.6780/7)} = 0.31 \text{ litres}$$

Table 4.1 Calculation of the standard deviation of the plasma volumes (in litres) of eight healthy adult males (same data as in Example 4.1). Mean, $\bar{x} = 3.00$ litres.

	Plasma volume x	Deviation from the mean $x - \bar{x}$	Squared deviation $(x - \bar{x})^2$	Squared observation x^2
	2.75	−0.25	0.0625	7.5625
	2.86	−0.14	0.0196	8.1796
	3.37	0.37	0.1369	11.3569
	2.76	−0.24	0.0576	7.6176
	2.62	−0.38	0.1444	6.8644
	3.49	0.49	0.2401	12.1801
	3.05	0.05	0.0025	9.3025
	3.12	0.12	0.0144	9.7344
Totals	24.02	0.00	0.6780	72.7980

Interpretation of the standard deviation

Usually about 70% of the observations lie within one standard deviation of their mean, and about 95% lie within two standard deviations. These figures are based on a theoretical frequency distribution, called the normal distribution, which is described in Chapter 5. They may be used to derive reference ranges for the distribution of values in the population (see Chapter 5).

Change of units

Adding or subtracting a constant from the observations alters the mean by the same amount but leaves the standard deviation unaffected. Multiplying or dividing by a constant changes both the mean and the standard deviation in the same way.

For example, suppose a set of temperatures is converted from Fahrenheit to centigrade. This is done by subtracting 32, multiplying by 5, and dividing by 9. The new mean may be calculated from the old one in exactly the same way, that is by subtracting 32, multiplying by 5, and dividing by 9. The new standard deviation, however, is simply the old one multiplied by 5 and divided by 9, since the subtraction does not affect it.

Coefficient of variation

$$cv = \frac{s}{\bar{x}} \times 100\%$$

The **coefficient of variation** expresses the standard deviation as a percentage of the sample mean. This is useful when interest is in the size of the variation relative to the size of the observation, and it has the advantage that the coefficient of variation is independent of the units of observation. For example, the value of the standard deviation of a set of weights will be different depending on whether they are measured in kilograms or pounds. The coefficient of variation, however, will be the same in both cases as it does not depend on the unit of measurement.

4.4 CALCULATING THE MEAN AND STANDARD DEVIATION FROM A FREQUENCY DISTRIBUTION

Table 4.2 shows the distribution of the number of previous pregnancies of a group of women attending an antenatal clinic. Eighteen of the 100 women had no previous pregnancies, 27 had one, 31 had two, 19 had three, and five had four previous pregnancies. As, for example, adding 2 thirty-one times is

Table 4.2 Distribution of the number of previous pregnancies of a group of women aged 30–34 attending an antenatal clinic.

	No. of previous pregnancies					
	0	1	2	3	4	Total
No. of women	18	27	31	19	5	100

equivalent to adding the product (2×31), the total number of previous pregnancies is calculated by:

$$\Sigma x = (0 \times 18) + (1 \times 27) + (2 \times 31) + (3 \times 19) + (4 \times 5)$$
$$= 0 + 27 + 62 + 57 + 20 = 166$$

The average number of previous pregnancies is, therefore:

$$\bar{x} = 166/100 = 1.66$$

In the same way:

$$\Sigma x^2 = (0^2 \times 18) + (1^2 \times 27) + (2^2 \times 31) + (3^2 \times 19) + (4^2 \times 5)$$
$$= 0 + 27 + 124 + 171 + 80 = 402$$

The standard deviation is, therefore:

$$s = \sqrt{\frac{(402 - 166^2/100)}{99}} = \sqrt{\frac{126.44}{99}} = 1.13$$

If a variable has been grouped when constructing a frequency distribution, its mean and standard deviation should be calculated using the original values, not the frequency distribution. There are occasions, however, when only the frequency distribution is available. In such a case, approximate values for the mean and standard deviation can be calculated by using the values of the mid-points of the groups and proceeding as above.

4.5 SAMPLING VARIATION AND STANDARD ERROR

As discussed in Chapter 2, the sample is of interest not in its own right, but for what it tells the investigator about the population which it represents. The sample mean, $\bar{x}$, and standard deviation, s, are used to estimate the mean and standard deviation of the population, denoted by the Greek letters μ (mu) and σ (sigma) respectively.

The sample mean is unlikely to be exactly equal to the population mean. A different sample would give a different estimate, the difference being due to sampling variation. Imagine collecting many independent samples of the same size from the same population, and calculating the sample mean of each of them. A frequency distribution of these means (called the **sampling distribution**) could then be formed. It can be shown that:

1 the mean of this frequency distribution would be the population mean, and
2 the standard deviation would equal $\sigma/\sqrt{n}$. This is called the **standard error of the sample mean**, and it measures how precisely the population mean is estimated by the sample mean. The size of the standard error depends both on how much variation there is in the population and on the size of the sample. The larger the sample size n, the smaller is the standard error.

We seldom know the population standard deviation, σ, however, and so we use the sample standard deviation, s, in its place to estimate the standard error.

$$\text{s.e.} = \frac{s}{\sqrt{n}}$$

Example 4.3

The mean of the eight plasma volumes shown in Table 4.1 is 3.00 litres (Example 4.1) and the standard deviation is 0.31 litres (Example 4.2). The standard error of the mean is therefore estimated as:

$$s/\sqrt{n} = 0.31/\sqrt{8} = 0.11 \text{ litres}$$

Understanding standard deviations and standard errors

Example 4.4

Figure 4.1 shows the results of a game played with a class of 30 students to illustrate the concepts of sampling variation, the sampling distribution, and standard error. Blood pressure measurements for 250 airline pilots were used, and served as the population in the game. The distribution of these measurements is shown in Figure 4.1(a). The population mean, μ, was 78.2 mmHg, and the population standard deviation, σ, was 9.4 mmHg. Each value was written on a small disc and the 250 discs put into a bag.

Each student was asked to shake the bag, select ten discs, write down the ten diastolic blood pressures, work out their mean, $\bar{x}$, and return the discs to the bag. In this way 30 different samples were obtained, with 30 different sample means, each estimating the same population mean. The mean of these sample means was 78.23 mmHg, close to the population mean. Their distribution is shown in Figure 4.1(b). The standard deviation of the sample means was 3.01 mmHg, which agreed well with the theoretical value, $\sigma/\sqrt{n} = 9.4/\sqrt{10} = 2.97$ mmHg, for the standard error of the mean of a sample of size ten.

(a) Distribution of diastolic blood pressure for a population of 250 airline pilots

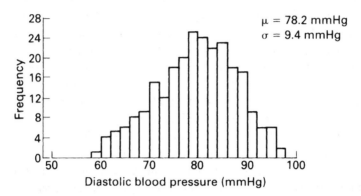

(b) Sampling distribution for 30 sample means, sample size = 10

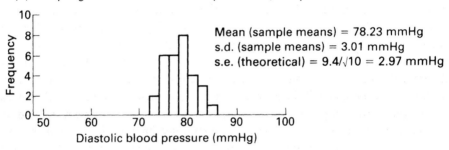

(c) Sampling distribution for 30 sample means, sample size = 20

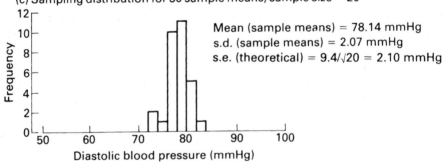

Fig. 4.1 Results of a game played to illustrate the concepts of sampling variation, the sampling distribution, and the standard error.

The exercise was repeated taking samples of size 20. The results are shown in Figure 4.1(c). The reduced variation in the sample means resulting from increasing the sample size from 10 to 20 can be clearly seen. The mean of the sample means was 78.14 mmHg, again close to the population mean. The standard deviation was 2.07 mmHg, again in good agreement with the theoretical value, $9.4/\sqrt{20} = 2.10$ mmHg, for the standard error of the mean of a sample of size 20.

In this game, we had the luxury of results from several different samples, and could draw the sampling distribution. Usually we are not in this position: we have just one sample that we wish to use to estimate the mean of a larger population, which it represents. We can draw the frequency distribution of the values in our sample (see, for example, Figure 3.3 of the histogram of haemoglobin levels of 70 women). Providing the sample size is not too small, this frequency distribution will be similar in appearance to the frequency distribution of the underlying population, with a similar spread of values. In particular, the sample standard deviation will be a fairly accurate estimate of the population standard deviation. As stated in Section 4.2, approximately, 95% of the sample values will lie within two standard deviations of the sample mean. Similarly, approximately 95% of all the values in the population will lie within this same amount of the population mean.

The sample mean will not be exactly equal to the population mean. The theoretical distribution called the **sampling distribution** gives us the spread of values we would get if we took a large number of additional samples; this spread depends on the amount of variation in the underlying population and on our sample size. The standard deviation of the sampling distribution is called the **standard error** and is equal to the standard deviation of the population, divided by the square root of n. This means that approximately 95% of the values in this theoretical sampling distribution of sample means lie within two standard errors of the population mean. This fact can be used to construct a range of likely values for the (unknown) population mean, based on the observed sample mean and its standard error. Such a range is called a **confidence interval**. Its method of construction is not described until Chapter 6 since it depends on using the normal distribution, described in Chapter 5. In summary:

- The standard deviation measures the amount of variability in the population.
- The standard error ($=$ standard deviation $/\sqrt{n}$) measures the amount of variability in the sample mean; it indicates how closely the population mean is likely to be estimated by the sample mean.
- Because standard deviations and standard errors are often confused it is very important that they are clearly labelled when presented in tables of results.

CHAPTER 5

The normal distribution

5.1 INTRODUCTION

Frequency distributions and their various shapes were discussed in Chapter 3. In practice it is found that a reasonable description of many variables is provided by the **normal distribution**, sometimes called the **Gaussian distribution** after its discoverer, Gauss. Its frequency distribution (defined by the **normal curve**) is symmetrical about the mean and bell-shaped; the bell is tall and narrow for small standard deviations and short and wide for large ones. Figure 5.1 illustrates the normal curve describing the distribution of heights of adult men in the United Kingdom. Other examples of variables that are approximately normally distributed are blood pressure, body temperature, and haemoglobin level. Examples of variables that are not normally distributed are triceps skinfold thickness and income, both of which are positively skewed. Sometimes *transforming* a variable, for example by

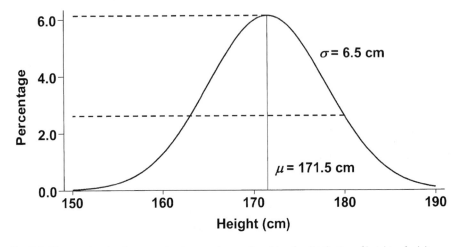

Fig. 5.1 Diagram showing the approximate normal curve describing the distribution of heights of adult men.

taking logarithms, will make its distribution more normal. This is described in Chapter 13, and methods to assess whether a variable is normally distributed are discussed in Chapter 12.

5.2 WHY THE NORMAL DISTRIBUTION IS IMPORTANT

The normal distribution is important not only because it is a good empirical description of the distribution of many variables, but because it occupies a central role in statistical analysis. This is because it can be shown that *the sampling distribution of a mean is normal*, even when the individual observations are not normally distributed, provided that the sample size is not too small. In other words, sample means will be normally distributed around the true population mean. A practical demonstration of this property can easily be had by carrying out a sampling game like Example 4.4, but with the 250 blood pressures replaced by a non-normally distributed variable, such as triceps skinfold thickness. The larger the sample selected in the game, the closer the sample mean will be to being normally distributed. The number needed to give a close approximation to normality depends on how non-normal the variable is, but in most circumstances a sample size of 15 or more is enough.

This finding is based on a remarkable and very useful result known as the **central limit theorem**. It means that calculations based on the normal distribution are used to derive confidence intervals, which were mentioned in Chapter 4, are defined fully in Chapter 6 and used throughout subsequent chapters. The normal distribution also underlies the calculation of *P*-values, which are used to test hypotheses and which are introduced in Chapter 7. The normal distribution is not only important in the analysis of numerical outcomes; we will see in parts C and D that statistical methods for proportions and rates are also based on approximations to the normal distribution.

For these reasons it is important to describe the principles of how to use the normal distribution in some detail before proceeding further. The precise mathematical equation which defines the normal distribution is included in the next section for reference only; this section can be skipped by the majority of readers. In practical terms, calculations are carried out either by a statistical package, or by using standard tables.

5.3 THE EQUATION OF THE NORMAL CURVE

The value of the normal curve with mean μ and standard deviation σ is:

$$y = \frac{1}{\sqrt{2\pi\sigma^2}} \exp\left(\frac{-(x-\mu)^2}{2\sigma^2}\right)$$

where y gives the height of the curve, x is any value on the horizontal axis, exp( ) is the exponential function (see Section 13.2 for an explanation of the exponential function) and $\pi = 3.14159$. The normal curve value y is expressed as a proportion and the total area under the curve sums to 1, corresponding to the whole population.

The vertical axis can be expressed as a percentage, as in Figure 5.1, by multiplying y by 100. The area under the curve then sums to 100%.

Example 5.1

The following give two examples of calculating the height of the curve in Figure 5.1, where $\mu = 171.5$ and $\sigma = 6.5$ cm.

1 When height $x = 171.5$ cm (the mean value) then $(x - \mu) = 0$. This means that the expression inside the bracket is zero. As $\exp(0) = 1$, the height of the curve is given by

$$y = \frac{1}{\sqrt{2\pi \times 6.5^2}} = 0.0614, \text{ or } 6.14\%$$

2 When height $x = 180$ cm, the exponential part of the equation is

$$\exp\left(-\frac{(180 - 171.5)^2}{2 \times 6.5^2}\right) = 0.4253$$

and the height of the curve is given by

$$y = \frac{0.4253}{\sqrt{2\pi \times 6.5^2}} = 0.0261, \text{ or } 2.61\%$$

These values are indicated by the horizontal dashed lines on the normal curve in Figure 5.1.

5.4 THE STANDARD NORMAL DISTRIBUTION

If a variable is normally distributed then a change of units does not affect this. Thus, for example, whether height is measured in centimetres or inches it is normally distributed. Changing the mean simply moves the curve along the horizontal axis, while changing the standard deviation alters the height and width of the curve.

In particular, by a suitable change of units any normally distributed variable can be related to the **standard normal distribution** whose mean is zero and whose standard deviation is 1. This is done by subtracting the mean from each observation and dividing by the standard deviation. The relationship is:

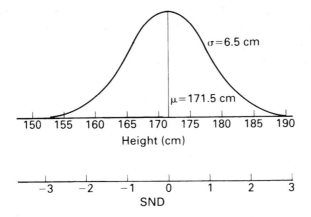

Fig. 5.2 Relationship between normal distribution in original units of measurement and in standard normal deviates. SND = (height − 171.5)/6.5. Height = 171.5 + (6.5 × SND).

$$\text{SND, } z = \frac{x - \mu}{\sigma}$$

where x is the original variable with mean μ and standard deviation σ, and z is the corresponding **standard normal deviate** (SND), alternatively called the **z-score**. This is illustrated for the distribution of adult male heights in Figure 5.2. The equation of the **standard normal distribution** is:

$$y = \frac{\exp(-z^2/2)}{\sqrt{2\pi}}$$

The possibility of converting any normally distributed variable into an SND means that calculations based on the standard normal distribution may be converted to corresponding calculations for any values of the mean and standard deviation. These calculations may be done either by using a computer, or by consulting tables of probability values for the normal distribution. The two most commonly provided sets of tables are (i) the area under the frequency distribution curve, and (ii) the so-called percentage points.

5.5 AREA UNDER THE CURVE OF THE NORMAL DISTRIBUTION

The standard normal distribution can be used to determine the proportion of the population that has values in some specified range or, equivalently, the probability that an individual observation from the distribution will lie in the specified range.

This is done by calculating the *area under the curve*. Calculation of areas under the normal curve requires a computer. It can be shown that the area under the whole of the normal curve is exactly 1; in other words the probability that an observation lies somewhere in the whole of the range is 1, or 100%.

Calculation of the proportion of the population in different ranges will be illustrated for the distribution shown in Figure 5.1 of the heights of adult men in the United Kingdom, which is approximately normal with mean $\mu = 171.5$ cm and standard deviation $\sigma = 6.5$ cm.

Area in upper tail of distribution

The proportion of men who are taller than 180 cm may be derived from the proportion of the area under the normal frequency distribution curve that is above 180 cm. The corresponding SND is:

$$z = \frac{180 - 171.5}{6.5} = 1.31$$

so that the proportion may be derived from the proportion of the area of the standard normal distribution that is above 1.31. This area is illustrated in Figure 5.3(a) and can be found from a computer or from Table A1 in the Appendix. The rows of the table refer to z to one decimal place and the columns to the second decimal place. Thus the area above 1.31 is given in row 1.3 and column 0.01 and is 0.0951. We conclude that a fraction 0.0951, or equivalently 9.51%, of adult men are taller than 180 cm.

Area in lower tail of distribution

The proportion of men shorter than 160 cm, for example, can be similarly estimated:

$$z = \frac{160 - 171.5}{6.5} = -1.77$$

The required area is illustrated in Figure 5.3(b). As the standard normal distribution is symmetrical about zero the area below $z = -1.77$ is equal to

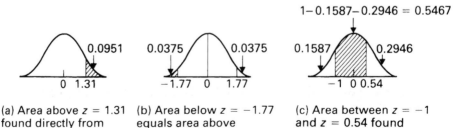

(a) Area above $z = 1.31$ found directly from Table A1

(b) Area below $z = -1.77$ equals area above $z = 1.77$ by symmetry

(c) Area between $z = -1$ and $z = 0.54$ found by subtraction

Fig. 5.3 Examples of the calculation of areas of the standard normal distribution.

the area above $z = 1.77$ and is 0.0375. Thus 3.75% of men are shorter than 160 cm.

Area of distribution between two values

The proportion of men with a height between, for example, 165 cm and 175 cm is estimated by finding the proportions of men shorter than 165 cm and taller than 175 cm and subtracting these from 1. This is illustrated in Figure 5.3(c).

1 SND corresponding to 165 cm is:

$$z = \frac{165 - 171.5}{6.5} = -1$$

Proportion below this height is 0.1587.

2 SND corresponding to 175 cm is:

$$z = \frac{175 - 171.5}{6.5} = 0.54$$

Proportion above this height is 0.2946.

3 Proportion of men with heights between 165 cm and 175 cm

$= 1 -$ proportion below 165 cm $-$ proportion above 175 cm

$= 1 - 0.1587 - 0.2946 = 0.5467$ or 54.67%

Value corresponding to specified tail area

Table A1 can also be used the other way round, that is starting with an area and finding the corresponding z value. For example, what height is exceeded by 5% or 0.05 of the population? Looking through the table the closest value to 0.05 is found in row 1.6 and column 0.04 and so the required z value is 1.64. The corresponding height is found by inverting the definition of SND to give:

$$x = \mu + z\sigma$$

and is $171.5 + 1.64 \times 6.5 = 182.2$ cm.

5.6 PERCENTAGE POINTS OF THE NORMAL DISTRIBUTION, AND REFERENCE RANGES

The SND expresses the value of a variable in terms of the number of standard deviations it is away from the mean. This is shown on the scale of the original variable in Figure 5.4. Thus, for example, $z = 1$ corresponds to a value which is one standard deviation above the mean and $z = -1$ to one standard deviation below the mean. The areas above $z = 1$ and below $z = -1$ are both 0.1587 or 15.87%. Therefore 31.74% ($2 \times 15.87\%$) of the distribution is further than one standard deviation from the mean, or equivalently 68.26% of the distribution lies within one standard deviation of the mean. Similarly, 4.55% of the distribution is further than two standard deviations from the mean, or equivalently 95.45% of the distribution lies within two standard deviations of the mean. This is the justification for the practical interpretation of the standard deviation given in Section 4.3.

Exactly 95% of the distribution lies between -1.96 and 1.96 (Fig 5.5a). Therefore the z value 1.96 is said to be the 5% **percentage point** of the normal distribution, as 5% of the distribution is further than 1.96 standard deviations from the mean (2.5% in each tail). Similarly, 2.58 is the 1% percentage point. The commonly used percentage points are tabulated in Table A2. Note that they could also be found from Table A1 in the way described above.

The percentage points described here are known as **two-sided** percentage points, as they cover extreme observations in both the upper and lower tails of the distribution. Some tables give **one-sided** percentage points, referring to just one tail of the distribution. The one-sided $a\%$ point is the same as the two-sided $2a\%$

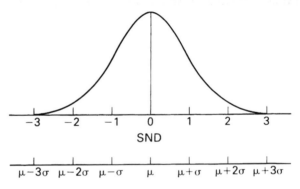

Fig. 5.4 Interpretation of SND in terms of a scale showing the number of standard deviations from the mean.

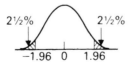

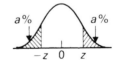

(a) 1.96 is the one-sided 2½%
point or the two-sided
5% point

(b) z is the one-sided $a\%$
point or the two-sided $2a\%$
point

Fig. 5.5 Percentage points of the normal distribution.

point (Figure 5.5b). For example, 1.96 is the one-sided 2.5% point, as 2.5% of the standard normal distribution is above 1.96 (or equivalently 2.5% is below -1.96) and it is the two-sided 5% point. This difference is discussed again in Section 7.3 in the context of hypothesis tests.

These properties mean that, for a normally distributed population, we can derive the range of values within which a given proportion of the population will lie. The 95% **reference range** is given by the mean -1.96 s.d. to mean $+1.96$ s.d., since 95% of the values in a population lie in this range. We can also define the 90% reference range and the 99% reference range in the same way, as mean -1.64 s.d. to mean $+1.64$ s.d. and mean -2.58 s.d. to mean $+2.58$ s.d., respectively.

5.7 USING *Z*-SCORES TO COMPARE DATA WITH REFERENCE CURVES

SNDs and *z*-scores are also used as a way of comparing the values of a variable with those of **reference curves**. The analysis is then carried out using the *z*-scores rather than the original values. For example, this is commonly carried out for anthropometric data, where **growth charts** are used to assess where an individual's weight (or height) lies compared to standard values for their age and sex, and the analysis is in terms of weight-for-age, height-for-age or weight-for-height *z*-scores. This use of *z*-scores is described in Section 13.4, in the chapter on transformations.

CHAPTER 6

Confidence interval for a mean

6.1 INTRODUCTION

In Chapter 4 we explained the idea of sampling variation and the *sampling distribution* of the mean. We showed that the mean of this sampling distribution equals the population mean, μ, and its standard deviation equals $\sigma/\sqrt{n}$, where σ is the population standard deviation, and n is the sample size. We introduced the concept that this standard deviation, which is called the *standard error* of the sample mean, measures how precisely the population mean is estimated by the sample mean. We now describe how we can use the sample mean and its standard error to give us a range of likely values for the population mean, which we wish to estimate.

6.2 LARGE SAMPLE CASE (NORMAL DISTRIBUTION)

In Chapter 4, we stated that approximately 95% of the sample means in the distribution obtained by repeated sampling would lie within two standard errors above or below the population mean. By drawing on the finding presented in Chapter 5, that provided that the sample size is not too small, this sampling distribution is a **normal distribution**, *whether or not* the underlying population distribution is normal, we can now be more precise. We can state that 95% of the sample means would lie within 1.96 standard errors above or below the population mean, since 1.96 is the two-sided 5% point of the standard normal distribution. This means that there is a 95% probability that a particular sample mean ($\bar{x}$) lies within 1.96 standard errors above or below the population mean (μ), which we wish to estimate:

$$\text{Prob}(\bar{x} \text{ is in the range } \mu - 1.96 \times \text{s.e. to } \mu + 1.96 \times \text{s.e.}) = 95\%$$

In practice, this result is used to estimate from the observed sample mean ($\bar{x}$) and its standard error (s.e.) a range within which the population mean is likely to lie. The statement:

'$\bar{x}$ is in the range $\mu - 1.96 \times$ s.e. to $\mu + 1.96 \times$ s.e.'

is equivalent to the statement:

'μ is in the range $\bar{x} - 1.96 \times$ s.e. to $\bar{x} + 1.96 \times$ s.e.'

Therefore there is a 95% probability that the interval between $\bar{x} - 1.96 \times$ s.e. and $\bar{x} + 1.96 \times$ s.e. contains the (unknown) population mean. This interval is called a 95% **confidence interval** (CI) for the population mean, and $\bar{x} - 1.96 \times$ s.e. and $\bar{x} + 1.96 \times$ s.e. are called upper and lower 95% **confidence limits** for the population mean, respectively.

When the sample is large, say n greater than 60, not only is the sampling distribution of sample means well approximated by the normal distribution, but the *sample standard deviation, s, is a reliable estimate of the population standard deviation, σ,* which is usually also not known. The standard error of the sample mean, $\sigma/\sqrt{n}$, can therefore be estimated by $s/\sqrt{n}$.

> Large-sample 95% CI $= \bar{x} - (1.96 \times s/\sqrt{n})$ to $\bar{x} + (1.96 \times s/\sqrt{n})$

Confidence intervals for percentages other than 95% are calculated in the same way using the appropriate percentage point, z', of the standard normal distribution in place of 1.96 (see Chapter 5). For example:

> Large-sample 90% CI $= \bar{x} - (1.64 \times s/\sqrt{n})$ to $\bar{x} + (1.64 \times s/\sqrt{n})$
>
> Large-sample 99% CI $= \bar{x} - (2.58 \times s/\sqrt{n})$ to $\bar{x} + (2.58 \times s/\sqrt{n})$

Example 6.1

As part of a malaria control programme it was planned to spray all the 10 000 houses in a rural area with insecticide and it was necessary to estimate the amount that would be required. Since it was not feasible to measure all 10 000 houses, a random sample of 100 houses was chosen and the sprayable surface of each of these was measured.

The mean sprayable surface area for these 100 houses was 24.2 m^2 and the standard deviation was 5.9 m^2. It is unlikely that the mean surface area of this sample of 100 houses ($\bar{x}$) exactly equals the mean surface area of all 10 000 houses (μ). Its precision is measured by the standard error $\sigma/\sqrt{n}$, estimated by $s/\sqrt{n} = 5.9/\sqrt{100} = 0.6$ m^2. There is a 95% probability that the sample mean of 24.2 m^2 differs from the population mean by less than 1.96 s.e. $= 1.96 \times 0.6 = 1.2$ m^2. The 95% confidence interval is:

$$95\% \text{ CI} = \bar{x} - 1.96 \times \text{s.e. to } \bar{x} + 1.96 \times \text{s.e.}$$
$$= 24.2 - 1.2 \text{ to } 24.2 + 1.2 = 23.0 \text{ to } 25.4 \text{ m}^2$$

It was decided to use the upper 95% confidence limit in budgeting for the amount of insecticide required as it was preferable to overestimate rather than underestimate the amount. One litre of insecticide is sufficient to spray $50\,\text{m}^2$ and so the amount budgeted for was:

$$10\,000 \times 254/50 = 5080 \text{ litres}$$

There is still a possibility, however, that this is too little insecticide. The interval 23.0 to $25.4\,\text{m}^2$ gives the likely range of values for the mean surface area of all 10 000 houses. There is a 95% probability that this interval contains the population mean but a 5% probability that it does not, with a 2.5% probability ($0.5 \times 5\%$) that the estimate based on the upper confidence limit is too small. A more cautious estimate for the amount of insecticide required would be based on a wider confidence interval, such as 99%, giving a smaller probability (0.5%) that too little would be estimated.

6.3 INTERPRETATION OF CONFIDENCE INTERVALS

We stated in Chapter 2 that our aim in many statistical analyses is to use the sample to make inferences about the population from which it was drawn. Confidence intervals provide us with a means of doing this (see Fig. 6.1).

It is tempting to interpret a 95% CI by saying that 'there is a 95% probability that the population mean lies within the CI'. Formally, this is not quite correct because the population mean (μ) is a fixed unknown number: it is the confidence

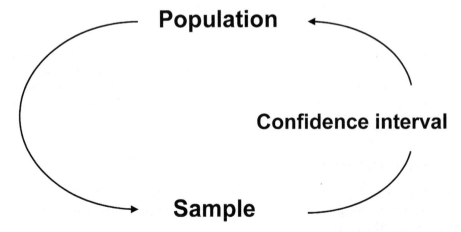

Fig. 6.1 Use of confidence intervals to make inferences about the population from which the sample was drawn.

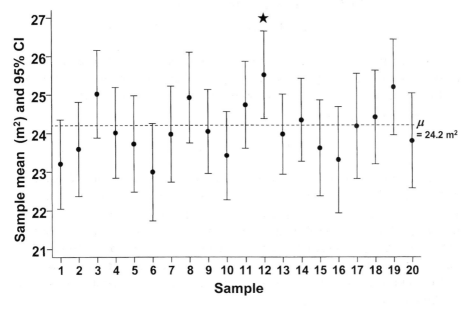

Fig. 6.2 Mean sprayable areas, with 95% confidence intervals, from 20 samples of 100 houses in a rural area. The star indicates that the CI does not contain the population mean.

interval that will vary between samples. In other words, if we were to draw several independent, random samples from the same population and calculate 95% confidence intervals from each of them, then on average 19 of every 20 (95%) such confidence intervals would contain the true population mean, and one of every 20 (5%) would not.

Example 6.2

A further 19 samples, each of 100 houses, were taken from the 10 000 houses described in Example 6.1. The mean sprayable surface and its standard error were calculated from each sample, and these were used to derive 95% confidence intervals. The means and 95% CIs from all 20 samples are shown in Figure 6.2. The mean in the whole population ($\mu = 24.2\,\mathrm{m}^2$) is shown by a horizontal dashed line. The sample means vary around the population mean μ, and one of the twenty 95% confidence intervals (indicated by a star) does not contain μ.

6.4 SMALLER SAMPLES

In the calculation of confidence intervals so far described the sample size (n) has been assumed to be large (greater than 60). When the sample size is not large, two aspects may alter:

1 the sample standard deviation, s, which is itself subject to sampling variation, may not be a reliable estimate for σ;

2 when the distribution in the population is not normal, the distribution of the sample mean may also be non-normal.

The second of these effects is of practical importance only when the sample size is very small (less than, say, 15) and when the distribution in the population is extremely non-normal. Because of the central limit theorem (see Chapter 5), it is usually only the first point, the sampling variation in s, which invalidates the use of the normal distribution in the calculation of confidence intervals. Instead, a distribution called the t distribution is used. Strictly speaking, this is valid only if the population is normally distributed, but the use of the t distribution has been shown to be justified, except where the population is extremely non-normal. (This property is called **robustness**.) What to do in cases of severe non-normality is described later in this chapter.

Confidence interval using t distribution

The earlier calculation of a confidence interval using the normal distribution was based on the fact that $(\bar{x} - \mu)/(\sigma/\sqrt{n})$ is a value from the standard normal distribution, and that for large samples we could use s in place of σ. In fact, $(\bar{x} - \mu)/(s/\sqrt{n})$ is a value not from the standard normal distribution but from a distribution called the **t distribution** with $(n-1)$ **degrees of freedom**. This distribution was introduced by W. S. Gossett, who used the pen-name 'Student', and is often called Student's t distribution. Like the normal distribution, the t distribution is a symmetrical bell-shaped distribution, but it is more spread out, having longer tails (Figure 6.3).

The exact shape of the t distribution depends on the degrees of freedom (d.f.), $n-1$, of the sample standard deviation s; the fewer the degrees of freedom, the more the t distribution is spread out. The percentage points are tabulated for various degrees of freedom in Table A3 in the Appendix. For example, if the sample size is 8, the degrees of freedom are 7 and the two-sided 5% point is 2.36. In this case the 95% confidence interval using the sample standard deviation s would be

$$95\% \text{ CI} = x - 2.36 \, s/\sqrt{n} \text{ to } x + 2.36 \, s/\sqrt{n}$$

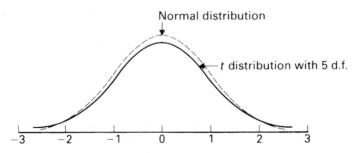

Fig. 6.3 t distribution with 5 degrees of freedom compared to the normal distribution.

In general a confidence interval is calculated using t', the appropriate percentage point of the t distribution with $(n - 1)$ degrees of freedom.

$$\text{Small-sample CI} = \bar{x} - (t' \times s/\sqrt{n}) \text{ to } \bar{x} + (t' \times s/\sqrt{n})$$

For small degrees of freedom the percentage points of the t distribution are appreciably larger in value than the corresponding percentage points of the normal distribution. This is because the sample standard deviation s may be a poor estimate of the population value σ, and when this uncertainty is taken into account the resulting confidence interval is considerably wider than if σ were reliably known. For large degrees of freedom the t distribution is almost the same as the standard normal distribution, since s is a good estimate of σ. The bottom row of Table A3 in the Appendix gives the percentage points for the t distribution with an infinite number (∞) of degrees of freedom and it may be seen by comparison with Table A2 that these are the same as for the normal distribution.

Example 6.3

The following are the numbers of hours of relief obtained by six arthritic patients after receiving a new drug:

$$2.2, 2.4, 4.9, 2.5, 3.7, 4.3 \text{ hours}$$
$$\bar{x} = 3.3 \text{ hours}, s = 1.13 \text{ hours}, n = 6, \text{d.f.} = n - 1 = 5$$
$$s/\sqrt{n} = 0.46 \text{ hours}$$

The 5% point of the t distribution with 5 degrees of freedom is 2.57, and so the 95% confidence interval for the average number of hours of relief for arthritic patients in general is:

$$3.3 - 2.57 \times 0.46 \text{ to } 3.3 + 2.57 \times 0.46 = 3.3 - 1.2 \text{ to } 3.3 + 1.2 = 2.1 \text{ to } 4.5 \text{ hours}$$

Severe non-normality

When the distribution in the population is markedly non-normal (see Section 12.2), it may be desirable to **transform** the scale on which the variable x is measured so as to make its distribution on the new scale more normal (see Chapter 13). An alternative is to calculate a **non-parametric** confidence interval or to use **bootstrap** methods (see Chapter 30).

6.5 SUMMARY OF ALTERNATIVES

Table 6.1 summarizes which procedure should be used in constructing a confidence interval. There is no precise boundary between approximate normality and non-normality but, for example, a reverse J-shaped distribution (Fig. 3.6b) is

Table 6.1 Recommended procedures for constructing a confidence interval. (z' is the percentage point from the *normal* distribution, and t' the percentage point from the t distribution with $(n-1)$ degrees of freedom.)

(a) Population standard deviation σ unknown.

Sample size	Population distribution	
	Approximately normal	Severely non-normal*
60 or more	$\bar{x} - (z' \times s/\sqrt{n})$ to $\bar{x} + (z' \times s/\sqrt{n})$	$\bar{x} - (z' \times s/\sqrt{n})$ to $\bar{x} + (z' \times s/\sqrt{n})$
Less than 60	$\bar{x} - (t' \times s/\sqrt{n})$ to $\bar{x} + (t' \times s/\sqrt{n})$	see Chapter 30

(b) Population standard deviation σ known.

Sample size	Population distribution	
	Approximately normal	Severely non-normal*
15 or more	$\bar{x} - (z' \times \sigma/\sqrt{n})$ to $\bar{x} + (z' \times \sigma/\sqrt{n})$	$\bar{x} - (z' \times \sigma/\sqrt{n})$ to $\bar{x} + (z' \times \sigma/\sqrt{n})$
Less than 15	$\bar{x} - (z' \times \sigma/\sqrt{n})$ to $\bar{x} + (z' \times \sigma/\sqrt{n})$	see Chapter 30

*It may be preferable to transform the scale of measurement to make the distribution more normal (see Chapter 13).

severely non-normal, and a skewed distribution (Fig. 3.5b or c) is moderately non-normal.

In rare instances the population standard deviation, σ, is known and therefore not estimated from the sample. When this occurs the standard normal distribution percentage points are used to give the confidence interval regardless of sample size, provided the population distribution is not severely non-normal (in which case see the preceding paragraph).

6.6 CONFIDENCE INTERVALS AND REFERENCE RANGES

It is important to understand the distinction between the **reference range** (which was defined in Section 5.6) and confidence intervals, defined in this chapter. Although they are often confused, each has a different use and a different definition.

A 95% reference range is given by:

$$95\% \text{ reference range} = \mu - 1.96 \times \text{s.d. to } \mu + 1.96 \times \text{s.d.}$$

where μ is the mean of the distribution and s.d. is its standard deviation. A large sample 95% confidence interval is given by:

$$95\% \text{ CI} = \bar{x} - 1.96 \times \text{s.e. to } \bar{x} + 1.96 \times \text{s.e.}$$

where s.e. is the standard error of the distribution: s.e. $= \text{s.d.}/\sqrt{n}$.

The reference range tells us about the variability between individual observations in the population: providing that the distribution is approximately normal

95% of individual observations will lie within the reference range. In contrast, as explained earlier in this chapter, the 95% CI tells us a range of plausible values for the population mean, given the sample mean. Since the sample size n must be > 1, the confidence interval will always be narrower than the reference range.

CHAPTER 7

Comparison of two means: confidence intervals, hypothesis tests and *P*-values

7.1 INTRODUCTION

In Chapter 6 we described how to use a sample mean and its standard error to give us a range of likely values, called a *confidence interval*, for the corresponding population mean. We now extend these ideas to situations where we wish to compare the mean outcomes in two **exposure** (or **treatment**) **groups**. We will label the two groups 0 and 1, and the two means $\bar{x}_0$ and $\bar{x}_1$, with group 1 denoting individuals *exposed* to a risk factor, and group 0 denoting those *unexposed*. In clinical trials, group 1 will denote the *treatment* group and group 0 the *control* group. For example:

- In a study of the determinants of birthweight, we may wish to compare the mean birthweight of children born to smokers (the exposed group, 1) with that for children born to non-smokers (the unexposed group, 0).
- In a clinical trial of a new anti-hypertensive drug, the comparison of interest might be mean systolic blood pressure after 6 months of treatment, between patients allocated to receive the new drug (the treatment group, 1) and those allocated to receive standard therapy (the control group, 0).

The two group means, $\bar{x}_1$ and $\bar{x}_0$, are of interest not in their own right, but for what they tell us more generally about the effect of the exposure on the outcome of interest (or in the case of a clinical trial, of the treatment), in the population from which the groups are drawn. More specifically, we wish to answer the following related questions.

1 What does the *difference* between the two group means in our sample ($\bar{x}_1$ and $\bar{x}_0$) tell us about the difference between the two group means in the population? In other words, what can we say about how much better (or worse) off are exposed individuals compared to unexposed? This is addressed by calculating a

confidence interval for the range of likely values for the difference, following a similar approach to that used for a single mean (see Chapter 6).

2 Do the data provide evidence that the exposure actually affects the outcome, or might the observed difference between the sample means have arisen by chance? In other words, are the data consistent with there being zero difference between the means in the two groups in the population? We address this by carrying out a **hypothesis** (or *significance*) **test** to give a **P-value**, which is the probability of recording a difference between the two groups at least as large as that in our sample, if there was no effect of the exposure in the population.

In this chapter we define the sampling distribution of the difference in means comparing the two groups, and then describe how to use this to calculate a confidence interval for the true difference, and how to calculate the test statistic and *P*-value for the related hypothesis test. The methods used are based on either the *normal* or *t* distributions. The rules for which distribution to use are similar to those for the one-sample case. For large samples, or known standard deviations, we use the normal distribution, and for small samples we use the *t* distribution.

The majority of this chapter is concerned with comparing mean outcomes measured in two separate groups of individuals. In some circumstances, however, our data consist instead of *pairs* of outcome measurements. How to compare **paired measurements** is covered in Section 7.6. For example:

- We might wish to carry out a study where the assessment of an anti-hypertensive drug is based on comparing blood pressure measurements in a group of hypertensive men, before and after they received treatment. For each man, we therefore have a pair of outcome measures, blood pressure after treatment and blood pressure before treatment. It is important to take this pairing in the data into account when assessing how much on average the treatment has affected blood pressure.

- Another example would be data from a matched case–control study (see Section 21.4), in which the data consist of case–control pairs rather than of two independent groups of cases and controls, with a control specifically selected to match each case on key variables such as age and sex.

7.2 SAMPLING DISTRIBUTION OF THE DIFFERENCE BETWEEN TWO MEANS

Before we can construct a confidence interval for the difference between two means, or carry out the related hypothesis test, we need to know the sampling distribution of the difference. The difference, $\bar{x}_1 - \bar{x}_0$, between the mean outcomes in the exposed and unexposed groups in our sample provides an estimate of the underlying difference, $\mu_1 - \mu_0$, between the mean outcomes in the exposed and unexposed groups in the population. Just as discussed for a single mean (see Chapter 6), this sample difference will not be exactly equal to the population difference. It is subject to *sampling variation*, so that a different sample from the same population would give a different value of $\bar{x}_1 - \bar{x}_0$. *Providing that each of the means, $\bar{x}_1$ and $\bar{x}_0$, is normally distributed*, then:

1 the sampling distribution of the difference $(\bar{x}_1 - \bar{x}_0)$ is normally distributed;

2 the mean of this sampling distribution is simply the difference between the two population means, $\mu_1 - \mu_0$;

3 the standard error of $(\bar{x}_1 - \bar{x}_0)$ is based on a combination of the standard errors of the individual means:

$$\text{s.e.} = \sqrt{(s.e._1^2 + s.e._0^2)} = \sqrt{\left(\frac{\sigma_1^2}{n_1} + \frac{\sigma_0^2}{n_0}\right)}$$

This is estimated using the sample standard deviations, s_1 and s_0. Note that when we calculate the difference between the means in the two groups we *combine* the uncertainty in $\bar{x}_1$ with the uncertainty in $\bar{x}_0$.

7.3 METHODS BASED ON THE NORMAL DISTRIBUTION (LARGE SAMPLES OR KNOWN STANDARD DEVIATIONS)

Confidence interval

When both groups are large (say, greater than 30), or in the rare instances when the population standard deviations are known, then methods for comparing means are based on the normal distribution. We calculate 95% confidence intervals for the difference in the population as:

Large samples

$\text{CI} = (\bar{x}_1 - \bar{x}_0) - (z' \times \text{s.e.})$ to $(\bar{x}_1 - \bar{x}_0) + (z' \times \text{s.e.})$

$\text{s.e.} = \sqrt{(s_1^2/n_1 + s_0^2/n_0)}$

or

Known σ's

$\text{CI} = (\bar{x}_1 - \bar{x}_0) - (z' \times \text{s.e.})$ to $(\bar{x}_1 - \bar{x}_0) + (z' \times \text{s.e.})$

$\text{s.e.} = \sqrt{(\sigma_1^2/n_1 + \sigma_0^2/n_0)}$

In these formulae z' is the appropriate percentage point of the normal distribution. For example, when calculating a 95% confidence interval we use $z' = 1.96$.

Example 7.1

To investigate whether smoking reduces lung function, forced vital capacity (FVC, a test of lung function) was measured in 100 men aged 25–29, of whom 36 were smokers and 64 non-smokers. Results of the study are shown in Table 7.1.

Table 7.1 Results of a study to investigate the association between smoking and lung function.

Group	Number of men	Mean FVC (litres)	s	s.e. of mean FVC
Smokers (1)	$n_1 = 36$	$\bar{x}_1 = 4.7$	$s_1 = 0.6$	s.e.$_1 = 0.6/\sqrt{36} = 0.100$
Non-smokers (0)	$n_0 = 64$	$\bar{x}_0 = 5.0$	$s_0 = 0.6$	s.e.$_0 = 0.6/\sqrt{64} = 0.075$

The mean FVC in smokers was 4.7 litres compared with 5.0 litres in non-smokers. The difference in mean FVC, $\bar{x}_1 - \bar{x}_0$, is therefore 4.7 − 5.0, that is −0.3 litres. The s.d. in both groups was 0.6 litres. The standard error of the difference in mean FVC is calculated from the individual standard errors, which are shown in the right hand column of the table, as follows:

$$\text{s.e.} = \sqrt{(\text{s.e.}_1^2 + \text{s.e.}_0^2)} = \sqrt{(0.1^2 + 0.075^2)} = 0.125 \text{ litres}$$

The 95% confidence interval for the population difference in mean FVC is therefore:

$$95\% \text{ CI} = -0.3 - (1.96 \times 0.125) \text{ to } -0.3 + (1.96 \times 0.125)$$
$$= -0.545 \text{ litres to } -0.055 \text{ litres}$$

Both the lower and upper confidence limits are negative, and both therefore correspond to a reduced FVC among smokers compared to non-smokers. With 95% confidence, the reduction in mean FVC in smokers, compared to non-smokers, lies between 0.055 litres (a relatively small reduction) and 0.545 litres (a reduction likely to have obvious effects).

z-test

The confidence interval gives a range of likely values for the difference in mean outcome between exposed and unexposed groups in the population. With reference to Example 7.1, we now address the related issue of whether the data provide evidence that the exposure (smoking) actually affects the mean outcome (FVC), or whether they are consistent with smoking having no effect. In other words, might the *population* difference between the two groups be zero? We address this issue by carrying out a **hypothesis** (or **significance**) test.

A hypothesis test begins by postulating that, *in the population*, mean FVC is the same in smokers and non-smokers, so that any observed difference between the sample means is due to sampling variation. This is called the **null hypothesis**. The next step is to calculate the probability, *if the null hypothesis were true*, of getting a difference between the two group means as large or larger than the difference than that was observed. This probability is called a **P-value**. The idea is that the *smaller* the P-value, the *stronger* is the evidence against the null hypothesis.

We use the fact that the sampling distribution of $(\bar{x}_1 - \bar{x}_0)$ is *normal* to derive the P-value. If the null hypothesis is true, then the mean of the sampling distribution, $\mu_1 - \mu_0$, is zero. Our **test statistic** is the z-score, or **standard normal deviate** (see Chapter 5) corresponding to the observed difference between the means:

$$z = \frac{\text{difference in means}}{\text{standard error of difference in means}} = \frac{\bar{x}_1 - \bar{x}_0}{\text{s.e.}}$$

The formulae for the z-test are as follows:

Large samples

$$z = \frac{\bar{x}_1 - \bar{x}_0}{\text{s.e.}} = \frac{\bar{x}_1 - \bar{x}_0}{\sqrt{(s_1^2/n_1 + s_0^2/n_0)}}$$

or

Known $\sigma's$

$$z = \frac{\bar{x}_1 - \bar{x}_0}{\text{s.e.}} = \frac{\bar{x}_1 - \bar{x}_0}{\sqrt{(\sigma_1^2/n_1 + \sigma_0^2/n_0)}}$$

The **test statistic** z measures by how many standard errors the mean difference $(\bar{x}_1 - \bar{x}_0)$ differs from the null value of 0. In this example,

$$z = \frac{-0.3}{0.125} = -2.4$$

The difference between the means is therefore 2.4 standard errors below 0, as illustrated in Figure 7.1. The probability of getting a difference of -2.4 standard errors or less (the area under the curve to the left of -2.4) is found using a computer or using Table A1; it is 0.0082. This probability is known as the **one-sided P-value**. By convention, we usually use **two-sided P-values**; our assessment of the probability that the result is due to chance is based on how extreme the *size* of the departure is from the null hypothesis, and not its direction. We therefore include the probability that the difference might (by chance) have been in the opposite direction: mean FVC might have been greater in smokers than non-smokers. Because the normal distribution is symmetrical, this probability is also 0.0082. The 'two-sided' P-value is thus found to be $0.0164 (= 0.0082 + 0.0082)$, as shown in Figure 7.1.

This means that the probability of observing a difference at least as extreme as 2.4, if the null hypothesis of no difference is correct, is 0.0164, or 1.64%. In other words, if the null hypothesis were true, then sampling variation would yield such a large difference in the mean FVC between smokers and non-smokers in only about 16 in every 1000 similar-sized studies that might be carried out. Such a P-value provides evidence *against* the null hypothesis, and suggests that smoking affects FVC.

At this point, you may wish to skip forward to Chapter 8, which gives a fuller description of how to interpret P-values, and how to use P-values and confidence intervals to interpret the results of statistical analyses.

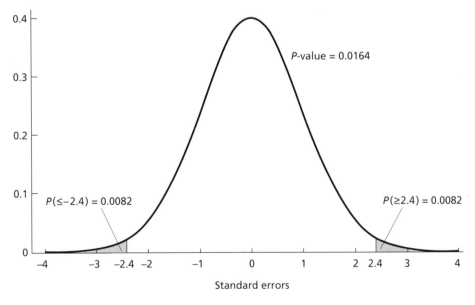

Fig. 7.1 Probability that the size of a standard normal deviate (z) is 2.4 standard errors or larger.

7.4 METHODS BASED ON THE t DISTRIBUTION (SMALL SAMPLES, EQUAL STANDARD DEVIATIONS)

We saw in Chapter 6 that for small samples we must also allow for the sampling variation in the standard deviation, s, when deriving a confidence interval for a mean. Similar considerations arise when we wish to compare means between small samples. Methods based on the t distribution rather than the normal distribution are used. These require that the population distributions are normal but, as with confidence intervals for a single mean, they are robust against departures from this assumption. When comparing two means, the validity of these methods also depends on the *equality* of the two population standard deviations. In many situations it is reasonable to assume this equality. If the sample standard deviations are very different in size, however, say if one is more than twice as large as the other, then an alternative must be used. This is discussed below in Section 7.5.

Confidence interval

The formula for the standard error of the difference between the means is simplified to:

$$\text{s.e.} = \sqrt{(\sigma^2/n_1 + \sigma^2/n_0)} \text{ or } \sigma\sqrt{(1/n_1 + 1/n_0)}$$

where σ is the common standard deviation. There are two sample estimates of σ from the two samples, s_1 and s_0 and these are combined to give a common estimate, s, of the population standard deviation, with degrees of freedom equal to $(n_1 - 1) + (n_0 - 1) = n_1 + n_0 - 2$.

$$s = \sqrt{\left[\frac{(n_1 - 1)s_1^2 + (n_0 - 1)s_0^2}{(n_1 + n_0 - 2)}\right]}$$

This formula gives greater weight to the estimate from the larger sample as this will be more reliable. The standard error of the difference between the two means is estimated by:

$$\text{s.e.} = s\sqrt{(1/n_1 + 1/n_0)}$$

The confidence interval is calculated using t', the appropriate percentage point of the t distribution with $(n_1 + n_0 - 2)$ degrees of freedom:

$$\text{CI} = (\bar{x}_1 - \bar{x}_0) - (t' \times \text{s.e.}) \text{ to } (\bar{x}_1 - \bar{x}_0) + (t' \times \text{s.e.}),$$
$$\text{d.f.} = (n_1 + n_0 - 2)$$

Example 7.2

Table 7.2 shows the birth weights of children born to 14 heavy smokers (group 1) and to 15 non-smokers (group 0), sampled from live births at a large teaching hospital. The calculations needed to derive the confidence interval are:

difference between the means, $\bar{x}_1 - \bar{x}_0 = 3.1743 - 3.6267 = -0.4524$

$$\text{standard deviation, } s = \sqrt{\left[\frac{13 \times 0.4631^2 + 14 \times 0.3584^2}{15 + 14 - 2}\right]} = 0.4121 \text{ kg}$$

standard error of the difference, s.e. $= 0.4121 \times \sqrt{(1/14 + 1/15)} = 0.1531 \text{ kg}$

degrees of freedom, d.f. $= 14 + 15 - 2 = 27;\ t' = 2.05$

The 5% percentage point of the t distribution with 27 degrees of freedom is 2.05, and so the 95% confidence interval for the difference between the mean birth weights is:

$$-0.4524 - (2.05 \times 0.1531) \text{ to } -0.4524 + (2.05 \times 0.1531) = -0.77 \text{ to } -0.14 \text{ kg}$$

Table 7.2 Comparison of birth weights (kg) of children born to 14 heavy smokers with those of children born to 15 non-smokers.

Heavy smokers (group 1)	Non-smokers (group 0)
3.18	3.99
2.74	3.89
2.90	3.60
3.27	3.73
3.65	3.31
3.42	3.70
3.23	4.08
2.86	3.61
3.60	3.83
3.65	3.41
3.69	4.13
3.53	3.36
2.38	3.54
2.34	3.51
	2.71
$\bar{x}_1 = 3.1743$	$\bar{x}_0 = 3.6267$
$s_1 = 0.4631$	$s_0 = 0.3584$
$n_1 = 14$	$n_0 = 15$

With 95% confidence, mean birth weight is between 0.14 and 0.77 kg lower for children born to heavy smokers than for those born to non-smokers.

t test

In small samples we allow for the sampling variation in the standard deviations by using the t distribution for our test of the null hypothesis. This is called a *t* **test**, sometimes also known as an **unpaired *t* test**, to distinguish it from the **paired *t* test** for paired measurements, described in Section 7.6. The t value is calculated as:

$$t = \frac{\bar{x}_1 - \bar{x}_0}{\text{s.e.}} = \frac{\bar{x}_1 - \bar{x}_0}{s\sqrt{(1/n_1 + 1/n_0)}}, \quad \text{d.f.} = n_1 + n_0 - 2$$

where, as before

$$s = \sqrt{\left[\frac{(n_1 - 1)s_1^2 + (n_0 - 1)s_0^2}{(n_1 + n_0 - 2)}\right]}$$

The corresponding P-value is derived in exactly the same way as for the z distribution. This is best done using a computer, rather than tables, as it is impractical to have sets of tables for all the different possible degrees of freedom. However, an approximate P-value corresponding to different values of the test statistic t may be derived from Table A4 (see Appendix), which tabulates this for a selection of degrees of freedom. It can be seen that unless the number of degrees of freedom is small the P-value based on the normal distribution (right hand column) does not differ greatly from that based on the t distribution (main part of table).

Example 7.2 (continued)
The calculations for the t-test to compare the birth weights of children born to 14 heavy smokers with those of children born to 15 non-smokers, as shown in Table 7.2, are as follows:

$$t = \frac{(3.1743 - 3.6267)}{0.4121\sqrt{(1/14 + 1/15)}} = -\frac{0.4524}{0.1531} = -2.95,$$

$$\text{d.f.} = 14 + 15 - 2 = 27, \quad P = 0.0064$$

As the test is two-sided, the *P*-value corresponding to *minus* 2.95 is the same as that corresponding to *plus* 2.95. Table A4 shows that the *P*-value corresponding to $t = 3.0$ with 25 degrees of freedom is 0.006. The *precise* *P*-value of 0.0064 was derived using a computer. As explained in more detail in Chapter 8, a *P*-value of 0.0064 provides fairly strong evidence against the null hypothesis. These data therefore suggest that smoking during pregnancy reduces the birthweight of the baby.

7.5 SMALL SAMPLES, UNEQUAL STANDARD DEVIATIONS

When the population standard deviations of the two groups are different, and the sample size is not large, the main possibilities are:

1 seek a suitable change of scale (a *transformation*, see Chapter 13) which makes the standard deviations similar so that methods based on the *t* distribution can be used. For example, if the standard deviations seem to be proportional in size to the means, then taking logarithms of the individual values may be appropriate;

2 use *non-parametric* methods based on ranks (*see* Section 30.2);

3 use either the Fisher–Behrens or the Welch tests, which allow for unequal standard deviations (consult Armitage & Berry 2002);

4 estimate the difference between the means using the original measurements, but use bootstrap methods to derive confidence intervals (see Section 30.3).

7.6 PAIRED MEASUREMENTS

In some circumstances our data consist of *pairs* of measurements, as described in the introduction to the chapter. These pairs may be two outcomes measured on the same individual under different exposure (or treatment) circumstances. Alternatively, the pairs may be two individuals matched during sample selection to share certain key characteristics such as age and sex, for example in a matched case–control study or in a clinical trial with matched controls (see Chapter 21). Our analysis needs to take this pairing in the data into account: this is done by considering the *differences* between each pair of outcome observations. In other words we turn our data of pairs of outcomes into a single sample of differences.

Confidence interval

The confidence interval for the mean of these differences is calculated using the methods explained for a single mean in Chapter 6, and depending on the sample size uses either the normal or the *t* distribution. In brief, the confidence interval for the difference between the means is:

Large samples (60 or more pairs)

$$\text{CI} = \bar{x} - (z' \times \text{s.e.}) \text{ to } \bar{x} + (z' \times \text{s.e.})$$

or

Small samples (less than 60 pairs)

$$\text{CI} = \bar{x} - (t' \times \text{s.e.}) \text{ to } \bar{x} + (t' \times \text{s.e.})$$

where for large samples z' is the chosen percentage point of the normal distribution and for small samples t' is the chosen percentage point of the t distribution with $n - 1$ degrees of freedom. (See Table 6.1 for more details.)

Example 7.3

Consider the results of a clinical trial to test the effectiveness of a sleeping drug in which the sleep of ten patients was observed during one night with the drug and one night with a placebo. The results obtained are shown in Table 7.3. For each patient a pair of sleep times, namely those with the drug and with the placebo, was recorded and the difference between these calculated. The average number of additional hours slept with the drug compared with the placebo was $\bar{x} = 1.08$, and the standard deviation *of the differences* was $s = 2.31$ hours. The standard error of the differences is $s/\sqrt{n} = 2.31/\sqrt{10} = 0.73$ hours.

Table 7.3 Results of a placebo-controlled clinical trial to test the effectiveness of a sleeping drug.

Patient	Hours of sleep		Difference
	Drug	Placebo	
1	6.1	5.2	0.9
2	6.0	7.9	−1.9
3	8.2	3.9	4.3
4	7.6	4.7	2.9
5	6.5	5.3	1.2
6	5.4	7.4	−2.0
7	6.9	4.2	2.7
8	6.7	6.1	0.6
9	7.4	3.8	3.6
10	5.8	7.3	−1.5
Mean	$\bar{x}_1 = 6.66$	$\bar{x}_0 = 5.58$	$\bar{x} = 1.08$

Since we have only ten pairs we use the t distribution with 9 degrees of freedom. The 5% point is 2.26, and so the 95% confidence interval is:

$$95\% \text{ CI} = 1.08 - (2.26 \times 0.73) \text{ to } 1.08 + (2.26 \times 0.73) = -0.57 \text{ to } 2.73 \text{ hours.}$$

With 95% confidence, we therefore estimate the drug to increase average sleeping times by between -0.51 and 2.73 hours. This small study is thus consistent with an effect of the drug which ranges from a small reduction in mean sleep time to a substantial increase in mean sleep time.

Note that the mean of the differences ($\bar{x}$) is the same as the difference between the means ($\bar{x}_1 - \bar{x}_0$). However, the standard error of $\bar{x}$ will be smaller than the standard error of ($\bar{x}_1 - \bar{x}_0$) because we have cancelled out the variation between individuals in their underlying sleep times by calculating *within-person* differences. In other words, we have accounted for the *between-person* variation (see Section 31.4), and so our confidence interval is narrower than if we had used an unpaired design of a similar size.

Hypothesis test

Hypothesis testing of paired means is carried out using either a paired z test or paired t test, depending on the same criteria as laid out for confidence intervals. We calculate the mean of the paired differences, and the test statistic is:

Large sample		Small sample
$z = \dfrac{\bar{x}}{\text{s.e.}} = \dfrac{\bar{x}}{s/\sqrt{n}}$	or	$t = \dfrac{\bar{x}}{\text{s.e.}} = \dfrac{\bar{x}}{s/\sqrt{n}}, \quad \text{d.f.} = n - 1$

where $\bar{x}$ is the mean of the paired differences, and n is the number of pairs.

Example 7.3 (continued)
In the above example in Table 7.3 the mean difference in sleep time is 1.08 hours and the standard error is 0.73 hours. A paired t test gives:

$$t = 1.08/0.73 = 1.48, \quad \text{d.f.} = 9$$

The probability of getting a t value as large as this in a t distribution with 9 degrees of freedom is 0.17, so there is no evidence against the null hypothesis that the drug does not affect sleep time. This is consistent with the interpretation of the 95% CI given earlier. An approximate *P*-value can be found from Table A4 (see Appendix), which shows that if the test statistic is 1.5 with 9 degrees of freedom then the *P*-value is 0.168. Further examples of the use of confidence intervals and *P*-values to interpret the results of statistical analyses are given in the next chapter.

CHAPTER 8

Using *P*-values and confidence intervals to interpret the results of statistical analyses

8.1 INTRODUCTION

In Chapter 7 we described how statistical methods may be used to examine the difference between the mean outcome in two exposure groups We saw that we present the results of analyses in two related ways, by reporting a *confidence interval* which gives a range of likely values for the difference in the population, and a *P-value* which addresses whether the observed difference in the sample could arise because of chance alone, if there were no difference in the population.

Throughout this book, we will repeat this process. That is, we will:

1 estimate the magnitude of the difference in disease outcome between exposure groups;

2 derive a confidence interval for the difference; and

3 derive a *P*-value to test the null hypothesis that there is no association between exposure and disease in the population.

In this chapter, we consider how to use *P*-values and confidence intervals to interpret the results of statistical analyses. We discuss hypothesis tests in more detail, explain how to interpret *P*-values and describe some common errors in their interpretation. We conclude by giving examples of the interpretation of the results of different studies.

8.2 TESTING HYPOTHESES

Suppose we believe that everybody who lives to age 90 or more is a non-smoker. We could investigate this hypothesis in two ways:

1 *Prove the hypothesis* by finding every single person aged 90 or over and checking that they are all non-smokers.

2 *Disprove the hypothesis* by finding just one person aged 90 or over who is a smoker.

In general, it is much easier to find evidence *against* a hypothesis than to be able to prove that it is correct. In fact, one view of science (put forward by the philosopher

Karl Popper) is that it is a process of *disproving* hypotheses. For example, Newton's laws of mechanics were accepted until Einstein showed that there were circumstances in which they did not work.

Statistical methods formalize this idea by looking for evidence against a very specific form of hypothesis, called a **null hypothesis**: that there is *no difference* between groups or *no association* between variables. Relevant data are then collected and assessed for their consistency with the null hypothesis. Links between exposures and outcomes, or between treatments and outcomes, are assessed by examining the strength of the evidence *against* the null hypothesis, as measured by a ***P*-value** (see Section 8.3).

Examples of null hypotheses might be:
● Treatment with beta-interferon has no effect on mean quality of life in patients with multiple sclerosis.
● Performing radical surgery on men aged 55 to 75 diagnosed with prostate cancer does not improve their subsequent mortality.
● Living close to power lines does not affect a child's risk of developing leukaemia.

In some circumstances, statistical methods are not required in order to reject the null hypothesis. For example, before 1990 the most common treatment for stomach ulcers was surgery. A pathologist noticed a particular organism (now known as *Helicobacter pylori*) was often present in biopsy samples taken from stomach ulcers, and grew the organism in culture. He then swallowed a glassful, following which he experienced acute gastritis, and found that the organism progressed to a chronic infection. No statistical analysis of this experiment was necessary to confidently deduce this causal link and reject the *null hypothesis* of no association (B.J. Marshall *et al*. 1985, *Med J Australia* **142**; 436–9), although this was confirmed through antibiotic trials showing that eradicating *H. pylori* cured stomach ulcers.

Similarly, when penicillin was first used as a treatment for pneumonia in the 1940s the results were so dramatic that no formal trial was necessary. Unfortunately such examples, where the results 'hit you straight between the eyes', are rare in medical research. This is because there is rarely such a one-to-one link between exposures and outcomes; there is usually much more inherent *variability* from person to person. Thus although we know that smoking causes lung cancer, we are aware that some heavy smokers will live to an old age, and also that some non-smokers will die prematurely. In other words, smoking increases the risk, but it does not by itself determine death; the outcome is *unpredictable* and is influenced by many other factors.

Statistical methods are used to assess the strength of evidence against a null hypothesis, taking into account this person-to-person variability. Suppose that we want to evaluate whether a new drug reduces cholesterol levels. We might study a group of patients treated with the new drug (the *treatment* group) and a comparable group treated with a *placebo* (the *control* group), and discover that cholesterol levels were on average 5 mg per decilitre lower among patients in the treatment group compared to those in the control group. Before concluding that the drug is effective, we would need to consider whether this could be a chance finding. We address this question by calculating a *test statistic* and its corresponding *P-value* (also known as a *significance level*). This is the probability of getting a difference of at least 5 mg between the mean cholesterol levels of patients in the treatment and control groups if the drug really has no effect. The *smaller* the P-value, the *stronger* the evidence against the null hypothesis that the drug has no effect on cholesterol levels.

8.3 GENERAL FORM OF CONFIDENCE INTERVALS AND TEST STATISTICS

Note that in all cases the **confidence interval** is constructed as the sample estimate (be it a mean, a difference between means or any of the other measures of exposure effect introduced later in the book), plus or minus its standard error multiplied by the appropriate percentage point. Unless the sample size is small, this percentage point is based on the normal distribution (e.g. 1.96 for 95% confidence intervals). The **test statistic** is simply the sample estimate divided by its standard error.

$$95\% \text{ CI} = \text{estimate} - (1.96 \times \text{s.e.}) \text{ to estimate} + (1.96 \times \text{s.e.})$$

$$\text{Test statistic} = \frac{\text{estimate}}{\text{s.e.}}$$

The standard error is *inversely* related to the sample size. Thus the larger the sample size, the smaller will be the standard error. Since the standard error determines the width of the confidence interval and the size of the test statistic, this also implies the following: for any particular size of difference between the two groups, the *larger* the sample size, the *smaller* will be the confidence interval and the *larger* the test statistic.

The *test statistic* measures by how many standard errors the estimate differs from the null value of zero. As illustrated in Figure 7.1, the test statistic is used to derive a **P-value**, which is defined as the probability of getting a difference at least as big as that observed if the null hypothesis is true. By convention, we usually use **two-sided P-values**; we include the possibility that the difference could have been of the same size but in the opposite direction. Figure 8.1 gives some examples of how the P-value decreases as the test statistic z gets further away from zero. The *larger* the test statistic, the *smaller* is the P-value. This can also be seen by examining the one-sided P-values (the areas in the upper tail of the standard normal distribution), which are tabulated for different values of z in Table A1 in the Appendix.

Note that we will meet other ways of deriving test statistics later in the book. For example, we introduce chi-squared tests for association in contingency tables

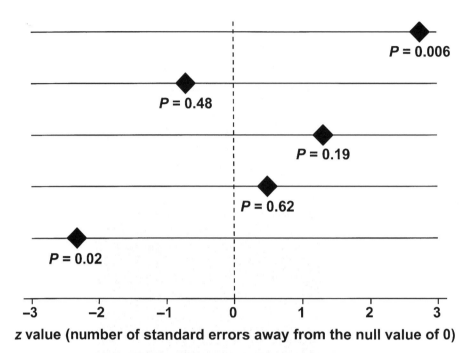

Fig. 8.1 Different *P*-values corresponding to the distance from the null value to the sample mean (expressed as standard errors). Adapted from original by Dr K. Tilling, with thanks.

in Chapter 17, and likelihood ratio tests for testing hypotheses in regression models in Chapters 28 and 29. The interpretation of *P*-values is the same, no matter how they are derived.

8.4 INTERPRETATION OF *P*-VALUES

The smaller the *P*-value, the lower the chance of getting a difference as big as the one observed if the null hypothesis were true. In other words, *the smaller the P-value, the stronger the evidence against the null hypothesis*, as illustrated in Figure 8.2. If the *P*-value is large (more than 0.1, say) then the data do not provide evidence against the null hypothesis, since there is a reasonable chance that the observed difference could simply be the result of sampling variation. If the *P*-value is small (less than 0.001, say) then a difference as big as that observed would be very unlikely to occur if the null hypothesis were true; there is therefore strong evidence against the null hypothesis.

It has been common practice to interpret a *P*-value by examining whether it is smaller than particular threshold values. In particular *P*-values less than 0.05 are often reported as '**statistically significant**' and interpreted as being small enough to justify rejection of the null hypothesis. This is why hypothesis tests have often been called **significance tests**. The 0.05 threshold is an arbitrary one that became commonly used in medical and psychological research, largely because *P*-values

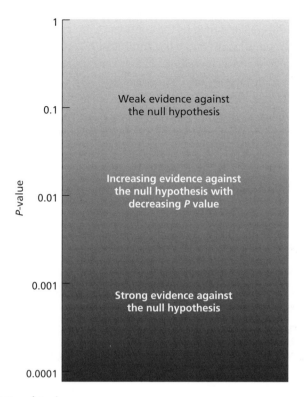

Fig. 8.2 Interpretation of *P*-values.

were determined by comparing the test statistic against tabulations of specific percentage points of distributions such as the *z* and *t* distributions, as for example in Table A3 (see Appendix). These days most statistical computer packages will report the precise *P*-value rather than simply whether it is less than 0.05, 0.01, etc. In reporting the results of a study, we recommend this precise *P*-value should be reported together with the 95% confidence interval, and the results of the analyses should be interpreted in the light of both. This is illustrated in Section 8.5.

It should be acknowledged that the 95% confidence level is based on the same arbitrary value as the 0.05 threshold: a *z* value of 1.96 corresponds to a *P*-value of 0.05. This means that if $P < 0.05$ then the 95% confidence interval will not contain the null value. However, interpretation of a confidence interval should not focus on whether or not it contains the null value, but on the range and potential importance of the different values in the interval.

It is also important to appreciate that the size of the *P*-value depends on the size of the sample, as discussed in more detail in Section 8.5. Three common and serious mistakes in the interpretation of *P*-values are:

1 Potentially medically important differences observed in small studies, for which the *P*-value is more than 0.05, are denoted as non-significant and ignored. To protect ourselves against this error, we should always consider the range of possible values for the difference shown by the confidence interval, as well as the *P*-value.

2 All statistically significant ($P < 0.05$) findings are assumed to result from real treatment effects, whereas by definition an average of one in 20 comparisons in which the null hypothesis is true will result in $P < 0.05$.

3 All statistically significant ($P < 0.05$) findings are assumed to be of medical importance whereas, given a sufficiently large sample size, even an extremely small difference in the population will be detected as different from the null hypothesis value of zero.

These issues are discussed in the context of examples in the following section and in the context of sample size and power in Chapter 35.

8.5 USING *P*-VALUES AND CONFIDENCE INTERVALS TO INTERPRET THE RESULTS OF A STATISTICAL ANALYSIS

We have now described two different ways of making inferences about differences in mean outcomes between two exposure (or treatment) groups in the target population from the sample results.

1 A confidence interval gives us the range of values within which we are reasonably confident that the population difference lies.

2 The *P*-value tells us the strength of the evidence against the null hypothesis that the true difference in the population is zero.

Since both confidence intervals and *P*-values are derived from the size of the difference and its standard error, they are of course closely related. For example, if the 95% confidence interval does not contain the null value, then we know the *P*-value must be smaller than 0.05. And vice versa; if the 95% confidence interval does include the null value, then the *P*-value will be greater than 0.05. Similarly if the 99% confidence interval does not contain the null value, then the *P*-value is less than 0.01. Because the standard error decreases with increasing sample size, the width of the confidence interval and the size of the *P*-value are as dependent on the sample size as on the underlying population difference. For a particular size of difference in the population, the *larger* the sample size the *narrower* will be the confidence interval, the *larger* the test statistic and the *smaller* the *P*-value.

Both confidence intervals and *P*-values are helpful in interpreting the results of medical research, as shown in Figure 8.3.

Example 8.1
Table 8.1 shows the results of five controlled trials of three different drugs to lower cholesterol levels in middle-aged men and women considered to be at high risk of a heart attack. In each trial patients were randomly assigned to receive either the drug (drug group) or an identical placebo (control group). The number of patients was the same in the treatment and control groups. Drugs A and B are relatively cheap, while drug C is an expensive treatment. In each case cholesterol levels were measured after 1 year, and the mean cholesterol in the control group was

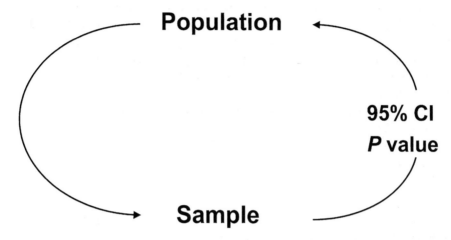

Fig. 8.3 Statistical methods to make inferences about the population from the sample.

Table 8.1 Results of five trials of drugs to lower serum cholesterol.

Trial	Drug	Cost	No. of patients per group	Mean cholesterol (mg/decilitre) in drug group	Mean cholesterol (mg/decilitre) in control group	Reduction (mg/decilitre)
1	A	Cheap	30	140	180	40
2	A	Cheap	3000	140	180	40
3	B	Cheap	40	160	180	20
4	B	Cheap	4000	178	180	2
5	C	Expensive	5000	175	180	5

180 mg/decilitre. The effect of treatment, measured by the difference in the mean cholesterol levels in the drug and control groups, varied markedly between the trials. We will assume that a mean reduction of 40 mg/decilitre confers substantial protection against subsequent heart disease, while a reduction of 20 mg/decilitre confers moderate protection.

What can we infer from these five trials about the effects of the drugs in the population? Table 8.2 shows the effects (measured by the difference in mean

Table 8.2 Results of five trials of drugs to lower serum cholesterol, presented as mean difference (drug group minus control group), s.e. of the difference, 95% confidence interval and *P*-value.

Trial	Drug	Cost	No. of patients per group	Difference in mean cholesterol (mg/decilitre)	s.e. of difference	95% CI for difference	*P*-value
1	A	Cheap	30	−40	40	−118.4 to 38.4	0.32
2	A	Cheap	3000	−40	4	−47.8 to −32.2	<0.001
3	B	Cheap	40	−20	33	−84.7 to 44.7	0.54
4	B	Cheap	4000	−2	3.3	−8.5 to 4.5	0.54
5	C	Expensive	5000	−5	2	−8.9 to −1.1	0.012

cholesterol between the drug and control groups), together with the standard error of the difference, the 95% confidence interval and the *P*-value.

Note that it is sufficient to display *P*-values accurate to two significant figures (e.g. 0.32 or 0.012). It is common practice to display *P*-values less than 1 in 1000 as '$P < 0.001$' (although other lower limits such as <0.0001 would be equally acceptable).

- In **trial 1 (drug A)**, mean cholesterol was reduced by 40 mg/decilitre. However, there were only 30 patients in each group. The 95% confidence interval shows us that the results of the trial are consistent with a difference ranging from an *increase* of 38.4 mg/decilitre (corresponding to an adverse effect of the drug) to a very large decrease of 118.4 mg/decilitre. The *P*-value shows that there is no evidence against the null hypothesis of no effect of drug A.
- In **trial 2 (also drug A)**, mean cholesterol was also reduced by 40 mg/decilitre. This trial was much larger, and the *P*-value shows that there was strong evidence against the null hypothesis of no treatment effect. The 95% confidence interval suggests that the effect of drug A in the population is a reduction in mean cholesterol of between 32.2 and 47.8 mg/decilitre. Given that drug A is cheap, this trial strongly suggests that it should be used routinely.

Note that the estimated effect of drug A was the same (a mean reduction of 40 mg/decilitre) in trials 1 and 2. However because trial 1 was small it provided no evidence against the null hypothesis of no treatment effect. This illustrates an extremely important point: in small studies *a large P-value does not mean that the null hypothesis is true*. This is summed up in the phrase '*Absence of evidence is not evidence of absence*'.

Because large studies have a better chance of detecting a given treatment effect than small studies, we say that they are *more powerful*. The concept of power is discussed in more detail in Chapter 35, on choice of sample size.

- In **trial 3 (drug B)**, the reduction in mean cholesterol was 20 mg/decilitre, but because the trial was small the 95% confidence interval is wide (from a reduction of 84.7 mg/decilitre to an increase of 44.7 mg/decilitre). The *P*-value is 0.54: there is no evidence against the null hypothesis that drug B has no effect on cholesterol levels.
- In **trial 4 (also drug B)**, mean cholesterol was reduced by only 2 mg/decilitre. Because the trial was large the 95% confidence interval is narrow (from a reduction of 8.5 mg/decilitre to an increase of 4.5 mg/decilitre). This trial therefore excludes any important effect of drug B. The *P*-value is 0.54: there is no evidence against the null hypothesis that drug B has no effect on cholesterol levels.

Note that there was no effect of drug B in either trial 3 or trial 4, and the *P*-values for the two trials were the same. However, examining the confidence intervals reveals that they provide very different information about the effect of drug B. Trial 3 (the small trial) is consistent with either a substantial benefit or a substantial harmful effect of drug B while trial 4 (the large trial) *excludes* any substantial effect of drug B (because the lower limit of the confidence interval corresponds to a reduction of only 8.5 mg per decilitre).

- Finally, **trial 5 (drug C)**, was a very large trial in which there was a 5 mg/decilitre reduction in mean cholesterol in the drug group, compared to the control group. The *P*-value shows that there was evidence against the null hypothesis of no effect of drug C. However, the 95% confidence interval suggests that the reduction in mean cholesterol in the population is at most 8.9 mg/decilitre, and may be as little as 1.1 mg/decilitre. Even though we are fairly sure that drug C would reduce cholesterol levels, it is very unlikely that it would be used routinely since it is expensive and the reduction is not of the size required clinically.

Even when the *P*-value shows strong evidence against the null hypothesis, it is vital to examine the confidence interval to ascertain the range of values for the difference between the groups that is consistent with our data. The *medical importance* of the estimated effect should always be considered, even when there is good statistical evidence against the null hypothesis.

For further discussion of these issues see Sterne and Davey Smith (2001), and Chapter 35 on choice of appropriate sample size.

CHAPTER 9

Comparison of means from several groups: analysis of variance

9.1 INTRODUCTION

When our exposure variable has more than two categories, we often wish to compare the mean outcomes from each of the groups defined by these categories. For example, we may wish to examine how haemoglobin measurements collected as part of a community survey vary with age and sex, and to see whether any sex difference is the same for all age groups. We can do this using **analysis of variance**. In general this will be done using a computer package, but we include details of the calculations for the simplest case, that of one-way analysis of variance, as these are helpful in understanding the basis of the methods. Analysis of variance may be seen as a generalization of the methods introduced in Chapters 6 to 8, and is in turn a special case of **multiple regression**, which is described in Chapter 11.

We start with one-way analysis of variance, which is appropriate when the subgroups to be compared are defined by just one exposure, for example in the comparison of means between different socioeconomic or ethnic groups. Two-way analysis of variance is also described and is appropriate when the subdivision is based on two factors such as age and sex. The methods can be extended to the comparison of subgroups cross-classified by more than two factors.

An exposure variable may be chosen for inclusion in an analysis of variance either in order to examine its effect on the outcome, or because it represents a source of variation that it is important to take into account. This is discussed in more detail in the context of multiple regression (Chapter 11).

This chapter may be omitted at a first reading.

9.2 ONE-WAY ANALYSIS OF VARIANCE

One-way analysis of variance is used to compare the mean of a numerical outcome variable in the groups defined by an exposure level with two or more categories. It is called one-way as the exposure groups are classified by just one variable. The method is based on assessing how much of the overall variation in the outcome is attributable to differences between the exposure group means:

hence the name analysis of variance. We will explain this in the context of a specific example.

Example 9.1

Table 9.1(a) shows the mean haemoglobin levels of patients according to type of sickle cell disease. We start by considering the variance of all the observations, ignoring their subdivision into groups. Recall from Chapter 4 that the variance is the square of the standard deviation, and equals the sum of squared deviations of the observations about the overall mean divided by the degrees of freedom:

$$\text{Variance, } s^2 = \frac{\Sigma(x - \bar{x})^2}{(n - 1)}$$

One-way analysis of variance partitions this **sum of squares** (SS $= \Sigma(x - \bar{x})^2$) into two distinct components.

1 The sum of squares due to differences between the group means.

2 The sum of squares due to differences between the observations within each group. This is also called the **residual** sum of squares.

The total degrees of freedom $(n - 1)$ are similarly divided. The between-groups SS has $(k - 1)$ d.f., and the residual SS has $(n - k)$ d.f., where k is the number of groups. The calculations for the sickle cell data are shown in Table 9.1(b) and the results laid out in an analysis of variance table in Table 9.1(c). Note that the subscript i refers to the group number so that n_1, n_2 and n_3 are the number of observations in each of the three groups, $\bar{x}_1, \bar{x}_2$ and $\bar{x}_3$ are their mean haemoglobin levels and s_1, s_2, and s_3 their standard deviations. Of the total sum of squares ($= 137.85$), 99.89 (72.5%) is attributable to between-group variation.

The fourth column of the table gives the amount of variation per degree of freedom, and this is called the **mean square** (MS). The test of the null hypothesis that the mean outcome does not differ between exposure groups is based on a comparison of the between-groups and within-groups mean squares. If the observed differences in mean haemoglobin levels for the different types of sickle cell disease were simply due to chance, the variation between these group means would be about the same size as the variation between individuals with the same type, while if they were real differences the between-groups variation would be larger. The mean squares are compared using the **F test**, sometimes called the **variance-ratio test**.

$$F = \frac{\text{Between-groups MS}}{\text{Within-groups MS}}, \quad \begin{aligned} \text{d.f.} &= \text{d.f.}_{\text{Between-groups}}, \ \text{d.f.}_{\text{Within-groups}} \\ &= k - 1, \ n - k \end{aligned}$$

where n is the total number of observations and k is the number of groups.

Table 9.1 One-way analysis of variance: differences in steady-state haemoglobin levels between patients with different types of sickle cell disease. Data from Anionwu *et al.* (1981) *British Medical Journal* **282**: 283–6.

(a) Data.

Type of sickle cell disease	No. of patients (n_i)	Haemoglobin (g/decilitre)		
		Mean ($\bar{x}_i$)	s.d. (s_i)	Individual values (x)
Hb SS	16	8.7125	0.8445	7.2, 7.7, 8.0, 8.1, 8.3, 8.4, 8.4, 8.5, 8.6, 8.7, 9.1, 9.1, 9.1, 9.8, 10.1, 10.3
Hb S/β-thalassaemia	10	10.6300	1.2841	8.1, 9.2, 10.0, 10.4, 10.6, 10.9, 11.1, 11.9, 12.0, 12.1
Hb SC	15	12.3000	0.9419	10.7, 11.3, 11.5, 11.6, 11.7, 11.8, 12.0, 12.1, 12.3, 12.6, 12.6, 13.3, 13.3, 13.8, 13.9

(b) Calculations.

$n \quad = \Sigma n_i = 16 + 10 + 15 = 41$, no. of groups $(k) = 3$
$\Sigma x = 7.2 + 7.7 + \ldots + 13.8 + 13.9 = 430.2$
$\Sigma x^2 = 7.2^2 + 7.7^2 + \ldots + 13.8^2 + 13.9^2 = 4651.80$

Total: $SS = \Sigma(x - \bar{x})^2 = \Sigma x^2 - (\Sigma x)^2/n = 4651.80 - 430.2^2/41 = 137.85$
     d.f. $= n - 1 = 40$

Between groups: $SS = \Sigma n_i(\bar{x}_i - \bar{x})^2$, more easily calculated as $\Sigma n_i \bar{x}_i^2 - (\Sigma x)^2/n$
         $= 16 \times 8.7125^2 + 10 \times 10.6300^2 + 15 \times 12.3000^2 - 430.2^2/41 = 99.89$
     d.f. $= k - 1 = 2$

Within groups: $SS = \Sigma(n_i - 1)s_i^2$
         $= 15 \times 0.8445^2 + 9 \times 1.2841^2 + 14 \times 0.9419^2 = 37.96$
     d.f. $= n - k = 41 - 3 = 38$

(c) Analysis of variance.

Source of variation	SS	d.f.	MS $=$ SS/d.f.	$F = \dfrac{\text{Between-groups MS}}{\text{Within-groups MS}}$
Between groups	99.89	2	49.94	49.9, $P < 0.001$
Within groups	37.96	38	1.00	
Total	137.85	40		

F should be about 1 if there are no real differences between the groups and larger than 1 if there are differences. Under the null hypothesis that the between-group differences are simply due to chance, this ratio follows an **F distribution** which, in contrast to most distributions, is specified by a pair of degrees of freedom: $(k - 1)$ degrees of freedom in the numerator and $(n - k)$ in the denominator. P-values for the corresponding test of the null hypothesis (that mean haemoglobin levels do not differ according to type of sickle-cell disease) are reported by statistical computer packages.

In Table 9.1(c), $F = 49.94/1.00 = 49.9$ with degrees of freedom (2,38): the corresponding P-value is < 0.001. There is thus strong evidence that mean steady-state haemoglobin levels differ between patients with different types of sickle cell disease, the mean being lowest for patients with Hb SS disease, intermediate for patients with Hb S/β-thalassaemia, and highest for patients with Hb SC disease.

Assumptions

There are two assumptions underlying the analysis of variance and corresponding F test. The first is that the outcome is normally distributed. The second is that the population value for the standard deviation between individuals is the same in each exposure group. This is estimated by the square root of the within-groups mean square. Moderate departures from normality may be safely ignored, but the effect of unequal standard deviations may be serious. In the latter case, transforming the data may help (see Chapter 13).

Relationship with the unpaired t test

When there are only two groups, the one-way analysis of variance gives exactly the same results as the t test. The F statistic (with $1, n - 2$ degrees of freedom) exactly equals the square of the corresponding t statistic (with $n - 2$ degrees of freedom), and the corresponding P-values are identical.

9.3 TWO-WAY ANALYSIS OF VARIANCE

Two-way analysis of variance is used when the data are classified in two ways, for example by age-group and sex. The data are said to have a **balanced design** if there are equal numbers of observations in each group and an **unbalanced design** if there are not. Balanced designs are of two types, **with replication** if there is more than one observation in each group and **without replication** if there is only one. Balanced designs were of great importance before the widespread availability of statistical computer packages, because they can be analysed using simple and elegant mathematical formulae. They also allow a division of the sum of squares into different components. However, they are of less importance now that calculations for analysis of variance are done using a computer.

Balanced design with replication

Example 9.2

Table 9.2 shows the results from an experiment in which five male and five female rats of each of three strains were treated with growth hormone. The aims were to find out whether the strains responded to the treatment to the same extent, and whether there was any sex difference. The measure of response was weight gain after seven days.

These data are classified in two ways, by strain and by sex. The design is balanced with replication because there are five observations in each strain–sex

Table 9.2 Differences in response to growth hormone for five male and five female rats from three different strains.

(a) Mean weight gains in grams with standard deviations in parentheses ($n = 5$ for each group).

Sex	Strain		
	A	B	C
Male	11.9 (0.9)	12.1 (0.7)	12.2 (0.7)
Female	12.3 (1.1)	11.8 (0.6)	13.1 (0.9)

(b) Two-way analysis of variance: balanced design with replication.

Source of variation	SS	d.f.	MS	$F = \dfrac{\text{MS effect}}{\text{MS residual}}$
Main effects				
Strain	2.63	2	1.32	1.9, $P = 0.17$
Sex	1.16	1	1.16	1.7, $P = 0.20$
Interaction				
Strain × sex	1.65	2	0.83	1.2, $P = 0.32$
Residual	16.86	24	0.70	
Total	22.30	29		

group. Two-way analysis of variance divides the total sum of squares into four components:

1 The sum of squares due to *differences between the strains*. This is said to be the **main effect** of the factor, strain. Its associated degrees of freedom are one less than the number of strains and equal 2.

2 The sum of squares due to *differences between the sexes*, that is the main effect of sex. Its degrees of freedom equal 1, one less than the number of sexes.

3 The sum of squares due to the **interaction** between strain and sex. An interaction means that the strain differences are not the same for both sexes and, equivalently, that the sex difference is not the same for the three strains. The degrees of freedom equal the product of the degrees of freedom of the two main effects, which is $2 \times 1 = 2$. The use of regression models to examine interaction between the effects of exposure variables is discussed in Section 29.5.

4 The *residual sum of squares* due to differences between the rats within each strain–sex group. Its degrees of freedom equal 24, the product of the number of strains (3), the number of sexes (2) and one less than the number of observations in each group (4).

The null hypotheses of no main effect of the two exposures and of no interaction are examined by using the *F* test to compare their mean squares with the residual mean square, as described for one-way analysis of variance. No evidence of any association was obtained in this experiment.

Balanced design without replication

In a balanced design without replication there is no residual sum of squares in the analysis of variance, since there is only one observation in each cell of the table showing the cross-classification of the two exposures. In such a case, it is assumed that there is no interaction between the effects of the two exposures, and the interaction mean square is used as an estimate of the residual mean square for calculating F statistics for the main effects. The two-way analysis of variance for a balanced design without replication is an extension of the **paired t test**, comparing the values of more than two variables measured on each individual. The two approaches give the same results when just two variables are measured, and the F value equals the square of the t value.

Unbalanced design

When the numbers of observations in each cell are not equal the design is said to be unbalanced. The main consequence, apart from the additional complexity of the calculations, is that it is not possible to disentangle the effects of the two exposures on the outcome. Instead, the *additional* sum of squares due to the effect of one variable, allowing for the effect of the other, may be calculated. These issues are explained in more detail in Chapter 11, which describes multiple linear regression.

Unbalanced data are common, and unavoidable, in survey investigations. The interpretation of clinical trials and laboratory experiments will be simplified if they have a balanced design, but even when a balanced design is planned this will not always succeed as, for example, people may withdraw or move out of the area half-way through a trial, or animals may die during the course of an experiment.

9.4 FIXED AND RANDOM EFFECTS

The effect of exposures can be defined in two ways, as **fixed effects** or as **random effects**. Factors such as sex, age-group and type of sickle cell disease are all *fixed effects* since their individual levels have specific values; sex is always male or female. In contrast, the individual levels of a *random* effect are not of intrinsic interest but are a sample of levels representative of a source of variation. For example, consider a study to investigate the variation in sodium and sucrose concentrations of home-prepared oral rehydration solutions, in which ten persons were each asked to prepare eight solutions. In this case, the ten persons are of interest only as representatives of the variation between solutions prepared by different persons. Persons is then a *random* effect. The method of analysis is the same for fixed and random effects in one-way designs and in two-way designs without replication, but not in two-way designs with replication (or in higher level designs). In the latter, if both effects are fixed, their mean squares are compared with the residual mean square as described above. If, on the other hand, both effects are random, their mean squares are compared with the interaction rather than the residual mean square. If one effect is random and the other fixed, it is the other way round; the random effect mean square is compared with the residual mean square, and the fixed effect mean square with the interaction. Analyses with random effects are described in more detail in Chapter 31.

CHAPTER 10

Linear regression and correlation

10.1 INTRODUCTION

Previous chapters have concentrated on the association between a numerical outcome variable and a categorical exposure variable with two or more levels. We now turn to the relationship between a numerical outcome and a *numerical* exposure. The method of linear regression is used to estimate the best-fitting straight line to describe the association. The method also provides an estimate of the correlation coefficient, which measures the closeness (strength) of the linear association. In this chapter we consider *simple* **linear regression** in which only one exposure variable is considered. In the next chapter we introduce *multiple regression* models for the effect of more than one exposure on a numerical outcome.

10.2 LINEAR REGRESSION

Example 10.1

Table 10.1 shows the body weight and plasma volume of eight healthy men. A **scatter plot** of these data (Figure 10.1) shows that high plasma volume tends to be

Table 10.1 Plasma volume, and body weight in eight healthy men. Sample size $n = 8$, mean body weight $\bar{x} = 66.875$, mean plasma volume $\bar{y} = 3.0025$.

Subject	Body weight (kg)	Plasma volume (litres)
1	58.0	2.75
2	70.0	2.86
3	74.0	3.37
4	63.5	2.76
5	62.0	2.62
6	70.5	3.49
7	71.0	3.05
8	66.0	3.12

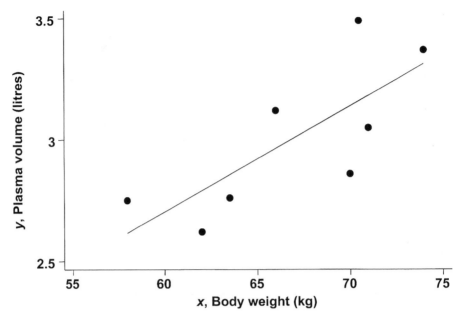

Fig. 10.1 Scatter diagram of plasma volume and body weight showing the best-fitting linear regression line.

associated with high weight and vice versa. Note that it is conventional to plot the exposure on the horizontal axis and the outcome on the vertical axis. In this example, it is obviously the dependence of plasma volume on body weight that is of interest, so plasma volume is the outcome variable and body weight is the exposure variable. Linear regression gives the equation of the straight line that best describes how the outcome y increases (or decreases) with an increase in the exposure variable x. The equation of the **regression line** is:

$$y = \beta_0 + \beta_1 x$$

where β is the Greek letter beta. We say that β_0 and β_1 are the **parameters** or **regression coefficients** of the linear regression: β_0 is the **intercept** (the value of y when $x = 0$), and β_1 the **slope** of the line (the increase in y for every unit increase in x; see Figure 10.2).

Estimation of the regression parameters

The best-fitting line is derived using the method of **least squares**: by finding the values for the parameters β_0 and β_1 that minimize the sum of the squared vertical distances of the points from the line (Figure 10.3). The parameters β_0 and β_1 are are estimated using the following formulae:

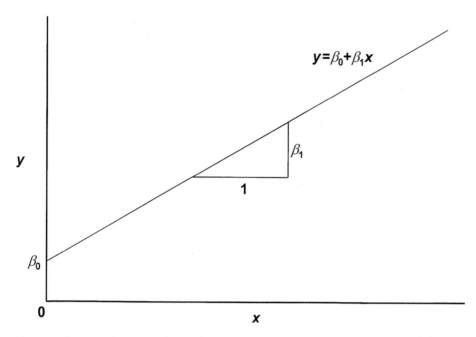

Fig. 10.2 The intercept and slope of the regression equation, $y = \beta_0 + \beta_1 x$. The intercept, β_0, is the point where the line crosses the y axis and gives the value of y for $x = 0$. The slope, β_1, is the increase in y corresponding to a unit increase in x.

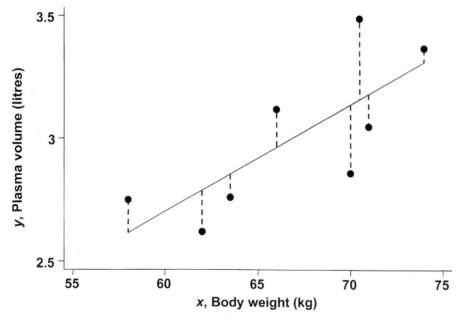

Fig. 10.3 Linear regression line, $y = \beta_0 + \beta_1 x$, fitted by least squares. β_0 and β_1 are calculated to minimize the sum of squares of the vertical deviations (shown by the dashed lines) of the points about the line; each deviation equals the difference between the observed value of y and the corresponding point on the line, $\beta_0 + \beta_1 x$.

$$\beta_1 = \frac{\Sigma(x - \bar{x})(y - \bar{y})}{\Sigma(x - \bar{x})^2} \quad \text{and} \quad \beta_0 = \bar{y} - \beta_1\bar{x}$$

Regression coefficients are sometimes known as 'beta-coefficients', and are labelled in this way by some statistical software packages. When the slope $\beta_1 = 0$ this corresponds to a horizontal line at a height of $\bar{y}$ and means that there is no association between x and y.

In this example:

$$\Sigma(x - \bar{x})(y - \bar{y}) = 8.96 \quad \text{and} \quad \Sigma(x - \bar{x})^2 = 205.38$$

So:

$$\beta_1 = 8.96/205.38 = 0.043615$$

and:

$$\beta_0 = 3.0025 - 0.043615 \times 66.875 = 0.0857$$

Thus the best-fitting straight line describing the association of plasma volume with body weight is:

$$\text{Plasma volume} = 0.0857 + 0.0436 \times \text{weight}$$

which is shown in Figures 10.1 and 10.3.

The regression line is drawn by calculating the co-ordinates of two points which lie on it. For example:

$$x = 60, \quad y = 0.0857 + 0.0436 \times 60 = 2.7$$

and

$$x = 70, \quad y = 0.0857 + 0.0436 \times 70 = 3.1$$

As a check, the line should pass through the point $(\bar{x}, \bar{y}) = (66.9, 3.0)$. Statistical software packages will usually allow the user to include the regression line in scatter plots.

The calculated values for β_0 and β_1 are estimates of the population values of the intercept and slope and are, therefore, subject to sampling variation. As with estimated differences between exposure group means (see Chapter 7) their precision is measured by their standard errors.

$$s.e.(\beta_0) = s\sqrt{\left[\frac{1}{n} + \frac{\bar{x}^2}{\Sigma(x - \bar{x})^2}\right]} \quad \text{and} \quad s.e.(\beta_1) = \frac{s}{\sqrt{\Sigma(x - \bar{x})^2}}$$

$$s = \sqrt{\left[\frac{\Sigma(y - \bar{y})^2 - \beta_1^2\Sigma(x - \bar{x})^2}{(n - 2)}\right]}$$

s is the **standard deviation of the points about the line**. It has $(n - 2)$ degrees of freedom (the sample size minus the number of regression coefficients). In this example $\Sigma(y - \bar{y})^2 = 0.6780$ and so:

$$s = \sqrt{\frac{0.6780 - 0.0436^2 \times 205.38}{6}} = 0.2189$$

$$s.e.(\beta_0) = 0.2189\sqrt{\left[\frac{1}{8} + \frac{66.9^2}{205.38}\right]} = 1.0237$$

and

$$s.e.(\beta_1) = \frac{0.2189}{\sqrt{205.38}} = 0.0153$$

Computer output

Linear regression models are usually estimated using a statistical computer package. Table 10.2 shows typical output; for our example, *plasvol* and *weight* were the names of the outcome and exposure variables respectively in the computer file. The output should be interpreted as follows.

1 The regression coefficient for *weight* is the same as the estimate of β_1 calculated earlier while the regression coefficient labelled 'Constant' corresponds to the estimate of the intercept (β_0).

Note that in this example the intercept is not a meaningful number: its literal interpretation is as the estimated mean plasma volume when weight $= 0$. The intercept can be made meaningful by **centring** the exposure variable: subtracting its mean so that the new exposure variable has mean $= 0$. The intercept in a linear regression with a centred exposure variable is equal to the mean outcome.

2 The standard errors also agree with those calculated above.

3 The *t* statistics in the fourth column are the values of each regression coefficient divided by its standard error. Each *t* statistic may be used to test the null hypothesis that the corresponding regression coefficient is equal to zero. The degrees

Table 10.2 Computer output for the linear regression of plasma volume on body weight (data in Table 10.1).

Plasvol	Coefficient	Std err	t	$P > |t|$	95% CI
Weight	0.0436	0.0153	2.857	0.029	0.0063 to 0.0810
Constant	0.0857	1.024	0.084	0.936	−2.420 to 2.591

of freedom are the sample size minus the number of regression coefficients, $n - 2$. The corresponding P-values are in the fifth column. In this example, the P-value for *weight* is 0.029: there is some evidence against the null hypothesis that there is no association between body weight and plasma volume. The P-value for the intercept tests the null hypothesis that the intercept is equal to zero: this is not usually an interesting null hypothesis but is reported because computer packages tend to present their output in a uniform manner.

4 The 95% confidence intervals are calculated as:

$$\text{CI} = \text{regression coefficient} - t' \times \text{s.e. to regression coefficient} + t' \times \text{s.e.}$$

where t' is the relevant percentage point of the t distribution with $n - 2$ degrees of freedom. In this example the 5% point of the t distribution with 6 d.f. is 2.45, and so (for example) the lower limit of the 95% CI for β_1 is $0.0436 - 2.45 \times 0.0153 = 0.0063$. In large samples the 5% point of the normal distribution (1.96) is used (d.f. $= \infty$ in Table A3, Appendix).

Assumptions

There are two assumptions underlying linear regression. The first is that, for any value of x, y is normally distributed. The second is that the magnitude of the scatter of the points about the line is the same throughout the length of the line. This scatter is measured by the standard deviation, s, of the points about the line as defined above. More formally, we assume that:

$$y = \beta_0 + \beta_1 x + e$$

where the **error**, e, is normally distributed with mean zero and standard deviation σ, which is estimated by s (the standard deviation of the points about the line). The vertical deviations (shown by the dotted lines) in Figure 10.3 are the estimated errors, known as **residuals**, for each pair of observations.

A change of scale may be appropriate if either of the two assumptions does not hold, or if the relationship seems non-linear (see Sections 11.5 and 29.6). It is important to examine the scatter plot to check that the association is approximately linear *before* proceeding to fit a linear regression. Ways to check the assumptions made in a linear regression are discussed in more detail in Section 12.3.

Prediction

In some situations it may be useful to use the regression equation to predict the value of y for a particular value of x, say x'. The **predicted value** is:

$$y' = \beta_0 + \beta_1 x'$$

and its standard error is:

$$\text{s.e.}(y') = s\sqrt{\left[1 + \frac{1}{n} + \frac{(x' - \bar{x})^2}{\Sigma(x - \bar{x})^2}\right]}$$

This standard error is least when x' is close to the mean, $\bar{x}$. In general, one should be reluctant to use the regression line for predicting values outside the range of x in the original data, as the linear relationship will not necessarily hold true beyond the range over which it has been fitted.

Example 10.1 (continued)

In this example, the measurement of plasma volume is time-consuming and so, in some circumstances, it may be convenient to predict it from the body weight. For instance, the predicted plasma volume for a man weighing 66 kg is:

$$0.0832 + 0.0436 \times 66 = 2.96 \text{ litres}$$

and its standard error equals:

$$0.2189\sqrt{\left[1 + \frac{1}{8} + \frac{(66 - 66.9)^2}{205.38}\right]} = 0.23 \text{ litres}$$

10.3 CORRELATION

As well as estimating the best-fitting straight line we may wish to examine the strength of the linear association between the outcome and exposure variables. This is measured by the **correlation coefficient**, r, which is estimated as:

$$r = \frac{\Sigma(x - \bar{x})(y - \bar{y})}{\sqrt{[\Sigma(x - \bar{x})^2 \Sigma(y - \bar{y})^2]}}$$

where x denotes the exposure, y denotes the outcome, and $\bar{x}$ and $\bar{y}$ are the corresponding means. Scatter plots illustrating different values of the correlation coefficient are shown in Figure 10.4. The correlation coefficient is always a number between -1 and $+1$, and equals zero if the variables are not associated. It is positive if x and y tend to be high or low together, and the larger its value the closer the association. The maximum value of 1 is obtained if the points in the scatter plot lie exactly on a straight line. Conversely, the correlation coefficient is negative if high values of y tend to go with low values of x, and vice versa. The correlation coefficient has the same sign as the regression coefficient β_1. When there is no correlation β_1 equals zero, corresponding to a horizontal regression line at height $\bar{y}$ (no association between x and y).

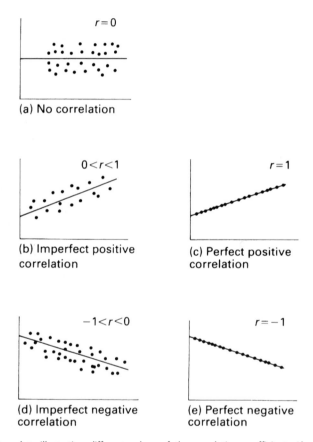

Fig. 10.4 Scatter plots illustrating different values of the correlation coefficient. Also shown are the regression lines.

Example 10.1 *(continued)*
In this example:

$$r = \frac{8.96}{\sqrt{(205.38 \times 0.6780)}} = 0.7591$$

Table 10.3 Computer output for the linear regression of the derived variable *stdplasvol* on *stdweight* (plasma volume and body weight divided by their standard deviations).

stdplasvol	Coefficient	Std err	t	$P > t$	95% CI
stdweight	0.7591	0.2657	2.86	0.029	0.1089 to 1.4094
Constant	0.2755	3.2904	0.08	0.936	−7.7759 to 8.3268

A useful interpretation of the correlation coefficient is that it is the *number of standard deviations that the outcome y changes for a standard deviation change in the exposure x*. In larger studies (sample size more than about 100), this provides a simple way to derive a confidence interval for the correlation coefficient, using standard linear regression. In this example, the standard deviation of body weight was 5.42 kg, and the standard deviation of plasma volume was 0.31 litres. If we divide each variable by its standard deviation we can create new variables, each of which has a standard deviation of 1. We will call these variables *stdplasvol* and *stdweight*: a change of 1 in these variables therefore corresponds to a change of one standard deviation in the original variables. Table 10.3 shows computer output from the regression of *stdplasvol* on *stdweight*. The regression coefficient for *stdweight* is precisely the same as the *correlation* coefficient calculated earlier. Note also that the *P*-values are identical to those in Table 10.2: the null hypothesis that the correlation $r = 0$ is identical to the null hypothesis that the regression coefficient $\beta_1 = 0$.

For large samples the confidence interval corresponding to the regression coefficient for the modified exposure variable (*stdweight* in Table 10.3) may be interpreted as a confidence interval for the correlation coefficient. In this very small study, however, the upper limit of the 95% CI is 1.4094, whereas the maximum possible value of the correlation is 1. For studies whose sample size is less than about 100, confidence intervals for the correlation coefficient can be derived using **Fisher's transformation**:

$$z_r = \frac{1}{2}\log_e\left(\frac{1+r}{1-r}\right)$$

See Section 13.2 for an explanation of logarithms and the exponential function. The standard error of the transformed correlation z_r is approximately $1/\sqrt{(n-3)}$, and so a 95% confidence interval for z_r is:

$$95\% \text{ CI} = z_r - 1.96/\sqrt{(n-3)} \text{ to } z_r + 1.96/\sqrt{(n-3)}$$

This can then be transformed back to give a confidence interval for *r* using the inverse of Fisher's transformation:

$$r = \frac{\exp(2z_r) - 1}{\exp(2z_r) + 1}$$

In this example, the transformed correlation between weight and plasma volume is $z_r = 0.5 \log_e (1.7591/0.2409) = 0.9941$. The standard error of z_r is $1/\sqrt{(8-3)} = 0.4472$. The 95% CI for z_r is:

$$95\% \text{ CI for } z_r = 0.9941 - 1.96 \times 0.4472 \text{ to } 0.9941 + 1.96 \times 0.4472$$
$$= 0.1176 \text{ to } 1.8706$$

Applying the inverse of Fisher's transformation to the upper and lower confidence limits gives a 95% CI for the correlation:

$$95\% \text{ CI for } r = 0.1171 \text{ to } 0.9536$$

10.4 ANALYSIS OF VARIANCE APPROACH TO SIMPLE LINEAR REGRESSION

We stated earlier that the regression coefficients β_0 and β_1 are calculated so as to minimize the sum of squared deviations of the points about the regression line. This can be compared to the overall variation in the outcome variable, measured by the **total sum of squares**

$$SS_{Total} = \Sigma(y - \bar{y})^2$$

This is illustrated in Figure 10.5 where the deviations about the line are shown by the dashed vertical lines and the deviations about the mean, $(y - \bar{y})$, are shown by the solid vertical lines. The sum of squared deviations about the best-fitting regression line is called the **residual sum of squares** ($SS_{Residual}$). This is less than SS_{Total} by an amount which is called the sum of squares *explained by the regression* of plasma volume on body weight, or simply the **regression sum of squares**

$$SS_{Regression} = SS_{Total} - SS_{Residual}$$

This splitting of the overall variation into two parts can be laid out in an analysis of variance table (see Chapter 9).

Example 10.1 (continued)
The analysis of variance results for the linear regression of plasma volume on body weight are presented in Table 10.4. There is 1 degree of freedom for the regression and $n - 2 = 6$ degrees of freedom for the residual.

If there were no association between the variables, then the regression mean square would be about the same size as the residual mean square, while if the variables were associated it would be larger. This is tested using an F test, with degrees

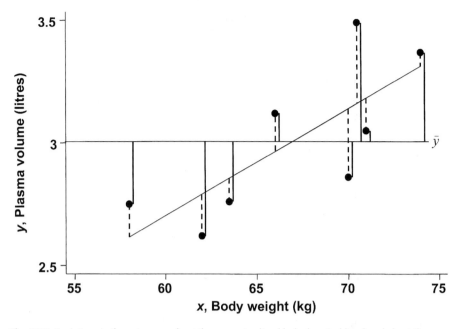

Fig. 10.5 Deviations in the outcome y about the regression line (dashed vertical lines) and about the mean $\bar{y}$ (solid vertical lines).

Table 10.4 Analysis of variance for the linear regression of plasma volume on body weight ($n = 8$).

Source of variation	Sum of squares (SS)	Degrees of freedom (d.f.)	Mean square (MS = SS/d.f.)	$F = \dfrac{\text{MS regression}}{\text{MS residual}}$
Regression	0.3907	1	0.3907	8.16, $P = 0.029$
Residual	0.2873	6	0.0479	
Total	0.6780	7	0.0969	

of freedom $(1, n - 2)$, as described in Chapter 9. The resulting P-value is identical to that from the t statistic in the linear regression output presented in Table 10.2.

10.5 RELATIONSHIP BETWEEN CORRELATION COEFFICIENT AND ANALYSIS OF VARIANCE TABLE

The analysis of variance table gives an alternative interpretation of the correlation coefficient. The square of the correlation coefficient, r^2, equals the regression sum of squares divided by the total sum of squares ($0.76^2 = 0.5763 = 0.3907/0.6780$). It is thus the *proportion of the total variation in plasma volume that has been explained by the regression*. In Example 10.1, we can say that body weight accounts for 57.63% of the total variation in plasma volume.

CHAPTER 11

Multiple regression

11.1 INTRODUCTION

Situations frequently occur in which we wish to examine the dependency of a numerical outcome variable on *several* exposure variables, not just one. This is done using **multiple linear regression**, a generalization of the methods for linear regression that were introduced in Chapter 10.

In general, there are two reasons for including extra exposure variables in a multiple regression analysis. The first is to estimate an exposure effect after allowing for the effects of other variables. For example, if two exposure groups differed in respect to other factors, such as age, sex, socioeconomic status, which were known to affect the outcome of interest, then it would be important to adjust for these differences before attributing any difference in outcome between the exposure groups to the exposure. This is described in Section 11.2 below, and is an example of the control of **confounding** factors, explained in more detail in Chapter 18. The second reason is that inclusion of exposure variables that are strongly associated with the outcome variable will reduce the residual variation and hence decrease the standard error of the regression coefficients for other exposure variables. This means that it will increase both the accuracy of the estimation of the other regression coefficients, and the likelihood that the related hypothesis tests will detect any real effects that exist. This latter attribute is called the power of the test and is described in detail in Chapter 35 ('Calculation of required sample size'). This second reason applies only when the outcome variable is numerical (and not, for example, when we use logistic regression to analyse the association of one or more exposure variables with a binary outcome variable, see Chapters 19 and 20).

Multiple regression can be carried out with any number of variables, although it is recommended that the number be kept reasonably small, as with larger numbers the interpretation becomes increasingly more complex. These issues are discussed in more detail in the chapters on regression modelling (Chapter 29) and strategies for analysis (Chapter 38).

11.2 MULTIPLE REGRESSION WITH TWO EXPOSURE VARIABLES

Example 11.1
All the methods will be illustrated using a study of lung function among 636 children aged 7 to 10 years living in a deprived suburb of Lima, Peru. The maximum volume of air that the children could breathe out in 1 second (Forced Expiratory Volume in 1 second, denoted as FEV_1) was measured using a spirometer. The age and height of the children were recorded, and their carers were asked about respiratory symptoms that the children had experienced in the last year.

Consider first the relationship of lung function (FEV_1) with the two exposure variables: age and height of the child. It seems likely that FEV_1 will increase with both height and age, and this is confirmed by scatter plots, which suggest that the relationship of FEV_1 with each of these is linear (Figure 11.1). The output from separate linear regression models for the association between FEV_1 and each of these two exposure variables is shown in Table 11.1.

As is apparent from the scatter plots, there is a strong association between FEV_1 and both age and height. The regression coefficients tell us that FEV_1 increases by 0.2185 litres for every year of age, and by 0.0311 litres for every centimetre of height. The regression lines are shown on the scatter plots in Figure 11.1. The correlations of FEV_1 with age and height are 0.5161 and 0.6376, respectively.

As might be expected, there is also a strong association between age and height (correlation $= 0.5946$). We may therefore ask the following questions:
- what is the association between age and FEV_1, having taken the association between height and FEV_1 into account?
- what is the association between height and FEV_1, having taken the association between age and FEV_1 into account?

Table 11.1 Computer output for two separate linear regression models for FEV_1.

(a) FEV_1 and age.

FEV_1	Coefficient	Std err	t	$P > |t|$	95% CI
Age	0.2185	0.0144	15.174	0.000	0.1902 to 0.2467
Constant	−0.3679	0.1298	−2.835	0.005	−0.6227 to −0.1131

(b) FEV_1 and height.

FEV_1	Coefficient	Std err	t	$P > |t|$	95% CI
Height	0.0311	0.00149	20.840	0.000	0.0282 to 0.0341
Constant	−2.2658	0.1855	−12.216	0.000	−2.6300 to −1.9016

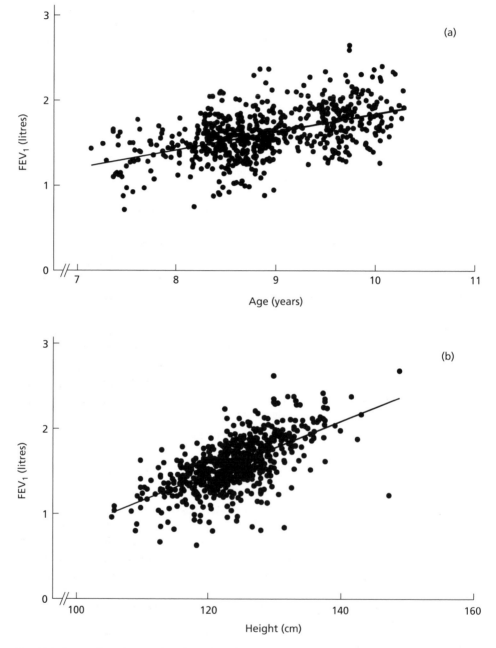

Fig. 11.1 Scatter plots showing the relationship of FEV_1 with (a) age and (b) height in 636 Peruvian children. Analyses and displays by kind permission of Dr M.E. Penny.

Often, we talk of the effect of a variable having **adjusted** or **controlled** for the effects of the other variable(s) in the model.

These questions may be answered by fitting a **multiple regression** model for the effects of height and age on FEV_1. The general form of a multiple regression model for the effects of two exposure variables (x_1 and x_2) on an outcome variable (y) is:

$$y = \beta_0 + \beta_1 x_1 + \beta_2 x_2$$

The **intercept** β_0 is the value of the outcome y when both exposure variables x_1 and x_2 are zero. In this example:

$$FEV_1 = \beta_0 + \beta_1 \times \text{age} + \beta_2 \times \text{height}$$

This model assumes that for any age, FEV_1 is linearly related to height, and correspondingly that for any height, FEV_1 is linearly related to age. Note that β_1 and β_2 will be different to the regression coefficients from the simple linear regressions on age and height separately, unless the two exposure variables are unrelated.

The way in which the regression coefficients are estimated is the same as for linear regression with a single exposure variable: the values of β_0, β_1 and β_2 are chosen to minimize the sum of squares of the differences $[y - (\beta_0 + \beta_1 x_1 + \beta_2 x_2)]$ or, in other words, the variation about the regression. In this example each observed FEV_1 is compared with ($\beta_0 + \beta_1 \times \text{age} + \beta_2 \times \text{height}$). The estimated regression coefficients are shown in Table 11.2.

The regression output tells us that the best-fitting model is:

$$FEV_1 = -2.3087 + 0.0897 \times \text{age} + 0.0250 \times \text{height}$$

After controlling for the association between FEV_1 and height, the regression coefficient for age is much reduced (from 0.2185 litres/year to 0.0897 litres/year). There is a smaller reduction in the regression coefficient for height: from 0.0311 litres/cm to 0.0250 litres/cm. The t statistics and corresponding P-values for age and height test the null hypotheses that, respectively, there is no association of

Table 11.2 Computer output showing the estimated regression coefficients from the multiple regression relating FEV_1 to age and height.

FEV_1	Coefficient	Std err	t	$P > \lvert t \rvert$	95% CI
Age	0.0897	0.0157	5.708	0.000	0.0588 to 0.1206
Height	0.0250	0.0018	13.77	0.000	0.0214 to 0.0285
Constant	−2.3087	0.1812	−12.743	0.000	−2.6645 to −1.9529

FEV_1 with age having controlled for its association with height, and no association of FEV_1 with height having controlled for its association with age.

Note that the P-values in this analysis are not really zero; they are simply too small to be displayed using the precision chosen by the software package. In this case the P-values should be interpreted and reported as < 0.001. There is thus strong evidence that age and height are each associated with FEV_1 after controlling for one another.

Analysis of variance for multiple regression

Example 11.1 (continued)

We can examine the extent to which the joint effects of age and height explain the variation in FEV_1 in an analysis of variance table (Table 11.3). There are now 2 degrees of freedom for the regression as there are two exposure variables. The F test for this regression is 244.3 with (2,633) degrees of freedom ($P < 0.0001$).

The regression accounts for 43.56% (25.6383/58.8584) of the total variation in FEV_1. This proportion equals R^2, where $R = \sqrt{0.4356} = 0.66$ is defined as the **multiple correlation coefficient**. R is always positive as no direction can be attached to a correlation based on more than one variable.

The sum of squares due to the regression of FEV_1 on both age and height comprises the sum of squares explained by age ($= 15.6802$, derived from the simple linear regression $FEV_1 = \beta_0 + \beta_1 \times \text{age}$) plus the *extra* sum of squares explained by height after controlling for age (Table 11.4). This provides an alternative means of testing the null hypothesis that there is no association of FEV_1 with height having controlled for its association with age. We derive an F statistic using the residual mean square from the multiple regression:

$$F = 9.9581/0.05248 = 189.75, \ \text{d.f} = (1,633), \ P < 0.0001$$

Again, there is clear evidence of an association of FEV_1 with height having controlled for its association with age. Note that the t statistic for height presented in the computer output shown in Table 11.2 is exactly the square root of the F statistic: $\sqrt{189.75} = 13.77$.

Reversing the order in which the variables are entered into the model allows us to test the null hypothesis that there is no association with age having controlled for height: this gives an F statistic 32.58, d.f $= (1,633)$, $P < 0.0001$. Again this corresponds to the t statistic in Table 11.2: $\sqrt{32.58} = 5.708$.

Table 11.3 Analysis of variance for the multiple regression relating FEV_1 to age and height.

Source of variation	SS	d.f.	MS	$F = \dfrac{\text{MS regression}}{\text{MS residual}}$
Regression on age and height of child	25.6383	2	12.8192	244.3, $P < 0.0001$
Residual	33.2201	633	0.05248	
Total	58.8584	635	0.09269	

Table 11.4 Individual contributions of age and height of the child to the multiple regression including both variables, when age is entered into multiple regression first.

Source of variation	SS	d.f.	MS	$F = \dfrac{MS\ regression}{MS\ residual}$
Age	15.6802	1	15.6082	
Height adjusting for age	9.9581	1	9.9581	189.75, $P < 0.0001$
Age and height	25.6383	2		

Note that these two orders of breaking down the combined regression sum of squares from Table 11.3 into the separate sums of squares do not give the same component sums of squares because the exposure variables (age and height) are themselves correlated. However, the regression coefficients and their corresponding standard errors in Table 11.2 are unaffected by the order in which the exposure variables are listed.

11.3 MULTIPLE REGRESSION WITH CATEGORICAL EXPOSURE VARIABLES

Until now, we have included only continuous exposure variables in regression models. In fact, it is straightforward to estimate the effects of binary or other categorical exposure variables in regression models. We now show how to do this, and how the results relate to methods introduced in previous chapters.

Regression with binary exposure variables

We start by considering a **binary exposure variable**, coded as 0 (unexposed) or 1 (exposed) in the dataset.

Example 11.1 (continued)
A variable that takes only the values 0 and 1 is known as an **indicator variable** because it indicates whether the individual possesses the characteristic or not. Computer output from the linear regression of FEV_1 on variable *male* in the data on lung function in Peruvian children is shown in Table 11.5. The interpretation of such output is straightforward.

1 The regression coefficient for the indicator variable is the difference between the mean in boys (variable *male* coded as 1) and the mean in girls (variable *male* coded as 0). The value of the t statistic (and corresponding P-value) for this coefficient is identical to that derived from the t test of the null hypothesis that the mean in girls is the same as in boys (see Chapter 7), and the confidence interval is identical to the confidence interval for the difference in means, also presented in Chapter 7.
2 The regression coefficient for the constant term is the mean in girls (the group for which the indicator variable is coded as 0).

To see why this is the case, consider the equation for this regression model. This states that on average:

Table 11.5 Computer output for the linear regression of FEV_1 on gender of the child.

FEV_1	Coefficient	Std err	t	$P > |t|$	95% CI
Male	0.1189	0.0237	5.01	0.000	0.0723 to 0.1655
Constant	1.5384	0.0163	94.22	0.000	1.5063 to 1.5705

$$FEV_1 = \beta_0 + \beta_1 \times \text{male}$$

Thus in girls, mean $FEV_1 = \beta_0 + \beta_1 \times 0 = \beta_0$ and so the estimated value of the intercept β_0 (the regression coefficient for the constant term) is the mean FEV_1 in girls. In boys, mean $FEV_1 = \beta_0 + \beta_1 \times 1 = \beta_0 + \beta_1$. Therefore:

$$\beta_1 = \text{mean } FEV_1 \text{ in boys} - \text{mean } FEV_1 \text{ in girls}$$

We may wish to ask whether the difference in mean FEV_1 between boys and girls is accounted for by differences in their age or height. This is done by including the three exposure variables together in a multiple regression model. The regression equation is:

$$FEV_1 = \beta_0 + \beta_1 \times \text{age} + \beta_2 \times \text{height} + \beta_3 \times \text{male}$$

Output for this model is shown in Table 11.6. The regression coefficient for variable male (β_3) estimates the difference in mean FEV_1 in boys compared to girls, *having allowed for the effects of age and height*. This is slightly increased compared to the mean difference before the effects of age and height were taken into account.

Table 11.6 Computer output for the multiple regression of FEV_1 on age, height and gender of the child.

FEV_1	Coefficient	Std err	t	$P > |t|$	95% CI
Age	0.0946	0.0152	6.23	0.000	0.0648 to 0.1244
Height	0.0246	0.0018	14.04	0.000	0.0211 to 0.0280
Male	0.1213	0.0176	6.90	0.000	0.0868 to 0.1559
Constant	−2.360	0.1750	−13.49	0.000	−2.704 to −2.0166

Regression with exposure variables with more than two categories

The effects of categorical exposures with more than two levels (for example age-group or extent of exposure to cigarette smoke) are estimated by introducing a series of indicator variables to describe the differences. First we choose a **baseline** group to which the other groups are to be compared: often this is the lowest coded value of the variable or the group representing the unexposed category. If the variable has k levels, $k - 1$ indicator variables are then included, corresponding to each non-baseline group. This is explained in more detail in the context of logistic regression, in the box in Section 19.3. The regression coefficients for the indicator variables then equal the differences in mean outcome, comparing each non-baseline group with the baseline.

11.4 GENERAL FORM OF THE MULTIPLE REGRESSION MODEL

The general form of a **multiple regression model** for the effects of p exposure variables is:

$$y = \beta_0 + \beta_1 x_1 + \beta_2 x_2 + \beta_3 x_3 + \ldots + \beta_p x_p + e$$

The quantity, $\beta_0 + \beta_1 x_1 + \beta_2 x_2 + \beta_3 x_3 + \ldots + \beta_p x_p$, on the right-hand side of the equation is known as the **linear predictor** of the outcome y, given particular values of the exposure variables x_1 to x_p. The *error*, e, is normally distributed with mean zero and standard deviation σ, which is estimated by the square root of the residual mean square.

11.5 MULTIPLE REGRESSION WITH NON-LINEAR EXPOSURE VARIABLES

It is often found that the relationship between the outcome variable and an exposure variable is non-linear. There are three possible ways of incorporating such an exposure variable in the multiple regression equation. The first method is to redefine the variable into distinct subgroups and include it as a categorical variable using indicator variables, as described in Section 11.3, rather than as a numerical variable. For example, age could be divided into five-year age-groups. The relationship with age would then be based on a comparison of the means of the outcome variable in each age-group (assuming that mean outcome is approximately constant in each age group) but would make no other assumption about the form of the relationship of mean outcome with age. At the initial stages of an analysis, it is often useful to include an exposure variable in both forms, as a numerical variable and grouped as a categorical variable. The difference between the two associated sums of squares can then be used to assess whether there is an important non-linear component to the relationship. For most purposes, a subdivision into 3–5 groups, depending on the sample size, is adequate to investigate non-linearity of the relationship. See Section 29.6 for more detail.

A second possibility is to find a suitable transformation for the exposure variable. For example, in a study of women attending an antenatal clinic conducted to identify variables associated with the birth weight of their baby, it was found that birth weight was linearly related to the logarithm of family income rather than to family income itself. The use of transformations is discussed more fully in Chapter 13. The third possibility is to find an algebraic description of the relationship. For example, it may be quadratic, in which case both the variable (x) and its square (x^2) would be included in the model. This is described in more detail in Section 29.6.

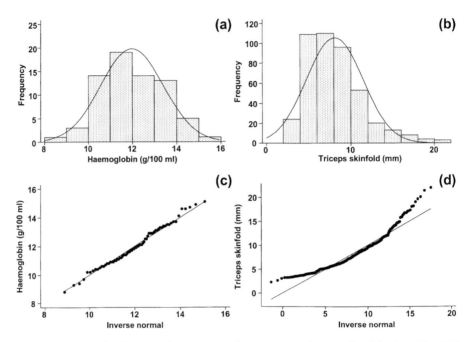

Fig. 12.1 Frequency distributions with inverse normal plots to assess the normality of the data. (a) and (c) Haemoglobin levels of 70 women (normally distributed, inverse normal plot linear). (b) and (d) Triceps skinfold measurements of 440 men (positively skewed, inverse normal plot non-linear).

Example 12.1

In Table 3.2 we presented measurements of haemoglobin (g/100 ml) in 70 women. The distribution of these measurements will be compared with that of triceps skinfold measurements made in 440 men. Histograms of these variables, together with the corresponding normal distribution curves with the same means and standard deviations, are shown in Figure 12.1(a) and (b). For haemoglobin the shape seems reasonably similar to that of the normal distribution, while that for triceps skinfold is clearly positively (right-) skewed.

Inverse normal plots

The precise shape of the histogram depends on the choice of groups, and it can be difficult to tell whether or not the bars at the extreme of the distribution are consistent with the normal distribution. A graphical technique that avoids these problems is the **inverse normal plot**. This is a scatter plot comparing the values of the observed distribution with the corresponding points of the normal distribution. The inverse normal plot is linear if the data are normally distributed and curved if they are not. The plot is constructed as follows:

1 The measurements are arranged in order, and the corresponding quantiles of the distribution are calculated as $1/(n+1)$, $2/(n+1)$, ... $n/(n+1)$. Table 12.1 illustrates the calculations for the haemoglobin data. It shows the

Table 12.1 Calculations of points for inverse normal plot of 70 haemoglobin measurements.

Observation no.	Haemoglobin (g/100 ml)	Quantile	Probit	Inverse normal = 11.98 + probit × 1.41
1	8.8	1/71 = 1.4%	−2.195	8.88
34	11.8	34/71 = 49.3%	−0.018	11.96
35	11.9	35/71 = 50.7%	0.018	12.01
70	15.1	70/71 = 98.6%	2.195	15.09

minimum (1st), median (34th and 35th) and maximum (70th) haemoglobin measurements, together with their corresponding quantiles.

2 For each measurement, the **probit** (the value of the standard normal distribution corresponding to its quantile) is derived using Table A6 in the Appendix or (more commonly) using a computer. For example, the value of the standard normal distribution corresponding to a quantile of 1.4% is −2.195, since 1.4% of the standard normal distribution lies *below* this value.

3 The corresponding points of the normal distribution with the same standard deviation and mean as the data are found by multiplying the probit by the standard deviation, then adding the mean. This is called the **inverse normal**:

$$\text{Inverse normal} = \text{mean} + \text{probit} \times \text{s.d.}$$

For the haemoglobin data, the mean is 11.98, and the standard deviation is 1.41 g/100 ml.

4 Finally, the original values are plotted against their corresponding inverse normal points. Figure 12.1(c) shows the haemoglobin levels plotted against their corresponding inverse normal points. If haemoglobin levels are normally distributed then they should lie along the line of identity (the line where $y = x$) shown on the plot. The plot is indeed linear, confirming the visual impression from the histogram that the haemoglobin data are normally distributed.

In contrast, Figure 12.1(d) shows the non-linear inverse normal plot corresponding to the positively skewed distribution of triceps skinfold measurements shown in Figure 12.1(b). The line is clearly curved, and illustrates the deficit of observations on the left and corresponding excess on the right.

Skewness and kurtosis

We now introduce two measures that can be used to assess departures from normality. In Chapter 4 we saw that the variance is defined as the average of the squared differences between each observation and the mean:

$$\text{Variance } s^2 = \frac{\Sigma(x - \bar{x})^2}{(n-1)}$$

Because the variance is based on the sum of the *squared* (power 2) differences between each observation and the sample mean, it is sometimes called the **second moment**, $m_2 = s^2$. The **third and fourth moments** of a distribution are defined in a similar way, based on the third and fourth powers of the differences:

$$\text{Third moment } m_3 = \frac{\Sigma(x - \bar{x})^3}{n} \quad \text{and} \quad \text{Fourth moment } m_4 = \frac{\Sigma(x - \bar{x})^4}{n}$$

The **coefficients of skewness** and **kurtosis** of a distribution are defined as:

$$\text{skewness} = m_3 m_2^{-\frac{3}{2}} \quad \text{and} \quad \text{kurtosis} = m_4 m_2^{-2}$$

For any symmetrical distribution, the coefficient of skewness is zero: positive values of the coefficient of skewness correspond to a right-skewed distribution while negative values correspond to a left-skewed distribution.

The coefficient of kurtosis measures how spread out are the values of a distribution. For the normal distribution the coefficient of kurtosis is 3. If the distribution is more spread out than the normal distribution then the coefficient of kurtosis will be greater than 3. For example, Figure 6.3 shows that compared to the normal distribution, the t distribution with 5 degrees of freedom is more spread out. The kurtosis of the t distribution with 5 d.f. is approximately 7.6.

Example 12.1 (continued)
For the 70 measurements of haemoglobin (g/100 ml) the coefficients of skewness and kurtosis were 0.170 and 2.51 respectively. This distribution shows little evidence of asymmetry, since the coefficient of skewness is close to zero. The coefficient of kurtosis shows that the spread of the observations was slightly less than would have been expected under the normal distribution. For the 440 measurements of triceps skinfold (mm) the coefficients of skewness and kurtosis were 1.15 and 4.68 respectively. This distribution is right-skewed and more spread out than the normal distribution.

Shapiro–Wilk test

We stated at the start of this section that although the assumption of normality underlies most of the statistical methods presented in this part of the book, formal tests of this assumption are rarely necessary. However, the assumption of a normal distribution may be of great importance if we wish to predict ranges within which a given proportion of the population should lie. For example, growth charts for babies and infants include lines within which it is expected that 90%, 99% and even 99.9% of the population will lie. Departures from normality may be very important if we wish to use the data to construct such charts.

The **Shapiro–Wilk test** (Shapiro and Wilk 1965, Royston 1993) is a general test of the assumption of normality, based on comparing the ordered sample values with those which would be expected if the distribution was normal (as done in the inverse normal plots introduced earlier). The mathematics of the test are a little complicated, but it is available in many statistical computer packages.

Example 12.1 (continued)
The *P*-values from the Shapiro–Wilk test were 0.612 for the haemoglobin measurements and < 0.0001 for the triceps measurements. As suggested by the quantile plots and coefficients of skewness and kurtosis, there is strong evidence against the assumption of normality for the triceps measurements, but no evidence against this assumption for the haemoglobin measurements.

12.3 REGRESSION DIAGNOSTICS

Examining residuals

In Chapters 10 and 11 we saw that linear and multiple regression models are fitted by minimizing the **residual sum of squares**:

$$SS_{residual} = \Sigma[y - (\beta_0 + \beta_1 x_1 + \beta_2 x_2 + \ldots)]^2$$

The differences $[y - (\beta_0 + \beta_1 x_1 + \beta_2 x_2 + \ldots)]$ between the observed outcome values and those predicted by the regression model (the dashed vertical lines in Figures 10.3 and 10.5) are called the **residuals**. As explained in Chapter 10, it is assumed that the residuals are normally distributed. This assumption can be examined using the methods introduced in the first part of this chapter.

Example 12.2
Figure 12.2(a) shows a histogram of the residuals from the multiple linear regression of FEV_1 on age, height and sex from the data on lung function in schoolchildren from Peru which were introduced in Chapter 11, while Figure 12.2(b) shows the corresponding inverse normal plot. The distribution appears reasonably close

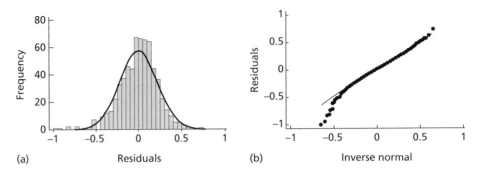

(a)   Residuals   (b)   Inverse normal

Fig. 12.2 (a) Histogram and (b) inverse normal plot of the residuals from the multiple linear regression of
FEV$_1$ on age, height and sex.

to normal except at the extreme left. The coefficients of skewness and kurtosis are
−0.52 and 4.68 respectively, confirming this impression.

The *P*-value from the Shapiro–Wilk test is less than 0.0001 so there is clear
evidence that the distribution is not normal. However, Figure 12.2 shows that the
departure from normality is fairly modest and is unlikely to undermine the results
of the analysis. For fairly large datasets such as this one the Shapiro–Wilk test is
extremely sensitive to departures from normality, while the central limit theorem
(see Chapter 5) means that the parameter estimates are likely to be normally
distributed even though the residuals are not.

A particular use of the residual plot is to detect unusual observations (**outliers**):
those for which the observed value of the outcome is a long way from that
predicted by the model. For example, we might check the data corresponding to
the extreme left of the distribution to make sure that these observations have not
resulted from coding errors in either the outcome or exposure variables. In
general, however, outliers should not be omitted simply because they are at the
extreme of the distribution. Unless we know they have resulted from errors they
should be included in our analyses. We discuss how to identify observations with a
substantial influence on the regression line later in this section.

Plots of residuals against fitted values

Having estimated the parameters of a regression model we can calculate the fitted
values (also called predicted values) for each observation in the data. For example,
the fitted values for the regression of FEV$_1$ on age, height and gender (see Table
11.6) are calculated using the regression equation:

$$\text{FEV}_1 = -2.360 + 0.0946 \times \text{age} + 0.0246 \times \text{height} + 0.1213 \times \text{male}$$

where the indicator variable *male* takes the value 0 in girls and 1 in boys. These
values can be calculated for every child in the dataset. If the model fits the data well

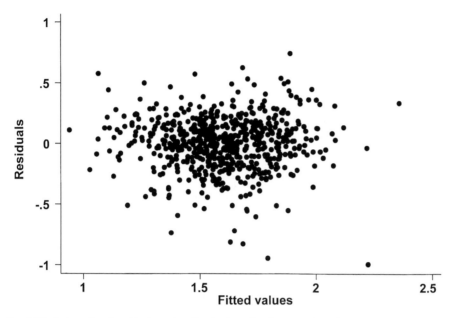

Fig. 12.3 Scatter plot of residuals against fitted values, for the regression of FEV_1 on age, height and gender.

then there should be no association between the fitted values and the residuals. This assumption can be examined in a scatter plot, as shown in Figure 12.3.

There is no strong pattern in Figure 12.3, but it does seem that the variability in the residuals increases a little with increasing fitted values, and that there may be a U-shaped relationship between the residuals and the fitted values. We might investigate this further by examining models which allow for quadratic or other non-linear associations between FEV_1 and age or height (see Section 29.6).

A common problem is that the variability (spread) of the residuals increases with increasing fitted values. This may indicate the need for a **log transformation** of the outcome variable (see Section 13.2).

Influence

A final consideration is whether individual observations have a large **influence** on the estimated regression line. In other words, would the omission of a particular observation make a large difference to the regression?

Example 12.3
Figure 12.4 is a scatter plot of a hypothetical outcome variable y against an exposure x. There appears to be clear evidence of an association between x and y: the slope of the regression line is 0.76, 95% CI $= 0.32$ to 1.19, $P = 0.004$. However, inspection of the scatter plot leads to the suspicion that the association

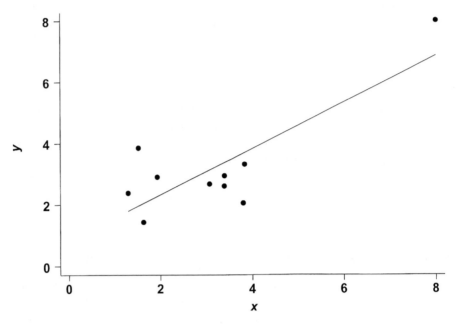

Fig. 12.4 Scatter plot of a hypothetical outcome variable y against an exposure x, in which there is a highly influential observation at the top right of the graph.

is mainly because of the point at the top right of the graph. The point is close to the regression line, so examining the residuals will not reveal a problem.

To assess the dependence of the regression on individual observations we calculate **influence** statistics. The most commonly used measure of influence is **Cook's D**. These statistics are listed, together with the residuals, in Table 12.2. It can be seen that observation 10 (the point on the top right of the graph) has much greater influence than the other observations. It would be appropriate to check whether this point arose because of an error in coding or data entry, or if there is some

Table 12.2 Data plotted in Figure 12.4, together with the influence statistic and residual for each observation.

Observation	y	x	Influence (Cook's D)	Residual
1	2.94	3.39	0.01	−0.43
2	3.32	3.83	0.01	−0.38
3	1.44	1.63	0.04	−0.61
4	2.05	3.80	0.15	−1.63
5	2.90	1.94	0.03	0.63
6	2.38	1.30	0.05	0.59
7	2.67	3.07	0.01	−0.45
8	3.85	1.53	0.39	1.89
9	2.60	3.38	0.03	−0.76
10	8.00	8.00	8.25	1.15

clear explanation for it being different from the rest of the population. As discussed earlier, observations should not be omitted from the regression purely because they have large residuals or have a large influence on the results. However, we might check whether similar conclusions are reached if an observation is omitted: and perhaps present results both including and excluding a highly influential observation.

Another useful plot is a scatter plot of influence against residuals (or squared residual) for each observation. Observations with large influence, large residuals or both may lead to further checks on the data, or attempts to fit different regression models. **Standardized residuals**, which are the residual divided by its standard error, are also of use in checking the assumptions made in regression models. These are discussed in more detail in Draper and Smith (1998) and Weisberg (1985).

What to do if the regression assumptions appear to be violated

The more checks we make, the more likely we are to find possible problems with our regression model. Evidence that assumptions are violated in one of the ways discussed here is *not* a reason to reject the whole analysis. It is very important to remember that provided that the sample size is reasonably large the results may well be robust to violation of assumptions. However, possible actions that might be taken include:
- checks for mistakes in data coding or data entry which have led to outlying or influential observations;
- exploration of non-linear relationships between the outcome and exposure variables;
- sensitivity analyses which examine whether conclusions change if influential observations are omitted;
- use of transformations as described in the next chapter;
- use of methods such as bootstrapping to derive confidence intervals independently of the assumptions made in the model about the distribution of the outcome variable. These are discussed in Chapter 30.

12.4 CHI-SQUARED GOODNESS OF FIT TEST

It is sometimes useful to test whether an observed frequency distribution differs significantly from a postulated theoretical one. This may be done by comparing the observed and expected frequencies using a chi-squared test. The form of the test is:

$$\chi^2 = \Sigma \frac{(O - E)^2}{E}$$

This is exactly the same as that for contingency tables, which is introduced in Chapter 17. Like the t distribution, the shape of the chi-squared distribution depends on the **degrees of freedom**. Here, these equal the number of groups in the frequency distribution minus 1, minus the number of parameters estimated from the data. In fitting a normal distribution, two parameters are needed, its mean, μ, and its standard deviation, σ. In some cases no parameters are estimated from the data, either because the theoretical model requires no parameters, as in Example 12.4 below, or because the parameters are specified as part of the model.

$$\text{d.f.} = \begin{array}{c} \text{number of groups} \\ \text{in frequency} \\ \text{distribution} \end{array} - \begin{array}{c} \text{number of} \\ \text{parameters} \\ \text{estimated} \end{array} - 1$$

Calculation of expected numbers

The first step in carrying out a chi-squared goodness of fit test is to estimate the parameters needed for the theoretical distribution from the data. The next step is to calculate the **expected numbers** in each category of the frequency distribution, by multiplying the total frequency by the probability that an individual value falls within the category.

$$\begin{array}{c} \text{Expected} \\ \text{frequency} \end{array} = \begin{array}{c} \text{total} \\ \text{frequency} \end{array} \times \begin{array}{c} \text{probability individual falls} \\ \text{within category} \end{array}$$

For discrete data, the probability is calculated by a straightforward application of the distributional formula. This is illustrated later in the book for the Poisson distribution (see Example 28.3).

Validity

The chi-squared goodness of fit test should not be used if more than a small proportion of the *expected* frequencies are less than 5 or if any are less than 2. This can be avoided by combining adjacent groups in the distribution.

Example 12.4
Table 12.3 examines the distribution of the final digit of the weights recorded in a survey, as a check on their accuracy. Ninety-six adults were weighed and their weights recorded to the nearest tenth of a kilogram. If there were no biases in recording, such as a tendency to record only whole or half kilograms, one would expect an equal number of 0s, 1s, 2s . . . and 9s for the final digit, that is 9.6 of each.

Table 12.3 Check on the accuracy in a survey of recording weight.

Final digit of weight	Observed frequency	Expected frequency	$\frac{(O-E)^2}{E}$
0	13	9.6	1.20
1	8	9.6	0.27
2	10	9.6	0.02
3	9	9.6	0.04
4	10	9.6	0.02
5	14	9.6	2.02
6	5	9.6	2.20
7	12	9.6	0.60
8	11	9.6	0.20
9	4	9.6	3.27
Total	96	96.0	9.84

The agreement of the observed distribution with this can be tested using the chi-squared goodness of fit test. There are ten frequencies and no parameters have been estimated.

$$\chi^2 = \Sigma \frac{(O-E)^2}{E} = 9.84, \text{ d.f.} = 10 - 0 - 1 = 9, \; P = 0.36$$

The observed frequencies therefore agree well with the theoretical ones, suggesting no recording bias.

Transformations

13.1 INTRODUCTION

The assumption of normality will not always be satisfied by a particular set of data. For example, a distribution may be positively skewed and this will often mean that the standard deviations in different groups will be very different. Or a relationship between the outcome and exposure variable(s) may not be linear, violating the assumptions of the linear and multiple regression methods introduced in this part of the book. We will now describe how such problems can often be overcome simply by transforming the data to a different scale of measurement. By far the most common choice is the logarithmic transformation, which will be described in detail. A summary of the use of other transformations will then be presented.

Finally, in the last section of the chapter, we describe the use of z-**scores** to compare data against **reference curves** in order to improve their *interpretability*. In particular, we explain why this is the standard approach for the analysis of **anthropometric data**.

13.2 LOGARITHMIC TRANSFORMATION

When a logarithmic transformation is applied to a variable, each individual value is replaced by its logarithm.

$$u = \log x$$

where x is the original value and u the transformed value. The meaning of logarithms is easiest to understand in reverse. We will start by explaining this for **logarithms to the base 10**.

If $x = 10^u$, then by definition 'u is the logarithm (base 10) of x'

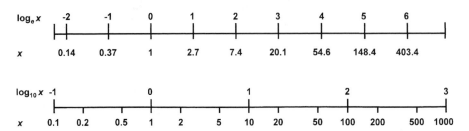

Fig. 13.1 The logarithmic transformation, using base 10 (lower line) and base e (upper line).

Thus, for example, since $100 = 10^2$, $2 = \log_{10}(100)$, and since $0.1 = 10^{-1}$, $-1 = \log_{10}(0.1)$. Different values of x and $\log_{10}(x)$ are shown in the lower part of Figure 13.1. The logarithmic transformation has the effect of stretching out the lower part of the original scale, and compressing the upper part. For example, on a logarithmic scale, the distance between 1 and 10 is the same as that between 10 and 100 and as that between 100 and 1000; they are all ten-fold differences.

Although logarithms to base 10 are most easily understood, statistical packages generally use **logarithms to base e**, where e is the 'natural constant':

$$e = 2.7182818$$

The function e^x is called the **exponential function** and is often written as $\exp(x)$.

> If $x = e^u$, then by definition 'u is the logarithm (base e) of x'

Logarithms to base e are also known as **natural logarithms**. For example, $7.389 = e^2$ so $2 = \log_e(7.389)$, $20.086 = e^3$ so $3 = \log_e(20.086)$, and $0.3679 = e^{-1}$ so $-1 = \log_e(0.3679)$. Different values of x and $\log_e(x)$ are shown in the upper part of Figure 13.1. Note that logarithms to base 10 are simply logarithms to base e multiplied by a constant amount:

$$\log_{10}(x) = \log_{10}(e) \times \log_e(x) = 0.4343 \times \log_e(x)$$

Throughout this book, we will use logarithms to base e (natural logarithms). We will omit the subscript, and refer simply to $\log(x)$*. The notation* $\ln(x)$ *is also used to refer to natural logarithms. For more on the laws of logarithms see Section 16.5, where we show how logarithmic transformations are used to derive confidence intervals for ratio measures such as risk ratios and odds ratios.*

Logarithmic transformations can only be used with positive values, since logarithms of negative numbers do not exist, and the logarithm of zero is minus infinity. There are sometimes instances, however, when a logarithmic transformation is indicated, as in the case of parasite counts, but the data contain some zeros as well as positive numbers. This problem can be solved by adding a constant to each value before transforming, although it must be remembered that the choice of the constant does affect the results obtained. One is a common choice. Note also that 1 must then also be subtracted after the final results have been converted back to the original scale.

Positively skewed distributions

Example 13.1
The logarithmic transformation will tend to normalize positively skewed distributions, as illustrated by Figure 13.2, which is the result of applying a logarithmic transformation to the triceps skinfold data presented in Figure 12.1(b). The histogram is now symmetrical and the inverse normal plot linear, showing that the transformation has removed the skewness and normalized the data. Triceps skinfold is said to have a **lognormal distribution**.

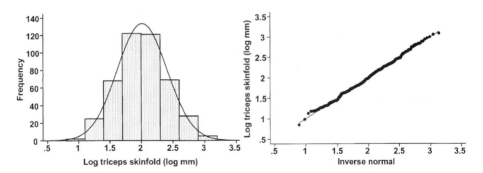

Fig. 13.2 Lognormal distribution of triceps skinfold measurements of 440 men. Compare with Figure 12.1 (b) and (d).

Unequal standard deviations

Example 13.2
The mechanics of using a logarithmic transformation will be described by considering the data of Table 13.1(a), which show a higher mean urinary β-thromboglobulin (β-TG) excretion in 12 diabetic patients than in 12 normal subjects. These means cannot be compared using a t test since the standard deviations of the two groups are very different. The right-hand columns of the table show the observations after a logarithmic transformation. For example, $\log_e(4.1) = 1.41$.

The transformation has had the effects both of equalizing the standard deviations (they are 0.595 and 0.637 on the logarithmic scale) and of removing skewness in each group (see Figure 13.3). The t test may now be used to examine

Table 13.1 Comparison of urinary β-thromboglobulin (β-TG) excretion in 12 normal subjects and in 12 diabetic patients. Adapted from results by van Oost, B.A., Veldhuyzen, B., Timmermans, A.P.M. & Sixma, J.J. (1983) Increased urinary β-thromboglobulin excretion in diabetes assayed with a modified RIA, Kit-Technique. *Thrombosis and Haemostasis* (Stuttgart) **49** (1): 18–20, with permission.

(a) Original and logged data.

	β-TG (ng/day/100 ml creatinine)		Log β-TG (log ng/day/100 ml creatinine)	
	Normals	Diabetics	Normals	Diabetics
	4.1	11.5	1.41	2.44
	6.3	12.1	1.84	2.49
	7.8	16.1	2.05	2.78
	8.5	17.8	2.14	2.88
	8.9	24.0	2.19	3.18
	10.4	28.8	2.34	3.36
	11.5	33.9	2.44	3.52
	12.0	40.7	2.48	3.71
	13.8	51.3	2.62	3.94
	17.6	56.2	2.87	4.03
	24.3	61.7	3.19	4.12
	37.2	69.2	3.62	4.24
Mean	13.53	35.28	2.433	3.391
s.d.	9.194	20.27	0.595	0.637
n	12	12	12	12

(b) Calculation of t test on logged data.

$$s = \sqrt{[(11 \times 0.595^2 + 11 \times 0.637^2)/22]} = 0.616$$

$$t = \frac{2.433 - 3.391}{0.616\sqrt{1/12 + 1/12}} = -3.81, \text{ d.f.} = 22, P = 0.001$$

(c) Results reported in original scale.

	Geometric mean β-TG	95% CI
Normals	exp(2.433) = 11.40	7.81 to 16.63
Diabetics	exp(3.391) = 29.68	19.81 to 44.49

differences in mean log β-TG between diabetic patients and normal subjects. The details of the calculations are presented in Table 13.1(b).

Geometric mean and confidence interval

Example 13.2 (continued)
When using a transformation, all analyses are carried out on the transformed values, *u*. It is important to note that this includes the calculation of any

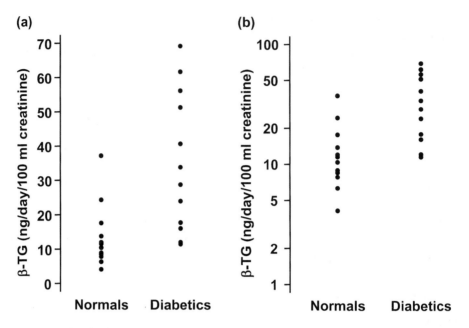

Fig. 13.3 β-Thromboglobulin data (Table 13.1) drawn using (a) a linear scale and (b) a logarithmic scale. Note that the logarithmic scale has been labelled in the original units.

confidence intervals. For example, the mean log β-TG of the normals was 2.433 log ng/day/100 ml. Its 95% confidence interval is:

$$95\% \text{ CI} = 2.433 - 2.20 \times 0.595/\sqrt{12} \text{ to } 2.433 - 2.20 \times 0.595/\sqrt{12}$$
$$= 2.055 \text{ to } 2.811 \text{ ng/day/100 ml}$$

Note that 2.20 is the 5% point of the t distribution with 11 degrees of freedom.

When reporting the final results, however, it is sometimes clearer to transform them back into the original units by taking **antilogs** (also known as **exponentiating**), as done in Table 13.1(c). The antilog of the mean of the transformed values is called the **geometric mean**.

$$\text{Geometric mean (GM)} = \text{antilog}(\bar{u}) = \exp(\bar{u}) = e^{\bar{u}}$$

For example, the geometric mean β-GT of the normal subjects is:

$$\text{Antilog}(2.433) = e^{2.433} = 11.39 \text{ ng/day/100 ml}$$

The geometric mean is always smaller than the corresponding arithmetic mean (unless all the observations have the same value, in which case the two measures are equal). Unlike the arithmetic mean, it is not overly influenced by the very large values in a skewed distribution, and so gives a better representation of the average in this situation.

Its confidence interval is calculated by exponentiating the confidence limits calculated on the log scale. For the normal subjects, the 95% confidence interval for the geometric mean therefore equals:

$$95\% \text{ CI} = \exp(2.055) \text{ to } \exp(2.811) = 7.81 \text{ to } 16.63 \text{ ng/day/100 ml}$$

Note that the confidence interval is not symmetric about the geometric mean. Instead the ratio of the upper limit to the geometric mean, $16.63/11.39 = 1.46$, is the same as the ratio of the geometric mean to the lower limit, $11.39/7.81 = 1.46$. This reflects the fact that a standard deviation on a log scale corresponds to a *multiplicative* rather than an *additive* error on the original scale. For the same reason, the antilog of the standard deviation is not readily interpretable, and is therefore not commonly used.

Non-linear relationship

Example 13.3
Figure 13.4(a) shows how the frequency of 6-thioguanine (6TG) resistant lymphocytes increases with age. The relationship curves upwards and there is greater scatter of the points at older ages. Figure 13.4(b) shows how using a log transformation for the frequency has both linearized the relationship and stabilized the variation.

In this example, the relationship curved upwards and the y variable (frequency) was transformed. The equivalent procedure for a relationship that curves downwards is to take the logarithm of the x value.

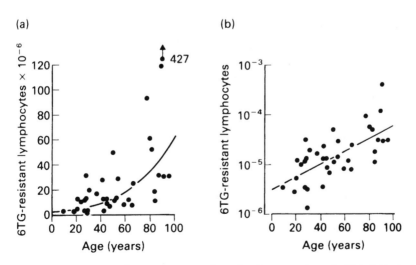

Fig. 13.4 Relationship between frequency of 6TG-resistant lymphocytes and age for 37 individuals drawn using (a) a linear scale, and (b) a logarithmic scale for frequency. Reprinted from Morley *et al. Mechanisms of Ageing and Development* **19**: 21–6, copyright (1982), with permission from Elsevier Science.

Analysis of titres

Many serological tests, such as the haemagglutination test for rubella antibody, are based on a series of doubling dilutions, and the strength of the most dilute solution that provides a reaction is recorded. The results are called **titres**, and are expressed in terms of the strengths of the dilutions: 1/2, 1/4, 1/8, 1/16, 1/32, etc. For convenience, we will use the terminology more loosely, and refer instead to the reciprocals of these numbers, namely 2, 4, 8, 16, 32, etc., as titres. Titres tend to be positively skewed, and are therefore best analysed using a logarithmic transformation. This is accomplished most easily by replacing the titres with their corresponding dilution numbers. Thus titre 2 is replaced by dilution number 1, titre 4 by 2, titre 8 by 3, titre 16 by 4, titre 32 by 5, and so on. This is equivalent to taking logarithms to the base 2 since, for example, $8 = 2^3$ and $16 = 2^4$.

$$u = \text{dilution number} = \log_2 \text{titre}$$

All analyses are carried out using the dilution numbers. The results are then transformed back into the original units by calculating 2 to the corresponding power.

Example 13.4

Table 13.2 shows the measles antibody levels of ten children one month after vaccination for measles. The results are expressed as titres with their corresponding dilution numbers. The mean dilution number is $\bar{u} = 4.4$. We antilog this by calculating $2^{4.4} = 21.1$. The result is the **geometric mean titre** and equals 21.1.

$$\text{Geometric mean titre} = 2^{\text{mean dilution number}}$$

Table 13.2 Measles antibody levels one month after vaccination.

Child no.	Antibody titre	Dilution no.
1	8	3
2	16	4
3	16	4
4	32	5
5	8	3
6	128	7
7	16	4
8	32	5
9	32	5
10	16	4

13.3 CHOICE OF TRANSFORMATION

As previously mentioned, the logarithmic transformation is by far the most frequently applied. It is appropriate for removing positive skewness and is used on a great variety of variables including incubation periods, parasite counts, titres, dose levels, concentrations of substances, and ratios. There are, however, alternative transformations for skewed data as summarized in Table 13.3. For example, the **reciprocal transformation** is stronger than the logarithmic, and would be appropriate if the distribution were considerably more positively skewed than lognormal, while the **square root transformation** is weaker. Negative skewness, on the other hand, can be removed by using a **power transformation**, such as a square or a cubic transformation, the strength increasing with the order of the power.

Table 13.3 Summary of different choices of transformations. Those removing positive skewness are called group A transformations, and those removing negative skewness group B.

Situation	Transformation
Positively skewed distribution (group A)	
Lognormal	Logarithmic ($u = \log x$)
More skewed than lognormal	Reciprocal ($u = 1/x$)
Less skewed than lognormal	Square root ($u = \sqrt{x}$)
Negatively skewed distribution (group B)	
Moderately skewed	Square ($u = x^2$)
More skewed	Cubic ($u = x^3$)
Unequal variation	
s.d. proportional to mean	Logarithmic ($u = \log x$)
s.d. proportional to mean^2	Reciprocal ($u = 1/x$)
s.d. proportional to $\sqrt{\text{mean}}$	Square root ($u = \sqrt{x}$)
Non-linear relationship	Transform: y variable and/or x variable
	Group A (y) Group B (x)
	Group B (y) Group A (x)
	Group A (y) Group A (x)
	Group B (y) Group B (x)

There is a similar choice of transformation for making standard deviations more similar, depending on how much the size of the standard error increases with increasing mean. (It rarely decreases.) Thus, the logarithmic transformation is appropriate if the standard deviation increases approximately in proportion to the mean, while the reciprocal is appropriate if the increase is steeper, and the square root if it is less steep.

Table 13.3 also summarizes the different sorts of simple non-linear relationships that might occur. The choice of transformation depends on the shape of the curve and whether the *y* variable or the *x* variable is to be transformed.

13.4 *z*-SCORES AND REFERENCE CURVES

In this section we consider a different type of transformation; namely the use of **z-scores** to compare data against **reference curves** in order to improve their *interpretability*. Their most common use is for the analysis of **anthropometric data**. For example, an individual's weight and height cannot be interpreted unless they are related to the individual's age and sex. More specifically they need to be compared to the distribution of weights (or heights) for individuals of the same age and sex in an appropriate reference population, such as the NCHS/WHO* growth reference data.

Recall from Section 5.4 that a *z*-score expresses how far a value is from the population mean, and expresses this difference in terms of the number of standard deviations by which it differs. In the context here, a *z*-score is used to compare a particular value with the mean and standard deviation for the corresponding reference data:

$$z\text{-}score = \frac{x - \mu}{\sigma}$$

where x is the observed value, μ is the mean reference value[†] and σ the standard deviation of the corresponding **reference data**. A *z*-score is therefore a value from the *standard normal distribution*.

---

*NCHS/WHO growth reference data for height and weight of US children collected by the National Center for Health Statistics and recommended by the World Health Organization for international use.

†The NCHS/WHO reference curves were developed by fitting two separate half normal distributions to the data for each group. Both distributions were centred on the median value for that age. One distribution was fitted so that its upper half matched the spread of values above the median, and the other so that its lower half matched the spread of values below the median. The upper half of the first curve was then joined together at the median with the lower half of the second curve. This means that the *z*-score calculations use the median value for that age, and the standard deviation corresponding to either the *upper* or the *lower* half of the distribution for that age, depending on whether the observed value is respectively *above* or *below* the median.

The analysis can then be carried out with the calculated *z*-scores as the outcome variable. Such a *z*-score value will have the same interpretation regardless of the age or sex of the individual. Thus, for example, individuals with weight-for-age *z*-scores of −2 or below compare approximately with the bottom 2% of the reference population, since 2.3% of the standard normal curve lies below −2 (see Appendix A1). This interpretation is true whatever the ages of the individuals.

Example 13.5

An example of an analysis based on *z*-scores is given in Figure 13.5, which shows the mean weight-for-age *z*-scores (based on the NCHS/WHO growth curves) during the first 5 years of life for children in the Africa, Asia and Latin America/Caribbean regions. A mean *z*-score of zero would imply that the average weight of children in the region is exactly comparable to the average weight of American children of the same age in the NCHS/WHO reference population. A mean *z*-score above zero would imply that children in the region were on average heavier than their reference counterparts, while a mean *z*-score below zero implies that on average they are lighter. The curves in Figure 13.5 illustrate how in all three regions there is rapid growth faltering that starts between 3 and 6 months of age, and that by one year of age in all three regions the average child is very considerably underweight compared to

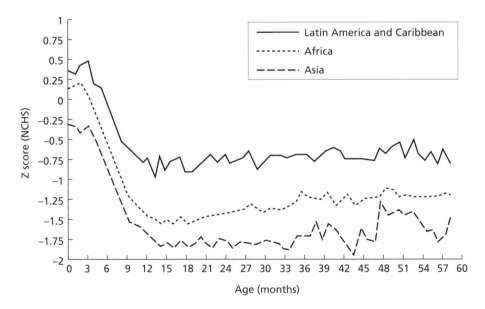

Fig. 13.5 Comparison of weight for age by region for children aged less than 5 years. Reprinted with permission from Shrimpton R, Victora CG, de Onis M, Lima RC, Bloessner M, Clugston G, Worldwide timing of growth faltering. *Pediatrics* 2001; **107**: E75

their counterparts in the reference population. It further shows that the level of disadvantage is most pronounced in Asia and least so in Latin America/Caribbean, with Africa in between.

See the report by the WHO Expert Committee on Physical Status (1995) for a detailed guide to the analysis and interpretation of anthropometric data.

PART C

ANALYSIS OF BINARY OUTCOMES

In this part of the book we describe methods that are used when the outcome is a **binary variable**; a variable where for each individual in the sample the value is one of two alternatives. For example, at the end of the study a subject may have experienced the particular disease (or event) of interest, or remained healthy. Other examples are that a patient dies or survives, or that a specimen is positive or negative.

Of particular interest is the **proportion** (p) of individuals in our sample who experience the event of interest. We use this sample proportion to estimate the **probability** or **risk** of the event in the population as a whole. For example, we might be interested in:

- the risk of death in the five years following diagnosis of prostate cancer;
- the risk of vertical transmission of HIV during pregnancy or childbirth in HIV-infected mothers given antiretroviral therapy during pregnancy.

Probabilities, risks and the related concept of the **odds** of an event are described in Chapter 14, together with the rules for calculating and manipulating probabilities. This lays the foundations for the rest of this part of the book. In Chapter 15, we derive the sampling distribution of a proportion, which is known as the **binomial distribution**, and show how it can be approximated by the normal distribution to give a confidence interval and z-test for a single proportion. In Chapter 16 we describe different ways to compare the occurrence of a binary outcome in two exposure groups; by examining the difference between the proportions, the ratio of the risks, or the ratio of the odds. In Chapter 17, we cover the use of chi-squared tests to examine associations between categorical exposure and outcome variables.

Confounding, which was briefly introduced in Chapter 11, is explained in detail in Chapter 18. It arises when there are differences between the exposure groups, in addition to the exposure itself, which are related to the outcome variable. We show how Mantel–Haenszel methods may be used to control for **confounding** using **stratification**; failure to do this would **bias** the interpretation of the comparison of the exposure groups.

In Chapter 19 we introduce **logistic regression** for the analysis of binary outcome variables, and describe how it can be used to compare two or more exposure groups. We extend this in Chapter 20, by explaining the control of confounding using logistic regression, and briefly describing other regression models for binary and categorical outcome variables. Finally, Chapter 21 introduces the special methods needed for **matched data**, in particular matched case–control studies.

CHAPTER 14

Probability, risk and odds (of disease)

14.1 INTRODUCTION

Probability has already been used several times in preceding chapters, its meaning being clear from the context. We now need to introduce it more formally and to give rules for manipulating it, before we can introduce methods for the analysis of binary outcome variables. We need to do this for two reasons:

1 There is a close link between the proportion of individuals in the sample who experience the event of interest defined by the binary outcome variable, and the definition of the **probability** or **risk** that an individual in the population as a whole will experience the outcome event (see Section 14.2).

2 We need to be able to carry out calculations involving probabilities in order to be able to derive the **binomial distribution** that describes the sampling distribution of a proportion. This is done in the next chapter.

14.2 DEFINING PROBABILITY

Frequentist definition: probability and risk

Although probability is a concept used in everyday life, and one with which we have an intuitive familiarity, it is difficult to define exactly. The **frequentist definition** is usually used in statistics. This states that the **probability** of the occurrence of a particular event equals the proportion of times that the event would (or does) occur in a large number of similar repeated trials. It has a value between 0 and 1, equalling 0 if the event can never occur and 1 if it is certain to occur. A probability may also be expressed as a percentage, taking a value between 0% and 100%. For example, suppose a coin is tossed thousands of times and in half the tosses it lands head up and in half it lands tail up. The probability of getting a head at any one toss would be defined as one-half, or 50%.

Similarly the probability of death in the five years following diagnosis of prostate cancer would be defined as the proportion of times that this would occur among a large number of men diagnosed with prostate cancer. This probability is then said to be the **risk** of death in the five years following diagnosis of prostate cancer.

Subjective (or Bayesian) definition

An alternative approach is to use a **subjective definition**, where the size of the probability simply represents one's degree of belief in the occurrence of an event, or in an hypothesis. This definition corresponds more closely with everyday usage and is the foundation of the **Bayesian** approach to statistics. In this approach, the investigator assigns a **prior probability** to the event (or hypothesis) under investigation. The study is then carried out, the data collected and the probability modified in the light of the results obtained, using Bayes' rule (see Section 14.4). The revised probability is called the **posterior probability**. The Bayesian approach to statistical inference is described in Chapter 33.

14.3 PROBABILITY CALCULATIONS

There are just two rules underlying the calculation of all probabilities. These are:
1 the **multiplicative rule** for the probability of the occurrence of *both* of two events, A and B, and;
2 the **additive rule** for the occurrence of *at least one of* event A or event B. This is equivalent to the occurrence of *either* event A *or* event B (or both).

We will illustrate these two rules in the context of the following example.

Example 14.1

Consider a couple who plan to have two children. There are four possible combinations for the sexes of these children, as shown in Table 14.1. Each combination is equally likely and so has a probability of 1/4.

Table 14.1 Possible combinations for the sexes of two children, with their probabilities.

First child	Second child	
	Boy 1/2	Girl 1/2
Boy 1/2	1/4 (boy, boy)	1/4 (boy, girl)
Girl 1/2	1/4 (girl, boy)	1/4 (girl, girl)

Multiplicative rule

In fact each of these probabilities of 1/4 derives from the individual probabilities of the sexes of each of the children. Consider in more detail the probability that *both children are girls*. The probability that the first child is a girl is 1/2. There is then a probability of 1/2 of this (i.e. 1/2 of 1/2 = 1/4) that the second child will also be a girl. Thus:

$$\text{Prob (both children are girls)} = \text{prob (first child is a girl)} \times$$
$$\text{prob (second child is a girl)}$$
$$= 1/2 \times 1/2 = 1/4$$

The general rule for the probability of *both* of two events is:

Prob (A *and* B) = prob (A) × prob (B given that A has occurred)

Prob (B given that A has occurred) is called a **conditional probability**, as it is the probability of the occurrence of event B conditional upon the occurrence of event A. If the likelihood of event B is unaffected by the occurrence or non-occurrence of event A, and *vice versa*, events A and B are said to be **independent** and the rule simplifies to:

Prob (A *and* B) = prob (A) × prob (B), if A and B are independent

The sexes of children are independent events as the probability that the next child is a girl is uninfluenced by the sexes of the previous children. An example with dependent events is the probability that a young girl in India is both anaemic and malnourished, since she is much more likely to be anaemic if she is malnourished than if she is not. We explore how **Bayes' rule** can help us understand relations between dependent events in Section 14.4.

Additive rule

We now turn to the **additive rule**, which is used for calculating the probability that at least one of event A or event B occurs. This is equivalent to either (i) A alone occurs, or (ii) B alone occurs, or (iii) both A *and* B occur. For example, consider the probability that the couple will have at least one girl if they have two children. We can see from Table 14.1 that this would happen in three of the four possible outcomes; it would not happen if both children were boys. The probability that the couple would have at least one girl is therefore 3/4. Note that it is *not* simply the *sum* of the probability that the first child is a girl *plus* the probability that the second child is a girl. Both these probabilities are 1/2 and would sum to 1 rather than the correct 3/4. This is because the possibility that both children are girls is included in each of the individual probabilities and has therefore been double-counted.

The **additive rule** for the calculation of the probability of occurrence of at least one of two events A and B is therefore:

$$\text{Prob}(A \text{ } or \text{ } B \text{ } or \text{ both}) = \text{prob}(A) + \text{prob}(B) - \text{prob}(\text{both})$$

In Example 14.1

$$\text{Prob}(\text{at least one girl}) = \text{prob}(\text{1st child is girl}) + \text{prob}(\text{2nd child is girl})$$
$$- \text{prob}(\text{both are girls})$$
$$= 1/2 + 1/2 - 1/4 = 3/4$$

From our example, it is also clear that an *alternative* formulation is:

$$\text{Prob}(A \text{ } or \text{ } B \text{ } or \text{ both}) = 1 - \text{prob}(A \text{ doesn't occur } and \text{ B doesn't occur})$$

since

$$\text{Prob}(\text{at least one girl}) = 1 - \text{prob}(\text{1st is not a girl and 2nd is not a girl})$$
or equivalently, $1 - \text{prob}(\text{both children are boys}) = 1 - 1/4 = 3/4$

14.4 BAYES' RULE

We will now introduce Bayes' rule, which is the basis of the **Bayesian** approach to statistics, introduced in Section 14.2 and described in Chapter 33. We saw above that the general rule for the probability of *both* of two events is

$$\text{Prob}(A \text{ } and \text{ } B) = \text{prob}(A) \times \text{prob}(B \text{ given } A)$$

where we have written the **conditional probability** prob (B given that A has occurred) more concisely as prob (B given A). We now show how this leads to **Bayes' rule** for relating conditional probabilities. Switching A and B in the above formula gives:

$$\text{Prob}(B \text{ } and \text{ } A) = \text{prob}(B) \times \text{prob}(A \text{ given } B)$$

Since the left hand sides of these two equations are exactly the same, that is the probability that both A and B occur, the right hand sides of the two equations must be equal:

$$\text{Prob}(A) \times \text{prob}(B \text{ given } A) = \text{prob}(B) \times \text{prob}(A \text{ given } B)$$

Rearranging this by dividing both sides of this equation by prob (A) gives **Bayes'**
rule for relating conditional probabilities:

$$\text{Prob (B given A)} = \frac{\text{prob (B)} \times \text{prob (A given B)}}{\text{prob (A)}}$$

This allows us to derive the probability of B given that A has happened from the
probability of A given that B has happened. The importance of this will become
clear in Chapter 33 on the Bayesian approach to statistics. Here, we will just
illustrate the calculation with an example.

Example 14.2
Suppose that we know that 10% of young girls in India are malnourished, and
that 5% are anaemic, and that we are interested in the relationship between the
two. Suppose that we also know that 50% of anaemic girls are also malnourished.
This means that the two conditions are not independent, since if they were then
only 10% (not 50%) of anaemic girls would also be malnourished, the same
proportion as the population as a whole. However, we don't know the relationship
the other way round, that is what percentage of malnourished girls are also
anaemic. We can use Bayes' rule to deduce this. Writing out the probabilities
gives:

$$\text{Probability (malnourished)} = 0.1$$
$$\text{Probability (anaemic)} = 0.05$$
$$\text{Probability (malnourished given anaemic)} = 0.5$$

Using Bayes rule gives:

$$\text{Prob (anaemic given malnourished)}$$
$$= \frac{\text{prob (anaemic)} \times \text{prob (manourished given anaemic)}}{\text{prob (malnourished)}}$$
$$= \frac{0.05 \times 0.5}{0.1} = 0.25$$

We can thus conclude that 25%, or one quarter, of malnourished girls are also
anaemic.

14.5 THE INDEPENDENCE ASSUMPTION

Standard statistical methods assume that the outcome for each individual is
independent of the outcome for other individuals. In other words, it is assumed
that the probability that the outcome occurs for a particular individual in the
sample is unrelated to whether or not it has occurred for the other individuals. An
example where this assumption is violated is when different individuals in the same

family (for example siblings) are sampled, because the outcome for an individual is on average more similar to that for their sibling than to the rest of the population. The data are then **clustered**, and special methods that allow for the clustering must be used. These are described in Chapter 31.

14.6 PROBABILITIES AND ODDS

In this section, we introduce the concept of odds and examine how they relate to probability. The **odds** of an event are commonly used in betting circles. For example, a bookmaker may offer odds of 10 to 1 that Arsenal Football Club will be champions of the Premiership this season. This means that the bookmaker considers the probability that Arsenal will *not* be champions is 10 times the probability that they will be. Most people have a better intuitive understanding of probability than odds, the only common use of odds being in gambling (see below). However, as we will see in Chapters 16 to 21, many of the statistical methods for the analysis of binary outcome variables are based on the odds of an event, rather than on its probability.

More formally, the **odds** of event A are defined as the probability that A *does* happen *divided* by the probability that it *does not* happen:

$$\text{Odds}(A) = \frac{\text{prob}(A \text{ happens})}{\text{prob}(A \text{ does not happen})} = \frac{\text{prob}(A)}{1 - \text{prob}(A)}$$

since $1 - \text{prob}(A)$ is the probability that A does not happen. By manipulating this equation, it is also possible to express the probability in terms of the odds:

$$\text{Prob}(A) = \frac{\text{Odds}(A)}{1 + \text{Odds}(A)}$$

Thus it is possible to derive the odds from the probability, and *vice versa*.

When bookmakers offer bets they do so in terms of the odds that the event *will not* happen, since the probability of this is usually greater than that of the event happening. Thus, if the odds on a horse in a race are 4 to 1, this means that the bookmaker considers the probability of the horse losing to be four times greater than the probability of the horse winning. In other words:

$$\text{Odds}(\text{horse loses}) = \frac{\text{prob}(\text{horse loses})}{\text{prob}(\text{horse wins})} = 4$$

Table 14.2 Values of the odds, for different values of the probability.

Probability	Odds
0	0
0.001	0.001001
0.005	0.005025
0.01	0.010101
0.05	0.052632
0.1	0.111111
0.2	0.25
0.5	1
0.9	9
0.95	19
0.99	99
0.995	199
0.999	999
1	∞

Using the equation above, it follows that prob (horse loses) $= 4/(1 + 4) = 0.8$, and the probability that it wins is 0.2.

Table 14.2 shows values of the odds corresponding to different values of the probability. It can be seen that the difference between the odds and the probability is small unless the probability is greater than about 0.1. It can also be seen that while probabilities must lie between 0 and 1, odds can take any value between 0 and infinity (∞). This is a major reason why odds are commonly used in the statistical analysis of binary outcomes. Properties of odds are summarized in the box below.

BOX 14.1 PROPERTIES OF THE ODDS

- Both prob (A) and $1 -$ prob (A) lie between 0 and 1. It follows that the odds lie between 0 (when prob (A) $= 0$) and ∞ (when prob (A) $= 1$)

- When the probability is 0.5, the odds are $0.5/(1 - 0.5) = 1$

- The odds are always bigger than the probability (since $1 -$ prob (A) is less than one)

- **Importantly**: When the probability is small (about 0.1 or less), the odds are very close to the probability. This is because for a small probability $[1 - \text{prob}(A)] \cong 1$ and so prob (A)$/[1 - \text{prob}(A)] \cong$ prob (A)

CHAPTER 15

Proportions and the binomial distribution

15.1 INTRODUCTION

In this chapter we start by introducing the notation for binary outcome variables that will be used throughout the book. These are outcomes where for each individual in the sample the outcome is one of two alternatives. For example, at the end of the study a subject may have experienced the particular disease (or event) of interest (D), or remained healthy (H). Throughout this part, we will label the two possible outcomes as D (disease) or H (healthy), regardless of the actual categories. Examples of other outcome variables are that a patient dies (D) or survives (H), or that a specimen is positive (D) or negative (H). It is *not* necessary that D refers to an adverse outcome; for example, in a smoking cessation study, our outcome may be that a participant has (D) or has not (H) successfully quit smoking after 6 months.

Of particular interest is the *proportion* (p) of individuals in our sample in category D, that is the number of subjects who experience the event (denoted by d) divided by the total number in the sample (denoted by n). The total who do not experience the event will be denoted throughout by $h = n - d$.

$$p = \frac{d}{n}$$

We use this **sample proportion** to estimate the **probability** or **risk** (see Section 14.2) that an individual in the *population* as a whole will be in category D rather than H.

Example 15.1

Suppose that in a trial of a new vaccine, 23 of 1000 children vaccinated showed signs of adverse reactions (such as fever or signs of irritability) within 24 hours of vaccination. The proportion exhibiting an adverse reaction was therefore:

$$p = 23/1000 = 0.023 \text{ or } 2.3\%$$

We would then advise parents of children about to be vaccinated that the vaccine is associated with an estimated 2.3% risk of adverse reactions. See Section 15.5 for how to calculate a confidence interval for such a proportion.

The (unknown) probability or risk that the outcome D occurs in the population is denoted by π (Greek letter pi; not related here to the mathematical constant 3.14159). Its estimation is, of course, subject to **sampling variation**, in exactly the same way as the estimation of a population mean from a sample mean, described in Section 4.5. In the following sections, we derive the sampling distribution of a proportion, which is known as the binomial distribution, and then show how it can be approximated by the normal distribution to give a confidence interval and z-test for a single proportion. Finally, we define two types of proportion that are of particular importance in medical research; cumulative incidence (risk) and prevalence.

15.2 BINOMIAL DISTRIBUTION: THE SAMPLING DISTRIBUTION OF A PROPORTION

The **sampling distribution of a proportion** is called the **binomial distribution** and can be calculated from the sample size, n, and the *population* proportion, π, as shown in Example 15.2. π is the probability that the outcome for any one individual is D.

Example 15.2

A man and woman each with sickle cell trait (AS; that is, heterozygous for the sickle cell [S] and normal [A] haemoglobin genes) have four children. What is the probability that none, one, two, three, or four of the children have sickle cell disease (SS)?

For each child the probability of being SS is the probability of having inherited the S gene from each parent, which is $0.5 \times 0.5 = 0.25$ by the multiplicative rule of probabilities (see Section 14.3). The probability of not being SS (i.e. of being AS or AA) is therefore 0.75. We shall call being SS category D and not being SS category H, so $\pi = 0.25$.

The probability that none of the children is SS (i.e. $d = 0$) is $0.75 \times 0.75 \times 0.75 \times 0.75 = 0.75^4 = 0.3164$ (0.75^4 means 0.75 multiplied together four times). This is by the multiplicative rule of probabilities.

The probability that exactly one child is SS (i.e. $d = 1$) is the probability that (first child SS; second, third, fourth not SS) or (second child SS; first, third, fourth not SS) or (third child SS; first, second, fourth not SS) or (fourth child SS; first, second, third not SS). Each of these four possibilities has probability 0.25×0.75^3 (multiplicative rule) and since they cannot occur together the probability of one or other of them occurring is $4 \times 0.25 \times 0.75^3 = 0.4219$, by the additive rule of probabilities (see Section 14.3).

Table 15.1 Calculation of the probabilities of the possible numbers of children who have inherited sickle cell (SS) disease, in a family of four children where both parents have the sickle cell trait. (The probability that an individual child inherits sickle cell disease is 0.25.)

No. of children			Probability
With SS (d)	Without SS (h)	No. of ways in which combination could occur	Prob $(d$ events$) = \dfrac{n!}{d!(n-d)!}\pi^d(1-\pi)^{n-d}$
0	4	1	$1 \times 1 \times 0.75^4 = 0.3164$
1	3	4	$4 \times 0.25 \times 0.75^3 = 0.4219$
2	2	6	$6 \times 0.25^2 \times 0.75^2 = 0.2109$
3	1	4	$4 \times 025^3 \times 0.75 = 0.0469$
4	0	1	$1 \times 0.25^4 \times 1 = 0.0039$
			Total $= 1.0000$

In similar fashion, one can calculate the probability that exactly two, three, or four children are SS by working out in each case the different possible arrangements within the family and adding together their probabilities. This gives the probabilities shown in Table 15.1. Note that the sum of these probabilities is 1, which it has to be as one of the alternatives must occur.

The probabilities are also illustrated as a probability distribution in Figure 15.1. This is the **binomial probability distribution** for $\pi = 0.25$ and $n = 4$.

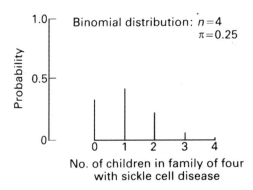

Fig. 15.1 Probability distribution of the number of children in a family of four with sickle cell disease where both parents have the sickle cell trait. The probability that a child inherits sickle cell disease is 0.25.

General formula for binomial probabilities

The general formula for the probability of getting exactly d events in a sample of n individuals when the probability of D for each individual is π is:

$$\text{Prob}\,(d \text{ events}) = \frac{n!}{d!(n-d)!}\pi^d(1-\pi)^{n-d}$$

The first part of the formula represents the number of possible ways in which d events could be observed in a sample of size n, and the second part equals the probability of each of these ways.
- The *exclamation mark* denotes the *factorial* of the number and means all the integers from the number down to 1 multiplied together. (0! is defined to equal 1.)
- π^d means π multiplied together d times or, in mathematical terminology, π to the power d. Any number to the power zero is defined to equal 1.
- Note that when π equals 0.5, $(1-\pi)$ also equals 0.5 and the second part of the formula simplifies to 0.5^n.

The interested reader may like to practise the application of the above formula by checking the calculations presented in Table 15.1. For example, applying the formula in the above example to calculate the probability that exactly two out of the four children are SS gives:

$$
\begin{aligned}
\text{Prob}\,(2 \text{ SS children}) &= \frac{4!}{2!(4-2)!}0.25^2(1-0.25)^{4-2} \\
&= \frac{4\times3\times2\times1}{2\times1\times2\times1}0.25^2(0.75)^2 \\
&= 6\times0.25^2\times0.75^2 = 0.2109
\end{aligned}
$$

The *first part of the formula* may be more easily calculated using the following expression, where $(n-d)!$ has been cancelled into $n!$

$$\frac{n!}{d!(n-d)!} = \frac{n\times(n-1)\times(n-2)\times\ldots\times(n-d+1)}{d\times(d-1)\times\ldots3\times2\times1}$$

For example, if $n = 18$ and $d = 5$, $(n-d+1) = 18-5+1 = 14$ and the expression equals:

$$\frac{18\times17\times16\times15\times14}{5\times4\times3\times2\times1} = \frac{1028160}{120} = 8568$$

Shape of the binomial distribution

Figure 15.2 shows examples of the binomial distribution for various values of π and n. These distributions have been illustrated for d, the number of events in the sample, although they apply equally to p, the proportion of events. For example, when the sample size, n, equals 5, the possible values for d are 0, 1, 2, 3, 4 or 5, and the horizontal axis has been labelled accordingly. The corresponding proportions are 0, 0.2, 0.4, 0.6, 0.8 and 1 respectively. Relabelling the horizontal axis with these values would give the binomial distribution for p. Note that, although p is a fraction, its sampling distribution is discrete and not continuous, since it may take only a limited number of values for any given sample size.

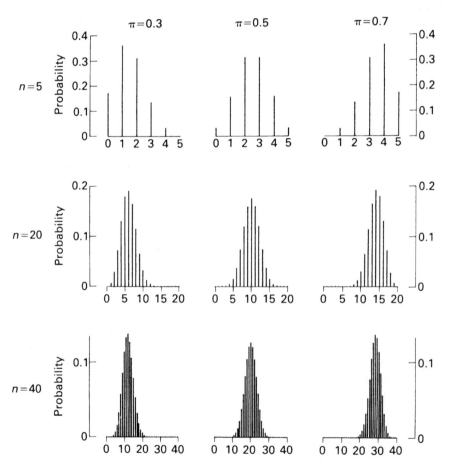

Fig. 15.2 Binomial distribution for various values of π and n. The horizontal scale in each diagram shows values of d.

15.3 STANDARD ERROR OF A PROPORTION

Since the binomial distribution is the **sampling distribution** for the number (or proportion) of D's, its mean equals the population mean and its standard deviation represents the **standard error**, which measures how closely the sample value estimates the population value. The population means and standard errors can be calculated from the binomial probabilities; the results are given in Table 15.2 for the number, proportion and percentage of events. The percentage is, of course, just the proportion multiplied by 100.

Table 15.2 Population mean and standard error for the number, proportion and percentage of D's in a sample.

	Observed value	Population mean	Standard error
Number of events	d	$n\pi$	$\sqrt{[n\pi(1-\pi)]}$
Proportion of events	$p = d/n$	π	$\sqrt{[\pi(1-\pi)/n]}$
Percentage of events	$100p$	100π	$100\sqrt{[\pi(1-\pi)/n]}$

15.4 NORMAL APPROXIMATION TO THE BINOMIAL DISTRIBUTION

As the sample size n increases the binomial distribution becomes very close to a **normal distribution** (see Figure 15.2), and this can be used to calculate confidence intervals and carry out hypothesis tests as described in the following sections. In fact the normal distribution can be used as a reasonable approximation to the binomial distribution if both $n\pi$ and $n - n\pi$ are 10 or more. This approximating normal distribution has the same mean and standard error as the binomial distribution (see Table 15.2).

15.5 CONFIDENCE INTERVAL FOR A SINGLE PROPORTION USING THE NORMAL DISTRIBUTION

The calculation and interpretation of confidence intervals was explained in detail in Chapters 6 and 8. Using the binomial distribution to derive a confidence interval for a proportion is complicated. Methods that do this are known as **exact methods** and are described in more detail by Altman *et al.* (2000), and by Clayton and Hills (1993). The usual approach is to use the approximation to the normal distribution with π estimated by p, the standard error estimated by $\sqrt{[p(1-p)/n]}$ (see Table 15.2), and methods similar to those described in Chapter 6 for means. This is valid providing that both np and $n - np$ are 10 or more, so that the normal approximation to the binomial distribution is sufficiently good. The confidence interval is:

$$CI = p - (z' \times \text{s.e.}) \text{ to } p + (z' \times \text{s.e.}),$$
$$\text{s.e.} = \sqrt{[p(1-p)/n]}$$

where z' is the appropriate percentage point of the standard normal distribution. For example, for a 95% confidence interval, $z' = 1.96$.

Example 15.3

In September 2001 a survey of smoking habits was conducted in a sample of 1000 teenagers aged 15–16, selected at random from all 15–16 year-olds living in Birmingham, UK. A total of 123 reported that they were current smokers. Thus the proportion of current smokers is:

$$p = 123/1000 = 0.123 = 12.3\%$$

The standard error of p is estimated by $\sqrt{[p(1-p)/n]} = \sqrt{0.123 \times 0.877/1000} = 0.0104$. Thus the 95% confidence interval is:

$$95\% \text{ CI} = 0.123 - (1.96 \times 0.0104) \text{ to } 0.123 + (1.96 \times 0.0104) = 0.103 \text{ to } 0.143$$

With 95% confidence, in September 2001 the proportion of 15–16 year-olds living in Birmingham who smoked was between 0.103 and 0.143 (or equivalently, between 10.3% and 14.3%).

15.6 z-TEST THAT THE POPULATION PROPORTION HAS A PARTICULAR VALUE

The approximating normal distribution (to the binomial sampling distribution) can also be used in a **z-test** of the null hypothesis that the population proportion equals a particular value, π. This is valid provided that both $n\pi$ and $n - n\pi$ are greater than or equal to 10. The z-test compares the size of the difference between the sample proportion and the hypothesized value, with the standard error. The formula is:

$$z = \frac{p - \pi}{s.e.(p)} = \frac{p - \pi}{\sqrt{[\pi(1 - \pi)/n]}}$$

In exactly the same way as explained in Chapter 8, we then derive a *P*-value, which measures the strength of the evidence against the null hypothesis that $p = \pi$.

Example 15.3 (continued)

In 1998 the UK Government announced a target of reducing smoking among children from the national average of 13% to 9% or less by the year 2010, with a fall to 11% by the year 2005. Is there evidence that the proportion of 15–16 year-old smokers in Birmingham at the time of our survey in 2001 was below the national average of 13% at the time the target was set?

The null hypothesis is that the population proportion is equal to 0.13 (13%). The sampling distribution for the number of smokers, if the null hypothesis is true, is therefore a binomial distribution with $\pi = 0.13$ and $n = 1000$. The standard error of p under the null hypothesis is:

$$\text{s.e.}(\pi) = \sqrt{[0.13(1 - 0.13)/1000]} = 0.106. \text{ Therefore } z = \frac{0.123 - 0.13}{0.106} = -0.658$$

The corresponding P-value is 0.51. There is no evidence that the proportion of teenage smokers in Birmingham in September 2001 was lower than the national 1998 levels.

Continuity correction

When either $n\pi$ or $n - n\pi$ are below 10, but both are 5 or more, the accuracy of hypothesis tests based on the normal approximation can be improved by the introduction of a **continuity correction** (see also Section 17.2). The continuity correction adjusts the numerator of the test statistic so that there is a closer fit between the P-value based on the z-test and the P-value based on an exact calculation using the binomial probabilities. This is illustrated in Figure 15.3 and Table 15.3, which show that incorporating a continuity correction and calculating the area under the normal curve above 8.5 gives a close approximation to the exact binomial probability of observing 9 events or more. In contrast the area of the normal curve above 9

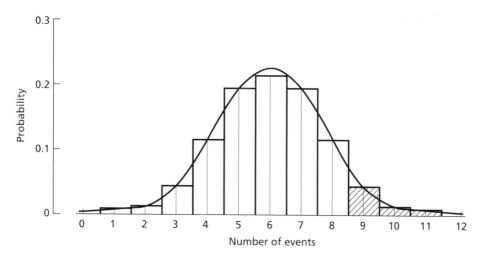

Fig. 15.3 Comparison of the binomial distribution ($n = 12, \pi = 0.5$) with the approximating normal distribution to illustrate the need for a continuity correction for small n. This shows that the area under the normal curve above 8.5 is closer to the shaded exact probabilities than the area above 9.

Table15.3 Comparisons of the different methods of calculating the probability of observing 9 or more events, when $n = 12$ and $\pi = 0.5$.

Probability of observing 9 or more events, when $n = 12$ and $\pi = 0.5$	
Calculated using binomial probabilities:	
9 events	$220 \times 0.5^{12} = 0.0537$
10 events	$66 \times 0.5^{12} = 0.0161$
11 events	$12 \times 0.5^{12} = 0.0029$
12 events	$1 \times 0.5^{12} = 0.0002$
Total of 9+ events	0.0729
Using approximating normal distribution:	
Based on area above 9	0.0418
With continuity correction, based on area above 8.5	0.0749

is not a good approximation. More details are not included here since continuity corrections are not often used in modern medical statistics. This is because they can't be extended to the regression models, described in Chapter 19 and later in the book, which are used to examine the effects of a *number* of exposure variables on a binary outcome.

15.7 INCIDENCE AND PREVALENCE

We now define two particular types of proportion that are of particular relevance in medical research. These are the cumulative incidence (or risk) of a disease event, and the prevalence of a disease.

Cumulative incidence (risk)

The **cumulative incidence** or **risk**, r, of a disease event is the probability that the disease event occurs during a specified period of time. It is estimated by the number of new cases of a disease during a specified period of time divided by the number of persons initially disease-free and therefore at risk of contracting the disease.

$$\text{Risk} = \text{cumulative incidence} = \frac{\text{number of new cases of disease in period}}{\text{number initially disease-free}}$$

For example, we might be interested in:
- the risk of death in the five years following diagnosis with prostate cancer;
- the risk of vertical transmission of HIV during pregnancy or childbirth in HIV-infected mothers given antiretroviral therapy during pregnancy.

Risks usually refer to adverse (undesirable) events, though this is not essential.

Example 15.4

Suppose we study 5000 individuals aged 45 to 54, with no existing cardiovascular disease. Ten years later, the same individuals are followed up and we find that 147 have died from or have developed coronary heart disease. Then the **risk** of coronary heart disease is the proportion of individuals who developed the disease: $147/5000 = 0.0294$, or 2.94%.

Prevalence

In contrast, the **prevalence** represents the burden of disease at a particular time, rather than the chance of future disease. It is based on the total number of existing cases among the whole population, and represents the probability that any one individual in the population is currently suffering from the disease.

$$\text{Prevalence} = \frac{\text{number of people with the disease at particular point in time}}{\text{total population}}$$

For example, we might be interested in:
- the prevalence of schistosomiasis among villagers living on the shore of Lake Malawi;
- the prevalence of chronic lower back pain among refuse collectors in Bristol, UK.

Example 15.5

Suppose we study a sample of 2000 individuals aged 15 to 50, registered with a particular general practice. Of these, 138 are being treated for asthma. Then the **prevalence** of diagnosed asthma in the practice population is the proportion of the sample with asthma: $138/2000 = 0.069$, or 6.9%.

Both cumulative incidence and prevalence are usually expressed as a percentage or, when small, as per 1000 population or per 10 000 or 100 000 population. In Chapter 22 we define the **incidence rate**, the measure used in longitudinal studies with variable lengths of follow up.

CHAPTER 16

Comparing two proportions

16.1 INTRODUCTION

In Chapter 15 we saw how the sampling distribution of a proportion can be approximated by the normal distribution to give a confidence interval and z-test for a single proportion. In this chapter we deal with the more common situation where we wish to compare the occurrence of a binary outcome variable between *two exposure (or treatment) groups*. We will use the same notation for these two groups as was introduced in Chapter 7 for the comparison of two means. Group 1 denotes individuals *exposed* to a risk factor, and group 0 denotes those *unexposed*. In clinical trials, group 1 denotes the *treatment* group, and group 0 the *control*, or *placebo* group (a **placebo** is a preparation made to be as similar as possible to the treatment in all respects, but with no effective action). For example,

- In a study of the effects of bacterial infection during pregnancy, we may wish to compare the risk of premature delivery for babies born to women infected during the first trimester (the exposed group, 1) with that for babies born to uninfected women (the unexposed group, 0).
- In a trial of a new influenza vaccine, the comparison of interest might be the proportion of participants who succumbed to influenza during the winter season in the vaccine group (the treatment group, 1), compared to the proportion in the placebo group (the control group, 0).

We start by showing how the data can be displayed in a **2 × 2 table**, with individuals in the sample classified according to whether they experienced the disease outcome (or not), and according to whether they were exposed (or not). We then explain three different measures for comparing the outcome between the two groups: the difference in the two proportions, the risk ratio and the odds ratio. We describe how to calculate a confidence interval and carry out a hypothesis test for each of them, and outline their relative advantages and disadvantages.

16.2 THE 2 × 2 TABLE, AND MEASURES OF EXPOSURE EFFECT

In Section 3.4, we described how the relationship between two categorical variables can be examined by cross-tabulating them in a **contingency table**. We noted that a useful convention is for the rows of the table to correspond to the exposure values and the columns to the outcomes. To compare the occurrence of a binary outcome variable between two exposure groups, we therefore display the data in a **2 × 2 table**. Table 16.1 shows the notation that we will use for the number of individuals in each group. As introduced in the last chapter, we use letter d to denote the number of subjects who experience the outcome event, h to denote the number of subjects who do not experience the outcome event, and n for the total number in the sample. In addition, we use the subscripts 1 and 0 to denote the exposed and unexposed groups respectively.

As explained in Section 3.4, it is recommended that the table also shows the proportion (or percentage) in each outcome category, within each of the exposure groups. Thus, if the exposure is the row variable (as here) then row percentages should be presented, while if it is the column variable then column percentages should be presented. Following the notation introduced in Chapter 15, the overall proportion is denoted by $p = d/n$, and the proportions in the exposed and unexposed groups are denoted by $p_1 = d_1/n_1$ and $p_0 = d_0/n_0$, respectively.

Example 16.1
Consider the following results from an influenza vaccine trial carried out during an epidemic. Of 460 adults who took part, 240 received influenza vaccination and 220 placebo vaccination. Overall 100 people contracted influenza, of whom 20 were in the vaccine group and 80 in the placebo group. We start by displaying the results of the trial in a 2 × 2 table (Table 16.2). In Table 16.2 the exposure is vaccination (the row variable) and the outcome is whether the subject contracts influenza (the column variable). We therefore also include *row* percentages in the

Table 16.1 Notation to denote the number of individuals in each group for the 2 × 2 table comparing a binary outcome variable between two exposure groups.

	Outcome		
Exposure	Experienced event: D (Disease)	Did not experience event: H (Healthy)	Total
Group 1 (exposed)	d_1	h_1	n_1
Group 0 (unexposed)	d_0	h_0	n_0
Total	d	h	n

Table 16.2 2 × 2 table showing results from an influenza vaccine trial.

	Influenza		
	Yes	No	Total
Vaccine	20 (8.3%)	220 (91.7%)	240
Placebo	80 (36.4%)	140 (63.6%)	220
Total	100 (21.7%)	360 (78.3%)	460

table. Overall, 21.7% of subjects contracted influenza. We can see that the percentage contracting influenza was much lower in the vaccine group (8.3%), than in the placebo group (36.4%). We can use these data to answer the following related questions.

1 How effective was the vaccine in preventing influenza in our trial? The size of this effect can be measured in three different ways:
   (a) The **difference** between the **risks** of contracting influenza in the vaccine group compared to the placebo group.
   (b) The **ratio** of the **risks** of contracting influenza in the vaccine group compared to the placebo group. This is also known as the **relative risk**.
   (c) The **ratio** of the **odds** of contracting (to not contracting) influenza in the vaccine group, compared to the placebo group.

2 What does the effect of the vaccine in our trial tell us about the size of its effect in preventing influenza more generally in the population? This is addressed by calculating a **confidence interval** for the size of the effect.

3 Do the data provide evidence that the vaccine actually affects the risk of contracting influenza, or might the observed difference between the two groups have arisen by chance? In other words, are the data consistent with there being no effect of the vaccine? We address this by carrying out a **hypothesis** (or **significance**) **test** to give a **P-value**, which is the probability of a difference between the two groups at least as large as that in our sample, if there was no effect of the vaccine in the population.

The use of confidence intervals and P-values to interpret the results of statistical analyses is discussed in detail in Chapter 8, and readers may wish to refer to that chapter at this point.

The three different measures for comparing a binary outcome between two exposure (or treatment) groups are summarized in Table 16.3, together with the results for the influenza vaccine trial. All three measures indicate a benefit of the vaccine. The risk difference is −0.281, meaning that the *absolute* risk of contracting influenza was 0.281 *lower* in the vaccine group compared to the placebo group. The risk ratio equals 0.228, meaning that the risk of contracting influenza in the vaccine group was only 22.8% of the risk in the placebo group. Equivalently, we could say the vaccine prevented 77.2% (100 − 22.8%) of influenza cases. This is called the **vaccine efficacy**; it is discussed in more detail in Chapter 37. The odds

Table 16.3 Three different measures for comparing a binary outcome between two exposure (or treatment) groups, together with the results for the vaccine trial data in Table 16.2.

Measure of comparison	Formula	Result for influenza vaccine trial
Risk difference	$p_1 - p_0$	$0.083 - 0.364 = -0.281$
Risk ratio (relative risk)	p_1/p_0	$0.083/0.364 = 0.228$
Odds ratio	$\dfrac{d_1/h_1}{d_0/h_0} = \dfrac{d_1 \times h_0}{d_0 \times h_1}$	$\dfrac{20/220}{80/140} = \dfrac{20 \times 140}{80 \times 220} = 0.159$

ratio in the trial was 0.292 meaning that the *odds* of contracting influenza in the vaccine group were 29.2% of the odds in the placebo group.

The following sections describe how to calculate confidence intervals and carry out hypothesis tests for each of these three measures. They also discuss their relative advantages and disadvantages. When to use which measure is also discussed in Chapter 37 ('Measures of association and impact').

16.3 RISK DIFFERENCES

We will start with the first of the three measures of effect, the difference between the two proportions. From now on we will refer to this as a **risk difference**, though the methods apply to any type of proportion. We will see how to derive a confidence interval for the difference, and carry out a test of the null hypothesis that there is no difference between the proportions in the population from which the sample was drawn. As in the case of a single proportion we will use methods based on the normal approximation to the sampling distribution of the two proportions. These will be illustrated in the context of the influenza vaccine trial described in Example 16.1 above.

Sampling distribution of the difference between two proportions

Before we can construct a confidence interval for the difference between two proportions, or carry out the related hypothesis test, we need to know the sampling distribution of the difference. The difference, $p_1 - p_0$, between the proportions in the exposed and unexposed groups in our sample provides an estimate of the underlying difference, $\pi_1 - \pi_0$, between the exposed and unexposed groups in the population. It is of course subject to *sampling variation*, so that a different sample from the same population would give a different value of $p_1 - p_0$. Note that:

1 The normal distribution is a reasonable approximation to the sampling distribution of the difference $p_1 - p_0$, provided $n_1 p_1$, $n_1 - n_1 p_1$, $n_0 p_0$ and $n_0 - n_0 p_0$ are each greater than 10, and will improve as these numbers get larger.

2 The mean of this sampling distribution is simply the difference between the two population means, $\pi_1 - \pi_0$.

3 The standard error of $p_1 - p_0$ is based on a combination of the standard errors of the individual proportions:

$$\text{s.e.}(p_1 - p_0) = \sqrt{[p_1(1 - p_1)/n_1 + p_0(1 - p_0)/n_0]} = \sqrt{[\text{s.e.}(p_1)^2 + \text{s.e.}(p_0)^2]}$$

The confidence interval for the difference between two proportions is given by:

$$\text{CI} = (p_1 - p_0) - z' \times \text{s.e.}(p_1 - p_0) \text{ to } (p_1 - p_0) + z' \times \text{s.e.}(p_1 - p_0)$$

where z' is the appropriate percentage point of the normal distribution.

Example 16.1 (continued)
The difference in proportions between the vaccine and placebo groups is $0.083 - 0.364 = -0.281$. Its standard error is:

$$\text{s.e.}(p_1 - p_0) = \sqrt{[0.083(1 - 0.083)/240 + 0.364(1 - 0.364)/220]} = 0.037$$

and so the approximate 95% confidence interval for this reduction is:

$$95\% \text{ CI} = -0.281 - (1.96 \times 0.037) \text{ to } -0.281 + (1.96 \times 0.037)$$
$$= -0.353 \text{ to } -0.208$$

That is, we are 95% confident that in the population the vaccine would reduce the risk of contracting influenza by between 0.208 and 0.353.

Test that the difference between two proportions is zero

The normal test to compare two sample proportions is based on:

$$z = \frac{p_1 - p_0}{\text{s.e.}(p_1 - p_0)}$$

The standard error used in the test is different to that used in the confidence interval because it is calculated assuming that the null hypothesis is true (i.e. that $\pi_1 = \pi_0 = \pi$). Under the null hypothesis that the population proportions are equal:

$$\text{s.e.}(p_1 - p_0) = \sqrt{[\pi(1 - \pi)(1/n_1 + 1/n_0)]}$$

π is estimated by the overall proportion in both samples, that is by:

$$p = \frac{d_0 + d_1}{n_0 + n_1} = \frac{d}{n}$$

The formula for the z-test is therefore:

$$z = \frac{p_1 - p_0}{\sqrt{[p(1-p)(1/n_1 + 1/n_0)]}}$$

This test is a valid approximation provided that either $n_1 + n_0$ is greater than 40 or $n_1 p$, $n_1 - n_1 p$, $n_2 p$ and $n_2 - n_2 p$ are all 10 or more. If this condition is not satisfied, but $n_1 p$, $n_1 - n_1 p$, $n_2 p$ and $n_2 - n_2 p$ are all 5 or more, then a modified version of the z-test incorporating a **continuity correction**, or the equivalent chi-squared test with a continuity correction, can be used (see Section 17.2). If none of these conditions are satisfied, the exact test described in Section 17.3 should be used.

Example 16.1 (continued)
The overall proportion that contracted influenza was 0.217 or 21.7%. Therefore:

$$z = \frac{(0.083 - 0.364)}{\sqrt{[0.217(1 - 0.217)(1/240 + 1/220)]}} = \frac{-0.281}{0.0385} = -7.299$$

The corresponding P-value is < 0.0001. Thus there is strong evidence that there was a reduction in the risk of contracting influenza following vaccination with the influenza vaccine.

16.4 RISK RATIOS

We now turn to the second measure of effect introduced in Section 16.2, the ratio of the two proportions. We will refer to this as the **risk ratio**, although the methods apply to ratios of any proportions, and not just those that estimate risks. The risk ratio is often abbreviated to **RR**, and is also known as the **relative risk**.

$$RR = \frac{p_1}{p_0} = \frac{d_1/n_1}{d_0/n_0}$$

Example 16.2
Table 16.4 shows hypothetical data from a study to investigate the association between smoking and lung cancer. 30 000 smokers and 60 000 non-smokers were followed for a year, during which time 39 of the smokers and 6 of the non-smokers developed lung cancer, giving risks of 0.13% and 0.01% respectively. Thus the risk of lung cancer was considerably higher among smokers than non-smokers.

Table 16.4 Hypothetical data from a cohort study to investigate the association between smoking and lung cancer. The calculations of risk ratio (RR) and risk difference are illustrated.

	Lung cancer	No lung cancer	Total	Risk
Smokers (exposed)	39	29 961	30 000	$p_1 - 39/30\,000 = 0.0013\ (0.13\%)$
Non-smokers (unexposed)	6	59 994	60 000	$p_0 - 6/60\,000 = 0.0001\ (0.01\%)$
Total	45	89 955	90 000	

Risk difference $= 0.13\% - 0.01\% = 0.12\%$
Risk ratio $= 0.0013/0.0001 = 13$

The risk ratio is:

$$\mathrm{RR} = \frac{p_1}{p_0} = \frac{0.0013}{0.0001} = 13$$

Interpreting the risk ratio

In an *epidemiological study*, comparing an exposed group with an unexposed, the risk ratio is a good indicator of the strength of the association between the exposure and the disease outcome. It equals:

$$\text{Risk ratio (RR)} = \frac{\text{risk in exposed group}}{\text{risk in unexposed group}}$$

In a *clinical trial* to assess the impact of a new treatment, procedure or preventive intervention on disease outcome or occurrence, the risk ratio equals:

$$\text{Risk ratio (RR)} = \frac{\text{risk in treatment group}}{\text{risk in control group}}$$

A risk ratio of 1 occurs when the risks are the same in the two groups and is equivalent to no association between the risk factor and the disease. A risk ratio greater than 1 occurs when the risk of the outcome is higher among those exposed to the factor (or treatment) than among the non-exposed, as in Example 16.2 above, with exposed referring to smoking. A risk ratio less than 1 occurs when the risk is lower among those exposed, suggesting that the factor (or treatment) may be protective. An example is the reduced risk of infant death observed among infants that are breast-fed compared to those that are not. The further the risk ratio is from 1, the stronger the association between exposure (or treatment) and outcome. Note that a risk ratio is always a positive number.

Relationship between risk ratios and risk differences

The risk ratio is more commonly used to measure of the strength of an association than is the difference in risks. This is because the amount by which an exposure (risk factor) multiplies the risk of an event is interpretable regardless of the size of the risk. For example, suppose we followed the population in Example 16.2 above for two years instead of one, and therefore observed exactly double the number of events in each group (here we are ignoring the small number of individuals lost to follow-up because they died in the first year). The risks are now 0.26% in smokers and 0.02% in non-smokers. The risk ratio is 0.26/0.02 = 13; exactly as before. However, the risk difference is now 0.26 − 0.02% = 0.24%, double that observed when there was only one year's follow-up. The use and interpretation of ratio and difference measures of the size of exposure effects is discussed in Chapter 37.

16.5 RISK RATIOS: CONFIDENCE INTERVALS AND HYPOTHESIS TESTS

Standard error and confidence interval for ratio measures

Until now, we have followed exactly the same procedure whenever we wish to calculate a confidence interval. We derive the standard error (s.e.) of the quantity, q, in which we are interested, and determine the multiplier z_α corresponding to the appropriate percentage point of the sampling distribution:

$$CI = q - z_\alpha \times \text{s.e. to } q + z_\alpha \times \text{s.e}$$

When the sampling distribution is normal, z_α is 1.96 for a 95% confidence interval and:

$$95\% \text{ CI} = q - 1.96 \times \text{s.e. to } q + 1.96 \times \text{s.e.}$$

For *ratio measures* such as risk ratios, this can lead to problems when the standard error is large and q is close to zero, because the lower limit of the confidence interval may come out negative despite the fact that the risk ratio is always positive. To overcome this problem, we adopt the following procedure:

1 Calculate the *logarithm* of the risk ratio, and its standard error. The formula for this standard error is derived using the **delta method** (see Box 16.1), and is:

$$\text{s.e.}(\log RR) = \sqrt{[1/d_1 - 1/n_1 + 1/d_0 - 1/n_0]}$$

Note that s.e.(log RR) should be interpreted as 'standard error of the log RR', and that throughout this book, all logs are to the base e (natural logarithms) unless explicitly denoted by $\log_{10}$ as being logs to the base 10. See Section 13.1 for an explanation of logarithms and the exponential function.

2 Derive a confidence interval for the *log risk ratio* in the usual way:

95% CI $(\log RR) = \log RR - 1.96 \times$ s.e.$(\log RR)$ to $\log RR + 1.96 \times$ s.e.$(\log RR)$

3 *Antilog the confidence limits* obtained, to convert this into a confidence interval for the risk ratio.

95% CI (RR) =
$\exp[\log RR - 1.96 \times$ s.e.$(\log RR)]$ to $\exp[\log RR + 1.96 \times$ s.e.$(\log RR)]$

4 Use the rules of logarithms and antilogs to make this simpler. The rules are:

Rules of logarithms:

$$\log(a) + \log(b) = \log(a \times b)$$
$$\log(a) - \log(b) = \log(a/b)$$

Rules of antilogs:

$\exp(a)$ means e^a; it is the antilog (exponential) function
$$\exp[\log(a)] = a$$
$$\exp(a + b) = \exp(a) \times \exp(b)$$
$$\exp(a - b) = \exp(a)/\exp(b)$$

Following these rules, and noting that $\exp(\log RR) = RR$, gives:

95% CI (RR) $= RR/\exp[1.96 \times$ s.e.$(\log RR)]$ to $RR \times \exp[1.96 \times$ s.e.$(\log RR)]$

The quantity $\exp[1.96 \times$ s.e. $(\log RR)]$ is known as an **error factor (EF)**; it is always greater than 1, because $\exp(x)$ is greater than 1 if x is greater than zero. The 95% confidence interval can therefore be written more simply as:

95% CI (RR) $= RR/EF$ to $RR \times EF$

Putting all of this together, the formula for the **95% confidence interval for the risk ratio** is:

95% CI (RR)$= RR/EF$ to $RR \times EF$,
where $EF = \exp[1.96 \times$ s.e.$(\log RR)]$
and s.e.$(\log RR) = \sqrt{[1/d_1 - 1/n_1 + 1/d_0 - 1/n_0]}$

BOX 16.1 DERIVATION OF THE FORMULA FOR THE STANDARD ERROR OF THE LOG(RISK RATIO)

This box is intended for those who wish to understand the mathematics behind the approximate formula for the *standard error of the log (risk ratio)* used in step 1 of the procedure described in Section 16.5, for calculating a confidence interval for the risk ratio.

The formula was derived using the **delta method**. This is a technique for calculating the standard error of a *transformed* variable from the mean and standard error of the original *untransformed* variable. In this Box, we briefly outline how this method is used to give (a) an approximate formula for the standard error of a *log transformed variable*, and in particular (b) the formula for the standard error of a *log transformed proportion*. We then show how this result can be used to derive (c) an approximate *formula for the standard error of the log(risk ratio)*.

(a) Deriving the formula for the standard error of a log transformed variable:

The delta method uses a mathematical technique known as a Taylor series expansion to show that:

$$\log(X) \simeq \log(\mu) + (X - \mu)(\log'(\mu))$$

where $\log'(\mu)$ denotes the first derivative of $\log(\mu)$, the slope of the graph of $\log(\mu)$ against μ. This approximation works provided that the variance of variable X is small compared to its mean.

As noted in Section 4.3, adding or subtracting a constant to a variable leaves its standard deviation (and variance) unaffected, and multiplying by a constant has the effect of multiplying the standard deviation by that constant (or equivalently multiplying the variance by the square of the constant). By applying these in the formula above, and further noting that $\log'(\mu) = 1/\mu$, we can deduce that

$$\text{s.e.}(\log(X)) \simeq \text{s.e.}(X) \times \log'(\mu) = \text{s.e.}(X)/\mu$$

(b) Formula for the standard error of the log(proportion):

Recall from Section 15.3 that the mean of the sampling distribution for a proportion is estimated by $p = d/n$ and the standard error by $\sqrt{[p(1-p)/n]}$. Therefore:

$$\text{s.e.}(\log p) \simeq \frac{\sqrt{[p(1-p)/n]}}{d/n} = \sqrt{[1/d - 1/n]}$$

(c) Formula for the standard error of the log(risk ratio):

$$\text{Risk ratio (RR)} = \frac{p_1}{p_0}$$

Using the rules of logarithms given above the log risk ratio is given by:

$$\log RR = \log(p_1) - \log(p_0)$$

Since the standard error of the difference between two variables is the square root of the sum of their variances (see Section 7.2), it follows that the standard error of $\log RR$ is given by:

$$\text{s.e.}(\log RR) = \sqrt{[\text{var}(\log(p_1)) + \text{var}(\log(p_0))]} = \sqrt{[1/d_1 - 1/n_1 + 1/d_0 - 1/n_0]}$$

Example 16.2 (continued)

Consider the data presented in Table 16.4, showing a risk ratio of 13 for the association between smoking and risk of lung cancer. The standard error of the log RR is given by:

$$\text{s.e.}(\log \text{RR}) = \sqrt{[(1/39 - 1/30000 + 1/6 - 1/60000)]} = 0.438$$

The error factor is given by:

$$\text{EF} = \exp(1.96 \times 0.438) = 2.362$$

The 95% confidence interval for the risk ratio is therefore:

$$95\% \text{ CI} = (13/2.362 \text{ to } 13 \times 2.362) = 5.5 \text{ to } 30.7$$

Test of the null hypothesis

If the null hypothesis of no difference between the risks in the two groups is true, then the $\text{RR} = 1$ and hence $\log \text{RR} = 0$. We use the log RR and its standard error to derive a z statistic and test the null hypothesis in the usual way:

$$z = \frac{\log RR}{\text{s.e.}(\log RR)}$$

Example 16.2 (continued)

In the smoking and lung cancer example,

$$z = 2.565/0.438 = 5.85$$

This corresponds to a *P*-value of < 0.0001. There is therefore strong evidence against the null hypothesis that the $\text{RR} = 1$.

Further analyses of risk ratios

The risk ratio is a measure that is easy to interpret, and the analyses based on risk ratios described in this chapter are straightforward. Perhaps surprisingly, however, more complicated analyses of associations between exposures and binary outcomes are rarely based on risk ratios. It is much more common for these to be based on *odds ratios*, as discussed in the next section, and used throughout

Chapters 17 to 21. In Section 20.4, we briefly describe how to conduct regression analyses based on risk ratios, rather than odds ratios, and why this is not usually the preferred method.

16.6 ODDS RATIOS

We now turn to the third and final measure of effect introduced in Section 16.2, the *ratio* of the *odds* of the outcome event in the exposed group compared to the odds in the unexposed group (or in the case of a clinical trial, in the treatment group compared to the control group). Recall from Section 14.6 that the odds of an outcome event D are defined as:

$$\text{Odds} = \frac{\text{prob(D happens)}}{\text{prob(D does not happen)}} = \frac{\text{prob(D)}}{1 - \text{prob(D)}}$$

The odds are *estimated* by:

$$\text{Odds} = \frac{p}{1-p} = \frac{d/n}{(1-d/n)} = \frac{d/n}{h/n} = \frac{d}{h}$$

i.e. by the number of individuals who experience the event divided by the number who do not experience the event. The **odds ratio** (often abbreviated to **OR**) is estimated by:

$$\text{OR} = \frac{\text{odds in exposed group}}{\text{odds in unexposed group}} = \frac{d_1/h_1}{d_0/h_0} = \frac{d_1 \times h_0}{d_0 \times h_1}$$

It is also known as the **cross-product ratio** of the 2×2 table.

Example 16.3
Example 15.5 introduced a survey of 2000 patients aged 15 to 50 registered with a particular general practice, which showed that 138 (6.9%) were being treated for asthma. Table 16.5 shows the number diagnosed with asthma according to their gender. Both the prevalence (proportion with asthma) and odds of asthma in women and men are shown, as are their ratios.

The odds ratio of 1.238 indicates that asthma is more common among women than men. In this example the odds ratio is close to the ratio of the prevalences; this is because the prevalence of asthma is low (6% to 8%). Properties of odds ratios are summarized in Box 16.2.

Table 16.5 Hypothetical data from a survey to examine the prevalence of asthma among patients at a particular general practice.

	Asthma	No asthma	Total	Prevalence	Odds
Women	81	995	1076	0.0753	0.0814
Men	57	867	924	0.0617	0.0657
Total	138	1862	2000	$RR = \dfrac{0.0753}{0.0617} = 1.220$	$OR = \dfrac{0.0814}{0.0657} = 1.238$

BOX 16.2   PROPERTIES OF ODDS RATIOS

The minimum possible value is zero, and the maximum possible value is infinity.

- An odds ratio of 1 occurs when the odds, and hence the proportions, are the same in the two groups and is equivalent to no association between the exposure and the disease.
- The odds ratio is always further away from 1 than the corresponding risk (or prevalence) ratio. Thus:

$$\text{if } RR > 1 \text{ then } OR > RR$$

$$\text{if } RR < 1 \text{ then } OR < RR$$

- For a rare outcome (one in which the probability of the event not occurring is close to 1) the odds ratio is approximately equal to the risk ratio (since the odds are approximately equal to the risk, see Section 14.6).
- The odds ratio for the occurrence of disease is the reciprocal of the odds ratio for non-occurrence.
- The odds ratio for exposure, that is the odds of disease in the exposed compared to the odds in the unexposed group, *equals* the odds ratio for disease, that is the odds of exposure in the disease compared to the odds in the healthy group. (This equivalence is fundamental for the analysis of case- control studies.)

Comparison of odds ratios and risk ratios

As mentioned in Section 16.2, both the risk difference and the risk ratio have immediate intuitive interpretations. It is relatively easy to explain that, for example, moderate smokers have twice the risk of cardiovascular disease than non-smokers ($RR = 2$). In contrast, interpretation of odds ratios often causes problems; except for gamblers, who tend to be extremely familiar with the meaning of odds (see Chapter 14).

Table 16.6 Values of the risk ratio when the odds ratio $= 2$, and the odds ratio when the risk ratio $= 2$, given different values of the risk in the unexposed group.

Odds ratio = 2		Risk ratio = 2	
Risk in the unexposed group	Corresponding risk ratio	Risk in the unexposed group	Corresponding odds ratio
0.001	1.998	0.001	2.002
0.005	1.99	0.005	2.010
0.01	1.980	0.01	2.020
0.05	1.905	0.05	2.111
0.1	1.818	0.1	2.25
0.5	1.333	0.3	3.5
0.9	1.053	0.4	6.0
0.95	1.026	0.45	11.0
0.99	1.005	0.5*	∞

*When π_0 is greater than 0.5, the risk ratio must be less than 2, since $\pi_1 = \text{RR} \times \pi_0$, and probabilities cannot exceed 1.

A common mistake in the literature is to interpret an odds ratio as if it were a risk ratio. For rare outcomes, this is not a problem since the two are numerically equal (see Box 16.2 and Table 16.6). However, for common outcomes, this is not the case; the interpretation of odds ratios diverges from that for risk ratios. Table 16.6 shows values of the risk ratio for an odds ratio of 2, and conversely the values of the odds ratio for a risk ratio of 2, for different values of the risk in the unexposed group. For example, it shows that if the risk in the exposed group is 0.5, then an odds ratio of 2 is equivalent to a risk ratio of 1.33. When the outcome is common, therefore, an odds ratio of (for example) 2 or 5 *must not* be interpreted as meaning that the risk is multiplied by 2 or 5.

As the risk in the unexposed group becomes larger, the maximum possible value of the risk ratio becomes constrained, because the maximum possible value for a risk is 1. For example, if the risk in the unexposed group is 0.33, the maximum possible value of the RR is 3. Because there is no upper limit for the odds, the OR is not constrained in this manner. Note that as the risk in the unexposed group increases the odds ratio becomes much larger than the risk ratio and, as explained above, should no longer be interpreted as the amount by which the risk factor multiplies the risk of the disease outcome.

The constraint on the value of the risk ratio can cause problems for statistical analyses using risk ratios when the outcome is not rare, because it can mean that the risk ratio differs between population strata. For example, in a low-risk stratum the risk of disease might be 0.2 (20%) in the unexposed group and 0.5 (50%) in the exposed group. The risk ratio in that stratum is therefore $0.5/0.2 = 2.5$. If the risk of disease in a high-risk stratum is 0.5 then the risk ratio can be at most 2 in that stratum, since the maximum possible risk of disease is 1, and $1/0.5 = 2$.

A further difficulty with risk ratios is that the interpretation of results may depend on whether the occurrence of an event, or its non-occurrence, is considered as the outcome. For odds ratios this presents no problems, since:

$$OR(disease) = 1/OR(healthy)$$

However no such relationship exists for risk ratios. For instance, consider the low-risk stratum in which the risk ratio is $0.5/0.2 = 2.5$. If the non-occurrence of disease (healthy) is considered as the outcome, then the risk ratio is $(1 - 0.5)/(1 - 0.2) = 0.5/0.8 = 0.625$. This is *not* the same as $1/2.5 = 0.4$.

Example 16.4

Consider a study in which we monitor the risk of severe nausea during chemotherapy for breast cancer. A new drug is compared with standard treatment. The hypothetical results are shown in Table 16.7.

The risk of severe nausea is 88% in the group treated with the new drug and 71% in the group given standard treatment, so the risk ratio is $0.88/0.71 = 1.239$, an apparently moderate increase in the prevalence of nausea. In contrast the odds ratio is 2.995, a much more dramatic increase. Note, however, that the risk ratio is constrained: it cannot be greater than $1/0.71 = 1.408$.

Suppose now that we consider our outcome to be *absence* of nausea. The risk ratio is $0.12/0.29 = 0.414$: the proportion of patients without severe nausea has more than halved. The odds ratio is 0.334: exactly the inverse of the odds ratio for nausea $(1/2.995 = 0.334)$.

Table 16.7 Risk of severe nausea following chemotherapy for breast cancer.

	Number with severe nausea	Number without severe nausea	Total
New drug	88 (88%)	12	100
Standard treatment	71 (71%)	29	100

Rationale for the use of odds ratios

In the recent medical literature, *the statistical analysis of binary outcomes is almost always based on odds ratios*, even though they are less easy to interpret than risk ratios (or risk differences). This is for the following three reasons:

1 When the **outcome is rare**, *the odds ratio is the same as the risk ratio*. This is because the *odds* of occurrence of a rare outcome are numerically equivalent to its *risk*. Analyses based on odds ratios therefore give the same results as analyses based on risk ratios.

2 When the **outcome is common**, risk ratios are *constrained* but odds ratios are not. Analyses based on risk ratios, particularly those examining the effects of more than one exposure variable, can cause computational problems and are difficult to interpret. In contrast, these problems do not occur in analyses based on odds ratios.

3 For odds ratios, the conclusions are identical whether we consider our outcome as the occurrence of an event, or the absence of the event.

Taken together, these mean that analyses of binary outcomes controlling for possible confounding (see Chapter 18), or which use regression modelling (see Chapters 19 to 21), usually report exposure effects as odds ratios, regardless of whether the outcome is rare or common.

In addition, odds ratios are the measure of choice in **case–control studies**. In fact, it is in this context that they were first developed and used. In case–control studies we recruit a group of people with the disease of interest (cases) and a random sample of people without the disease (the controls). The distribution of one or more exposures in the cases is then compared with the distribution in the controls. Because the controls usually represent an unknown fraction of the whole population, it is not possible to estimate the risk of disease in a case–control study, and so risk differences and risk ratios cannot be derived. The odds ratio can be used to compare cases and controls because the ratio of the *odds of exposure* (d_1/d_0) among the *diseased* group compared to the odds of exposure among the *healthy* group (h_1/h_0), is equivalent to the ratio of the odds of disease in exposed compared to unexposed:

$$OR = \frac{d_1/h_1}{d_0/h_0} = \frac{d_1 \times h_0}{d_0 \times h_1} = \frac{d_1/d_0}{h_1/h_0}$$

16.7 ODDS RATIOS: CONFIDENCE INTERVALS AND HYPOTHESIS TESTS

Confidence interval for the odds and the odds ratio

We saw in Section 16.5 how a confidence interval for the risk ratio is derived by calculating a confidence interval for the log risk ratio and then converting this to a confidence interval for the risk ratio. Confidence intervals for the odds, and the odds ratio, are calculated in exactly the same way. The results are shown in Table 16.8. Note that s.e.(log OR) should be interpreted as 's.e. of the log OR'. The formula for s.e.(log OR) is also known as **Woolf's formula**.

Table 16.8 Formulae for calculation of 95% confidence intervals for the odds and the odds ratio.

Odds	Odds ratio (OR)
95% CI = odds/EF to odds × EF,	95% CI = OR/EF to OR × EF,
where EF = exp [1.96 × s.e.(log odds)]	where EF = exp[1.96 × s.e.(log OR)]
and s.e.(log odds) = $\sqrt{[1/d + 1/h]}$	and s.e.(log OR) = $\sqrt{[1/d_1 + 1/h_1 + 1/d_0 + 1/h_0]}$

Example 16.3 (continued)

Consider the data from the asthma survey presented in Table 16.5. The standard error of the log OR is given by:

$$\text{s.e.}(\log OR) = \sqrt{[1/57 + 1/867 + 1/81 + 1/995]} = 0.179$$

The error factor is given by:

$$EF = \exp(1.96 \times 0.179) = 1.420$$

The 95% confidence interval for the odds ratio is therefore:

$$95\% \text{ CI} = 1.238/1.420 \text{ to } 1.238 \times 1.420 = 0.872 \text{ to } 1.759$$

With 95% confidence, the odds ratio in the population lies between 0.872 and 1.759.

Test of the null hypothesis

We use the log OR and its standard error to derive a z statistic and test the null hypothesis in the usual way:

$$z = \frac{\log OR}{\text{s.e.}(\log OR)}$$

The results are identical to those produced by simple logistic regression models (see Chapter 19).

Example 16.3 (continued)

The z statistic is given by $z = 0.214/0.179 = 1.194$. This corresponds to a P-value of 0.232. There is no clear evidence against the null hypothesis that the OR = 1, i.e. that the prevalence of asthma is the same in men and women.

CHAPTER 17

Chi-squared tests for 2 × 2 and larger contingency tables

17.1 INTRODUCTION

We saw in the last chapter that when both exposure and outcome variables have only two possible values (binary variables) the data can be displayed in a **2×2 table**. As described in Section 3.4, **contingency tables** can also be used to display the association between two categorical variables, one or both of which has more than two possible values. The categories for one variable define the rows, and the categories for the other variable define the columns. Individuals are assigned to the appropriate cell of the contingency table according to their values for the two variables. A contingency table is also used for discrete numerical variables, or for continuous numerical variables whose values have been grouped. These larger tables are generally called $r \times c$ **tables**, where r denotes the number of rows in the table and c the number of columns. If the variables displayed are an *exposure* and an *outcome*, then it is usual to arrange the table with exposure as the row variable and outcome as the column variable, and to display percentages corresponding to the *exposure* variable.

In this chapter, we describe how to use a **chi-squared (χ^2) test** to examine whether there is an association between the row variable and the column variable or, in other words, whether the distribution of individuals among the categories of one variable is independent of their distribution among the categories of the other. We explain this for 2 × 2 tables, and for larger $r \times c$ tables. When the table has only two rows and two columns the χ^2 test is equivalent to the z-test for the difference between two proportions. We also describe the **exact test** for a 2 × 2 table when the sample size is too small for the z-test or the χ^2 test to be valid. Finally, we describe the use of a χ^2 **test for trend**, for the special case where we have a binary outcome variable and several exposure categories, which have a natural order.

17.2 CHI-SQUARED TEST FOR A 2×2 TABLE

Example 17.1

Table 17.1 shows the data from the influenza vaccination trial described in the last chapter (see Example 16.1). Since the exposure is vaccination (the row variable), the table includes row percentages. We now wish to assess the strength of the evidence that vaccination affected the probability of contracting influenza.

Table 17.1 2 × 2 table showing results from an influenza vaccine trial.

(a) Observed numbers.

	Influenza		
	Yes	No	Total
Vaccine	20 (8.3%)	220 (91.7%)	240
Placebo	80 (36.4%)	140 (63.6%)	220
Total	100 (21.7%)	360 (78.3%)	460

(b) Expected numbers.

	Influenza		
	Yes	No	Total
Vaccine	52.2	187.8	240
Placebo	47.8	172.2	220
Total	100	360	460

The **chi-squared test** compares the observed numbers in each of the four categories in the contingency table with the numbers to be expected if there were no difference in efficacy between the vaccine and placebo. Overall 100/460 people contracted influenza and, if the vaccine and the placebo were equally effective, one would expect this same proportion in each of the two groups; that is 100/460 × 240 = 52.2 in the vaccine group and 100/460 × 220 = 47.8 in the placebo group would have contracted influenza. Similarly 360/460 × 240 = 187.8 and 360/460 × 220 = 172.2 would have escaped influenza. These expected numbers are shown in Table 17.1(b). They add up to the same row and column totals as the observed numbers. The chi-squared value is obtained by calculating

$$(\text{observed} - \text{expected})^2/\text{expected}$$

for each of the four cells in the contingency table and then summing them.

$$\chi^2 = \Sigma \frac{(O - E)^2}{E}, \text{d.f.} = 1 \text{ for a } 2 \times 2 \text{ table}$$

This is exactly the same formula as was given for the chi-squared goodness of fit test, which was described in Chapter 12. The greater the differences between the observed and expected numbers, the larger the value of x^2. The percentage points of the chi-squared distribution are given in Table A5 in the Appendix. The values depend on the degrees of freedom, which equal 1 for a 2 × 2 table (the number of rows minus 1 multiplied by the number of columns minus 1). In this example:

$$x^2 = \frac{(20 - 52.2)^2}{52.2} + \frac{(80 - 47.8)^2}{47.8} + \frac{(220 - 187.8)^2}{187.8} + \frac{(140 - 172.2)^2}{172.2}$$
$$= 19.86 + 21.69 + 5.52 + 6.02 = 53.09$$

53.09 is greater than 10.83, the 0.1% point for the chi-squared distribution with 1 degree of freedom so that the P-value for the test is < 0.001. This means that the probability is less than 0.001, or 0.1%, that such a large observed difference in the percentages contracting influenza could have arisen by chance, if there was no real difference between the vaccine and the placebo. Thus there is strong evidence against the null hypothesis of no effect of the vaccine on the probability of contracting influenza. It is therefore concluded that the vaccine is effective.

Quick formula

Using our standard notation for a 2 × 2 table (see Table 16.1), a quicker formula for calculating chi-squared on a 2 × 2 table is:

$$x^2 = \frac{n(d_1h_0 - d_0h_1)^2}{dhn_1n_0}, \text{d.f.} = 1$$

In the example,

$$x^2 = \frac{460 \times (20 \times 140 - 80 \times 220)^2}{100 \times 360 \times 240 \times 220} = 53.01$$

which, apart from rounding error, is the same as the value of 53.09 obtained above.

Relation with normal test for the difference between two proportions

The square of the z statistic (normal test) for the difference between two proportions and the chi-squared statistic for a 2 × 2 contingency table are in fact mathematically equivalent ($x^2 = z^2$), and the P-values from the two tests are identical. In Example 16.1 (Section 16.3) the z-test gave a value of -7.281 for the influenza vaccine data; $z^2 = (-7.281)^2 = 53.01$ which, apart from rounding error, is the same as the x^2 value of 53.09 calculated above.

We will show below that the chi-squared test can be extended to larger contingency tables. Note that the percentage points given in Table A5 for a chi-squared distribution with 1 degree of freedom correspond to the two-sided percentage points presented in Table A2 for the standard normal distribution (see Appendix). (The concepts of one- and two-sided tests do not extend to chi-squared tests with larger degrees of freedom as these contain multiple comparisons.)

Continuity correction

The chi-squared test for a 2 × 2 table can be improved by using a continuity correction, often called **Yates' continuity correction**. The formula becomes:

$$\chi^2 = \Sigma \frac{(|O - E| - 0.5)^2}{E}, \text{d.f.} = 1$$

resulting in a smaller value for χ^2. $|O - E|$ means the absolute value of $O - E$ or, in other words, the value of $O - E$ ignoring its sign.

In the example the value for χ^2 becomes:

$$\chi^2 = \frac{(32.2 - 0.5)^2}{52.2} + \frac{(32.2 - 0.5)^2}{47.8} + \frac{(32.2 - 0.5)^2}{187.8} + \frac{(32.2 - 0.5)^2}{172.2}$$
$$= 19.25 + 21.02 + 5.35 + 5.84 = 51.46, P < 0.001$$

compared to the uncorrected value of 53.09.

The rationale of the continuity correction is explained in Figure 15.3, where the normal and binomial distributions are superimposed. It makes little difference unless the total sample size is less than 40, or the expected numbers are small. However there is no analogue of the continuity correction for the Mantel–Haenszel and regression analyses described later in this part of the book. When the expected numbers are *very* small, then the exact test described in Section 17.3 should be used; see discussion on *validity* below.

Validity

When the expected numbers are very small the chi-squared test (and the equivalent z-test) is not a good enough approximation and the alternative exact test for a 2 × 2 table should be used (see Section 17.3). Cochran (1954) recommended the use of the **exact test** when:

1 the overall total of the table is less than 20, *or*
2 the overall total is between 20 and 40 and the smallest of the four *expected* numbers is less than 5.

Thus the chi-squared test is *valid* when the overall total is more than 40, regardless of the expected values, and when the overall total is between 20 and 40 provided all the expected values are at least 5.

17.3 EXACT TEST FOR 2×2 TABLES

The exact test to compare two proportions is needed when the numbers in the 2×2 table are very small; see the discussions concerning the validity of the z-test to compare two proportions (Section 16.3) and of the chi-squared test for a 2×2 table (Section 17.2 above). It is most easily described in the context of a particular example.

Example 17.2
Table 17.2 shows the results from a study to compare two treatment regimes for controlling bleeding in haemophiliacs undergoing surgery. Only one (8%) of the 13 haemophiliacs given treatment regime A suffered bleeding complications, compared to three (25%) of the 12 given regime B. These numbers are too small for the chi-squared test to be valid; the overall total, 25, is less than 40, and the smallest expected value, 1.9 (complications with regime B), is less than 5. The exact test is therefore indicated.

Table 17.2 Comparison of two treatment regimes for controlling bleeding in haemophiliacs undergoing surgery.

Treatment regime	Bleeding complications		Total
	Yes	No	
A (group 1)	1 (d_1)	12 (h_1)	13 (n_1)
B (group 0)	3 (d_0)	9 (h_0)	12 (n_0)
Total	4 (d)	21 (h)	25 (n)

The exact test is based on calculating the exact probabilities of the observed table and of more 'extreme' tables with the same row and column totals, using the following formula:

$$\text{Exact probability of } 2 \times 2 \text{ table} = \frac{d!\,h!\,n_1!\,n_0!}{n!\,d_1!\,d_0!\,h_1!\,h_0!}$$

where the notation is the same as that defined in Table 16.1. The exclamation mark denotes the *factorial* of the number and means all the integers from the number down to 1 multiplied together. (0! is defined to equal 1.) Many calculators have a key for factorial, although this expression may be easily computed by cancelling factors in the top and bottom. The exact probability of Table 17.2 is therefore:

$$\frac{4!21!13!12!}{25!1!3!12!9!} = \frac{4 \times 13 \times 12 \times 11 \times 10}{25 \times 24 \times 23 \times 22} = 0.2261$$

(21! being cancelled into 25!, for example, leaving $25 \times 24 \times 23 \times 22$).

In order to test the null hypothesis that there is no difference between the treatment regimes, we need to calculate not only the probability of the observed table but also the probability that a more extreme table could occur by chance. Altogether there are five possible tables that have the same row and column totals as the data. These are shown in Table 17.3 together with their probabilities, which total 1. The observed case is Table 17.3(b) with a probability of 0.2261.

Table 17.3 All possible tables with the same row and column totals as Table 17.2, together with their probabilities.

(a)		Total		(b)		Total
	0	13	13		1	12	13
	4	8	12		3	9	12
Total	4	21	25		Total	4	21	25
	$P = 0.0391$				$P = 0.2261$		

(c)		Total		(d)		Total
	2	11	13		3	10	13
	2	10	12		1	11	12
Total	4	21	25		Total	4	21	25
	$P = 0.4070$				$P = 0.2713$		

(e)		Total
	4	9	13
	0	12	12
Total	4	21	25
	$P = 0.0565$	

There are two approaches to calculating the *P*-value. In the first approach, more extreme is defined as less probable; more extreme tables are therefore 17.3(a) and 17.3(e) with probabilities 0.0391 and 0.0565 respectively. The total probability needed for the *P*-value is therefore $0.2261 + 0.0391 + 0.0565 = 0.3217$, and so there is clearly no evidence against the null hypothesis of no difference between the regimes.

P-value (approach I) = probability of observed table + probability of less probable tables

P-value (approach II) = 2 × (probability of observed table + probability of more extreme tables in the same direction)

The alternative approach is to restrict the calculation to extreme tables showing differences in the same direction as that observed, and then to double the resulting probability in order to cover differences in the other direction. In this example, the P-value thus obtained would be twice the sum of the probabilities of Tables 17.3(a) and 17.3(b), namely $2 \times (0.0391 + 0.2261) = 0.5304$. Neither method is clearly superior to the other, but the second method is simpler to carry out. Although the two approaches give different results, the choice is unlikely, in practice, to affect the assessment of whether the observed difference is due to chance or to a real effect.

17.4 LARGER CONTINGENCY TABLES

So far, we have dealt with 2×2 tables, which are used to display data classified according to the values of two binary variables. The chi-squared test can also be applied to larger tables, generally called $r \times c$ **tables**, where r denotes the number of rows in the table and c the number of columns.

$$\chi^2 = \Sigma \frac{(O - E)^2}{E}, \text{d.f.} = (r - 1) \times (c - 1)$$

There is no continuity correction or exact test for contingency tables larger than 2×2. Cochran (1954) recommends that the approximation of the chi-squared test is valid provided that less than 20% of the expected numbers are under 5 and none is less than 1. This restriction can sometimes be overcome by combining rows (or columns) with low expected numbers, providing that these combinations make biological sense.

There is no quick formula for a general $r \times c$ table. The expected numbers must be computed for each cell. The reasoning employed is the same as that described above for the 2×2 table. The general rule for calculating an expected number is:

$$E = \frac{\text{column total} \times \text{row total}}{\text{overall total}}$$

It is worth pointing out that the chi-squared test is only valid if applied to the actual numbers in the various categories. It must never be applied to tables showing just proportions or percentages.

Example 17.3

Table 17.4(a) shows the results from a survey to compare the principal water sources in three villages in West Africa. These data were also presented when we introduced cross-tabulations in Chapter 3. The numbers of households using a river, a pond, or a spring are given. We will treat the water source as outcome and village as exposure, so column percentages are displayed. For example, in village A, 40.0% of households use mainly a river, 36.0% a pond and 24.0% a spring. Overall, 70 of the 150 households use a river. If there were no difference between villages one would expect this same proportion of river usage in each village. Thus the expected numbers of households using a river in villages A, B and C, respectively, are:

$$\frac{70}{150} \times 50 = 23.3, \quad \frac{70}{150} \times 60 = 28.0 \quad \text{and} \quad \frac{70}{150} \times 40 = 18.7$$

The expected numbers can also be found by applying the general rule. For example, the expected number of households in village B using a river is:

$$\frac{\text{row total (B)} \times \text{column total (river)}}{\text{overall total}} = \frac{60 \times 70}{150} = 28.0$$

The expected numbers for the whole table are given in Table 17.4(b).

Table 17.4 Comparison of principal sources of water used by households in three villages in West Africa.

(a) Observed numbers.

| Village | Water source | | | |
	River	Pond	Spring	Total
A	20 (40.0%)	18 (36.0%)	12 (24.0%)	50 (100.0%)
B	32 (53.3%)	20 (33.3%)	8 (13.3%)	60 (100.0%)
C	18 (45.0%)	12 (30.0%)	10 (25.0%)	40 (100.0%)
Total	70 (46.7%)	50 (33.3%)	30 (20.0%)	150 (100.0%)

(b) Expected numbers.

| Village | Water source | | | |
	River	Pond	Spring	Total
A	23.3	16.7	10.0	50
B	28.0	20.0	12.0	60
C	18.7	13.3	8.0	40
Total	70	50	30	150

$$\chi^2 = \Sigma \frac{(O-E)^2}{E}$$

$$= (20-23.3)^2/23.3 + (18-16.7)^2/16.7 + (12-10.0)^2/10.0+$$
$$(32-28.0)^2/28.0 + (18-18.7)^2/18.7 + (20-20.0)^2/20.0+$$
$$(8-12.0)^2/12.0 + (12-13.3)^2/13.3 + (10-8.0)^2/8.0$$
$$= 3.53$$
$$\text{d.f.} = (r-1) \times (c-1) = 2 \times 2 = 4$$

The corresponding P-value (derived using a computer) is 0.47, so we can conclude that there is no evidence of a difference between the villages in the proportion of households using different water sources. Alternatively, we can see from the fourth row of Table A5 (see Appendix) that since 3.53 lies between 3.36 and 5.39, the P-value lies between 0.25 and 0.5.

17.5 ORDERED EXPOSURES: χ^2 TEST FOR TREND

We now consider the special case where we have a binary outcome variable and several exposure categories, which have a natural order. The standard chi-squared test for such data is a general test to assess whether there are differences among the proportions in the different exposure groups. The χ^2 **test for trend**, described now, is a more sensitive test that assesses whether there is an increasing (or decreasing) trend in the proportions over the exposure categories.

Example 17.4

Table 17.5 shows data from a study that examined the association between obesity and age at menarche in women. The outcome was whether the woman was aged < 12 years at menarche (event D) or aged > 12+ years (event H). The exposure, obesity, is represented by triceps skinfold, categorised into three groups. Although it is conventional that the exposure variable is the row variable, this is not an absolute rule. For convenience, we have not followed this convention, and have

Table 17.5. Relationship between triceps skinfold and early menarche. Data from a study on obesity in women (Beckles *et al.* (1985) *International Journal of Obesity* **9**: 127–35).

Age at menarche	Triceps skinfold group			Total
	Small	Intermediate	Large	
< 12 years (D)	15 (8.8%)	29 (12.8%)	36 (19.4%)	80
12+ years (H)	156 (91.2%)	197 (87.2%)	150 (80.6%)	503
Total	171 (100%)	226 (100%)	186 (100%)	583
Exposure group score (x)	0	1	2	
Odds of early menarche	0.10 (0.06 to 0.16)	0.15 (0.10 to 0.22)	0.24 (0.17 to 0.35)	
Log odds	−2.34 (−2.87 to −1.81)	−1.92 (−2.31 to −1.53)	−1.43 (−1.79 to −1.06)	

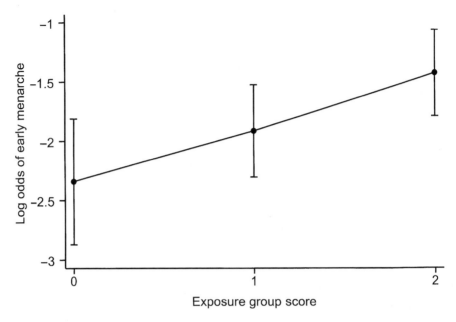

Fig. 17.1 Log odds of early menarche according to skinfold thickness group.

presented the exposure in the columns and the outcome in the rows. It can be seen that the proportion of women who had experienced early menarche increased with triceps skinfold size. This can be examined using the χ^2 **test for trend**.

The first step is to assign scores to the exposure groups. The usual choice is simply to number the columns 0, 1, 2, etc., as shown here (or equivalently 1, 2, 3, etc.). This is equivalent to assuming that the *log odds* goes up (or down) by equal amounts between the exposure groups, or in other words that there is a linear relationship between the two. The odds and log odds of early menarche are shown below the exposure scores, and the log odds with 95% confidence intervals are plotted in Figure 17.1. It is clear that the assumption of a linear increase in log odds, with exposure group is reasonable. The difference in log odds is $(-1.92 - -2.34) = 0.42$ between groups 1 and 0, and $(-1.43 - -1.92) = 0.49$ between groups 2 and 1.

Another possibility would have been to use the means or medians of the triceps skinfold measurements in each group. The assumption here would be a linear relationship between log odds and triceps skinfold measurement. The two approaches will give similar results if the differences between the means (or medians) are similar between the triceps skinfold groups.

The next step is to calculate three quantities for *each exposure group* in the table and to sum the results of each. These are:

1 dx, the product of the *observed* number, d, with outcome D, and the exposure group score, x;

2 nx, the product of the total, n, in the exposure group and its score, x; and

3 nx^2, the product of the total, n, in the exposure group and the square of its score, x^2.

Using N to denote the overall total and O the total observed number of events (the total of the top row), we then calculate:

$$U = \Sigma(dx) - \frac{O}{N}\Sigma(nx) \quad \text{and} \quad V = \frac{O(N-O)}{N^2(N-1)}[N\Sigma(nx^2) - (\Sigma nx)^2]$$

The increase in log odds ratio per group is estimated by U/V, with standard error $\sqrt{(1/V)}$. The formula for the chi-squared statistic is:

$$\chi^2_{trend} = \frac{U^2}{V}, \text{d.f.} = 1$$

This tests the null hypothesis that the linear increase in log odds per exposure group is zero.

There are various different forms for this test, most of which are algebraically equivalent. The only difference is that in some forms $(N-1)$ is replaced by N in the calculation of V. This difference is unimportant.

Example 17.4 (continued)

The calculations for the data presented in Table 17.5 are as follows:

$$\Sigma(dx) = 15 \times 0 + 29 \times 1 + 36 \times 2 = 101$$
$$\Sigma(nx) = 171 \times 0 + 226 \times 1 + 186 \times 2 = 598$$
$$\Sigma(nx^2) = 171 \times 0 + 226 \times 1 + 186 \times 4 = 970$$
$$O = 80, \ N = 583, \ N - O = 503$$
$$U = 101 - \left(\frac{80}{583} \times 598\right) = 18.9417$$
$$V = \left(\frac{80 \times 503}{583^2 \times 582}\right) \times (583 \times 970 - 598^2) = 42.2927$$

The increase in log odds ratio per group is $U/V = 0.445$: approximately an average of the differences between groups 1 and 0, and 2 and 1 (see above). Its standard error is $\sqrt{(1/V)} = 0.154$ and the 95% CI (derived in the usual way) is 0.146 to 0.749. This converts to an *odds ratio per exposure group* of 1.565 (95% CI 1.158 to 2.115). The chi-squared statistic is:

$$\chi^2_{trend} = \frac{(18.9417)^2}{42.2927} = 8.483, \quad \text{d.f.} = 1, \quad P = 0.0036.$$

There is therefore strong evidence that the odds of early menarche increased with increasing triceps skinfold.

This is a simple example of a **dose–response model** for the association between an exposure and a binary outcome. We show in Chapter 19 that a logistic regression model for this association gives very similar results. Note that the difference between the standard χ^2 value and the trend test χ^2 value provides a chi-squared value with $(c - 2)$ degrees of freedom to test for **departures from linear trend**, where c is the number of exposure groups. Such tests are described in more detail, in the context of regression modelling, in Section 29.6.

CHAPTER 18

Controlling for confounding: stratification

18.1 INTRODUCTION

Previous chapters in this part of the book have presented methods to examine the association between a binary outcome and two or more exposure (or treatment) groups. We have used confidence intervals and *P*-values to assess the likely size of the association, and the evidence that it represents a real difference in disease risk between the exposure groups. However, before attributing any difference in outcome between the exposure groups to the exposure itself, it is important to examine whether the exposure–outcome association has been affected by other factors that differ between the exposure groups and which also affect the outcome. Such factors are said to *confound* the association of interest. Failure to control for them can lead to **confounding bias**. This fundamental problem is illustrated by an example in the next section.

In this chapter, we describe the Mantel–Haenszel method that uses stratification to *control for confounding* when both the exposure and outcome are *binary* variables. In Chapter 11, on multiple regression for the analysis of numerical outcomes, we briefly described how regression models can be used to control for confounding. We will explain this in much more detail in Chapter 20 in the context of *logistic regression* for the analysis of binary outcomes.

18.2 CONFOUNDING

Example 18.1
Table 18.1 shows hypothetical results from a survey carried out to compare the prevalence of antibodies to leptospirosis in rural and urban areas of the West Indies, with rural residence as the exposure of interest.

Table 18.1 Results of a survey of the prevalence of leptospirosis in rural and urban areas of the West Indies.

	Leptospirosis antibodies			
Type of area	Yes	No	Total	Odds
Rural	60 (30%)	140 (70%)	200	0.429
Urban	60 (30%)	140 (70%)	200	0.429
Total	120	280	400	

Since the numbers of individuals with and without antibodies are identical in urban and rural areas, the odds ratio is exactly 1 and we would conclude that there is no association between leptospirosis antibodies and urban/rural residence. However, Table 18.2 shows that when the same sample is subdivided according to gender, the risk of having antibodies is higher in rural areas *for both males and females*. The disappearance of this effect when the genders are combined is caused by a combination of two factors:

1 Females in both areas are much less likely than males to have antibodies.
2 The samples from the rural and urban areas have different gender compositions. The proportion of males is 100/200 (50%) in the urban sample but only 50/200 (25%) in the rural sample.

Table 18.2 Association between antibodies to leptospirosis (the outcome variable) and rural/urban residence (the exposure variable), separately in males and females.

(a) Males.

	Antibodies			
Type of area	Yes	No	Total	Odds
Rural	36 (72%)	14 (28%)	50	2.57
Urban	50 (50%)	50 (50%)	100	1.00
Total	86	64	150	

$OR = 2.57/1 = 2.57$ (95% CI $= 1.21$ to 5.45), $P = 0.011$

(b) Females.

	Antibodies			
Type of area	Yes	No	Total	Odds
Rural	24 (16%)	126 (84%)	150	0.19
Urban	10 (10%)	90 (90%)	100	0.11
Total	34	216	250	

$OR = 0.19/0.11 = 1.71$ (95% CI $= 0.778$ to 3.78), $P = 0.176$

Gender is said to be a **confounding** variable because it is related both to the outcome variable (presence of antibodies) and to the exposure groups being compared (rural and urban). Ignoring gender in the analysis leads to a **bias** in the results. Analysing males and females separately provides evidence of a difference between the rural and urban areas for males but not for females (Table 18.2). However, we would like to be able to combine the information in the two tables to estimate the association between leptospirosis antibodies and urban/rural residence, *having allowed for* the association of each of these with gender. We describe how to do this in the next section.

In general confounding occurs when a confounding variable, C, is associated with the exposure, E, and also influences the disease outcome, D. This is illustrated in Figure 18.1. We are interested in the E–D association, but the E–C and C–D associations may bias our estimate of the E–D association unless we take them into account in our analysis.

In our example, failure to allow for gender masked an association with urban/rural residence. In other situations similar effects could suggest a difference or association where none exists, or could even suggest a difference the opposite way around to one that does exist. For example, in the assessment of whether persons suffering from schistosomiasis have a higher mortality rate than uninfected persons, it would be important to take age into account since both the risk of dying and the risk of having schistosomiasis increase with age. If age were not allowed for, schistosomiasis would appear to be associated with increased mortality, even if it were not, as those with schistosomiasis would be on average older and therefore more likely to die than younger uninfected persons.

Note that *a variable that is part of the causal chain leading from E to D is not a confounder*. That is, if E affects C, which in turn affects D, then we should not adjust for the effect of C in our analysis of the E–D association (unless we wish to estimate the effect of E on D which is not caused by the E–C association). For example, even though smoking during pregnancy is related both to socio-economic status and the risk of having a low birth-weight baby, it would be incorrect to control for it when examining socio-economic differences in the risk of low birth

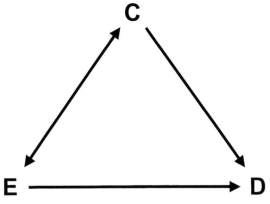

Fig. 18.1 Situation in which C may confound the affect of the E–D association.

weight, since it is on the causal path. Controlling for it in the analysis would lead to an underestimate of any socio-economic differences in risk. These issues are discussed in more detail in Section 38.5.

Note that in clinical trials (and other experimental studies), **randomization** is used to allocate individuals to the different treatment groups (see Chapter 34). Provided that such trials are large enough to ensure that chance differences between the groups are small, the problem of confounding is thus avoided, because the treatment and control groups will be similar in all respects other than those under trial.

18.3 STRATIFICATION TO CONTROL FOR CONFOUNDING

One way to solve the problem of confounding in the analysis is to restrict comparisons to individuals who have the same value of the confounding variable C. Among such individuals associations with C cannot bias the E–D association, because there is no variation in C. Thus in Example 18.1 above, the association between leptospirosis antibodies and urban/rural residence was examined separately for males and females. The subsets defined by the levels of C are called **strata**, and so this process is known as **stratification**. It leads to separate estimates of the odds ratio for the E–D association in each stratum. There is no reason why C should be a binary variable: for example we might allow for the confounding effects of age by splitting a sample of adults aged 15 to 50 years into seven five-year age groups.

Unless it appears that the association between the exposure and outcome varies markedly between the strata (see Section 18.5), we will usually wish to combine the evidence from the separate strata and summarize the association, **controlling** for the confounding effect of C. The simplest approach would be to calculate an average of the estimates of the odds ratios of the E–D association from the different strata. However, we know that, in general, strata in which there are more individuals will tend to have a more precise estimate of the association (i.e. one with a smaller standard error) than strata in which there are fewer individuals. We therefore calculate a **weighted average**, in which greater weight is given to the strata with more data.

$$\text{Weighted average OR} = \frac{\Sigma(w_i \times \text{OR}_i)}{\Sigma w_i}$$

where OR_i is the odds ratio in stratum i, and w_i is the weight it is given in the calculation of the weighted average odds ratio. This is also known as the **summary odds ratio**. Note that in a weighted average, the weights (w_i) are always positive numbers. The larger the value of w_i, the more OR_i influences the weighted average OR. Also note that if all the weights were equal to 1, then the weighted average OR would be equal to the mean OR.

The most widely used weighting scheme is that proposed by Mantel and Haenszel, as described in the next section.

18.4   MANTEL–HAENSZEL METHOD FOR 2 × 2 TABLES

Mantel–Haenszel methods can be used to combine the evidence from the separate strata, and summarize the association, **controlling** for the confounding effect of C. We will describe their use when *both* the outcome and exposure are *binary* variables. In this case, the stratified data will consist of c separate 2 × 2 tables, where c is the number of different values the confounding variable can take. Table 18.3 shows the notation we will use for the 2 × 2 table in stratum i. It is exactly the same as that in Table 16.1 for a single 2 × 2 table, but with the subscript i added, to refer to the stratum i. The estimate of the odds ratio for stratum i is:

$$OR_i = \frac{d_{1i} \times h_{0i}}{d_{0i} \times h_{1i}}$$

In Table 18.2, gender is the confounding variable; $c = 2$, and we have two tables of the association between rural/urban residence and presence of leptospirosis antibodies, one for males and one for females.

Table 18.3 Notation for the 2 × 2 table in stratum i.

	Experienced event: D (Disease)	Did not experience event: H (Healthy)	Total
Group 1 (exposed)	d_{1i}	h_{1i}	n_{1i}
Group 0 (unexposed)	d_{0i}	h_{0i}	n_{0i}
Total	d_i	h_i	n_i

Mantel–Haenszel estimate of the odds ratio controlled for confounding

The Mantel–Haenszel estimate of the summary odds ratio, which we shall denote as OR_{MH}, is a weighted average of the odds ratios from the separate strata, with weights:

$$w_i = \frac{d_{0i} \times h_{1i}}{n_i}$$

Since the numerator of the weight is the same as the denominator of the odds ratio (OR_i) in stratum i, $w_i \times OR_i = (d_{1i} \times h_{0i})/n_i$. Using these weights therefore leads to the following formula for the **Mantel–Haenszel estimate** of the odds ratio:

$$OR_{MH} = \frac{\Sigma(w_i \times OR_i)}{\Sigma w_i} = \frac{\Sigma \dfrac{d_{1i} \times h_{0i}}{n_i}}{\Sigma \dfrac{d_{0i} \times h_{1i}}{n_i}}$$

Following the notation of Clayton and Hills (1993), this can alternatively be written as:

$$OR_{MH} = Q/R, \text{where}$$
$$Q = \Sigma \frac{d_{1i} \times h_{0i}}{n_i} \text{ and } R = \Sigma \frac{d_{0i} \times h_{1i}}{n_i}$$

Example 18.1 (continued)

Table 18.4 shows the results of the calculations required to derive the Mantel–Haenszel odds ratio combining the data presented separately for males and females in Table 18.2 on the association between antibodies to leptospirosis (the outcome variable) and rural/urban residence (the exposure variable). This Mantel–Haenszel estimate of the odds ratio controlling for gender equals:

$$OR_{MH} = \frac{Q}{R} = \frac{20.64}{9.71} = 2.13$$

After controlling for the confounding effect of gender, the odds of leptospirosis antibodies are more than doubled in rural compared to urban areas. The summary OR (2.13) is, as expected, in between the odds ratios from the two strata, but is marginally closer to the OR for females (1.71) than it is to the OR for males (2.57). This is because the weight allocated to the estimate for females (5.04) is a little higher than that for males (4.67).

Table 18.4 Calculations required for deriving the Mantel–Haenszel OR, with associated confidence interval and P-value.

Stratum i	OR_i	$w_i = \dfrac{d_{0i} \times h_{1i}}{n_i}$	$w_iOR_i = \dfrac{d_{1i} \times h_{0i}}{n_i}$	V_i	d_{1i}	E_{1i}
Males ($i = 1$)	2.57	$\dfrac{50 \times 14}{150} = 4.67$	12.00	8.21	36	28.67
Females ($i = 2$)	1.71	$\dfrac{10 \times 126}{250} = 5.04$	8.64	7.08	24	20.40
Total		$R = 9.71$	$Q = 20.64$	$V = 15.29$	O=60	$E = 49.07$

Standard error and confidence interval of the Mantel–Haenszel OR

The 95% confidence interval for OR_{MH} is derived using the standard error of $\log OR_{MH}$, denoted by s.e.$_{MH}$, in exactly the same way as that for a single odds ratio (see Section 16.7):

$$95\% \text{ CI} = OR_{MH}/EF \text{ to } OR_{MH} \times EF,$$
$$\text{where the error factor } EF = \exp(1.96 \times \text{s.e.}_{MH})$$

The simplest formula for the **standard error of log OR_{MH}** (Clayton and Hills 1993) is:

$$\text{s.e.}_{MH} = \sqrt{[V/(Q \times R)]},$$
$$Q = \Sigma \frac{d_{1i} \times h_{0i}}{n_i}, \quad R = \Sigma \frac{d_{0i} \times h_{1i}}{n_i}, \quad V = \Sigma V_i = \Sigma \frac{d_i \times h_i \times n_{0i} \times n_{1i}}{n_i^2 \times (n_i - 1)}$$

V is the sum across the strata of the variances V_i for the number of exposed individuals experiencing the outcome event, i.e. the variances of the d_{1i}'s. Note that the formula for the variance V_i of d_{1i} for stratum i is based solely on the marginal totals of the table. It therefore gives the same value for each of the four cells in the table, implying they have equal variances. This is the case because once we know one cell value, we can deduce the others from the appropriate marginal totals.

Example 18.1 (continued)
Using the results of the calculations for Q, R and V shown in Table 18.4, we find that:

$$\text{s.e.}_{MH} = \sqrt{[V/(Q \times R)]} = \sqrt{[15.287/(20.640 \times 9.71)]} = 0.276$$

so that $EF = \exp(1.96 \times 0.276) = 1.72$, $OR_{MH}/EF = 2.13/1.72 = 1.24$ and $OR_{MH} \times EF = 2.13 \times 1.72 = 3.65$. The 95% CI is therefore:

$$95\% \text{ CI for } OR_{MH} = 1.24 \text{ to } 3.65$$

With 95% confidence, the odds of leptospirosis is between 1.24 and 3.65 times higher in rural than urban areas, having controlled for the confounding effect of gender.

Mantel–Haenszel χ^2 test

Finally, we test the null hypothesis that $OR_{MH} = 1$ by calculating the **Mantel–Haenszel χ^2 test statistic**:

$$\chi^2_{MH} = \frac{(\Sigma d_{1i} - \Sigma E_{1i})^2}{\Sigma V_i} = \frac{(O - E)^2}{V} = \frac{U^2}{V}; \; \text{d.f.} = 1$$

This is based on a comparison in each stratum of the number of exposed individuals *observed* to have experienced the event (d_{1i}), with the *expected* number in this category (E_{1i}) if there were no difference in the risks between exposed and unexposed. The expected numbers are calculated in exactly the same way as that described for the standard χ^2 test in Chapter 17:

$$E_{1i} = \frac{d_i \times n_{1i}}{n_i}$$

The formula has been simplified by writing O for the sum of the observed numbers, E for the sum of the expected numbers and U for the difference between them:

$$O = \Sigma d_{1i}, \; E = \Sigma E_{1i} \text{ and } U = O - E$$

Note that χ^2_{MH} has just *1 degree of freedom irrespective of how many strata are summarized*.

Example 18.1 (continued)

The calculations for the data presented in Table 18.2 are laid out in Table 18.4. A total $O = 60$ persons in rural areas had antibodies to leptospirosis compared with an expected total of $E = 49.07$, based on assuming no difference in prevalence between rural and urban areas. Thus the Mantel–Haenszel χ^2 statistic is:

$$\chi^2_{MH} = \frac{U^2}{V} = \frac{(60 - 49.07)^2}{15.29} = 7.82, \; \text{d.f.} = 1, \; P = 0.0052$$

After controlling for gender, there is good evidence of an increase in the prevalence of antibodies to leptospirosis among those living in rural compared to urban areas.

It may seem strange that this test appears to be based entirely on the observed and expected values of d_{1i} and not also on the other cells in the tables. This is not really the case, however, since once the value of d_{1i} is known the values of h_{1i}, d_{0i} and h_{0i} can be calculated from the totals of the table. If the Mantel–Haenszel test is applied to a single 2×2 table, the χ^2 value obtained is close to, but not exactly equal to, the standard χ^2 value. It is slightly smaller, equalling $(n-1)/n$ times the standard value. This difference is negligible for values of n of 20 or more, as required for the validity of the chi-squared test.

Validity of Mantel–Haenszel methods

The Mantel–Haenszel estimate of the odds ratio is valid even for small sample sizes. However, the formula that we have given for the standard error of log OR_{MH} will be inaccurate if the overall sample size is small. A more accurate estimate, which is more complicated to calculate, was given by Robins *et al.* (1986).

The **validity** of the Mantel–Haenszel χ^2 test can be assessed by the following 'rule of 5'. Two additional values are calculated for each table and summed over the strata. These are:

1 $\min(d_i, n_{1i})$, that is the smaller of d_i and n_{1i}, and
2 $\max(0, n_{1i} - h_i)$, which equals 0 if n_{1i} is smaller than or equal to h_i, and $(n_{1i} - h_i)$, if n_{1i} is larger than h_i.

Both sums must differ from the total of the expected values, E, by at least 5 for the test to be valid. The details of these calculations for the leptospirosis data are shown in Table 18.5. The two sums, 84 and 0, both differ from 70.933 by 5 or more, validating the use of the Mantel–Haenszel χ^2 test.

Table 18.5 Rule of 5, to check validity.

Stratum i	$\min(d_i, n_{1i})$,	$\max(0, n_{1i} - h_i)$	E_i
Males ($i = 1$)	$\min(86, 50) = 50$	$\max(0, -14) = 0$	57.333
Females ($i = 2$)	$\min(34, 150) = 34$	$\max(0, -116) = 0$	13.600
Total	84	0	70.933

18.5 EFFECT MODIFICATION

When we use Mantel–Haenszel methods to control for confounding we are making an important assumption; namely that the Exposure–Disease (E–D) association is really the same in each of the strata defined by the levels of the confounding variable, C. If this is not true, then it makes little sense to combine the odds ratios (the estimates of the effect of E on D) from the different strata. If the effect of E on D varies according to the level of C then we say that C modifies the effect of E on D: in other words there is **effect modification**. A number of different terms are used to describe effect modification:

- **Effect modification**: C modifies the effect of E on D.
- **Interaction**: there is interaction between the effects of E and C (on D).
- **Heterogeneity between strata**: the estimates of the E–D association differ between the strata.

Similarly, you may see tests for effect modification described as either **tests for interaction** or **tests of homogeneity** across strata.

Testing for effect modification

The use of regression models to examine effect modification (or equivalently interaction) is discussed in Section 29.5. This is the most flexible approach. When we are using Mantel–Haenszel methods to control for confounding, an alternative is to use a χ^2 test for effect modification. This is equivalently, and more commonly, called a χ^2 **test of heterogeneity**. Under the null hypothesis of no effect modification, all the individual stratum odds ratios would equal the overall summary odds ratio. In other words:

$$OR_i = \frac{d_{1i} \times h_{0i}}{d_{0i} \times h_{1i}} = OR_{MH}$$

Multiplying both sides of the equation by $d_{0i} \times h_{1i}$ and rearranging shows that, under the null hypothesis of no effect modification, the following set of differences would be zero:

$$(d_{1i} \times h_{0i} - OR_{MH} \times d_{0i} \times h_{1i}) = 0$$

The χ^2 **test of heterogeneity** is based on a weighted sum of the squares of these differences:

$$\chi^2 = \Sigma \frac{(d_{1i} \times h_{0i} - OR_{MH} \times d_{0i} \times h_{1i})^2}{OR_{MH} \times V_i \times n_i^2}, \ \text{d.f.} = c - 1$$

where V_i is as defined in Section 18.4, and c is the number of strata. The greater the differences between the stratum-specific odds ratios and OR_{MH}, the larger will be the heterogeneity statistic.

Example 18.1 (continued)
In our example, the odds ratios were 2.57 (95% CI 1.21 to 5.45) in males and 1.71 (95% CI 0.778 to 3.78) in females. Given that the confidence intervals easily overlapped, we would not expect to find evidence of effect modification (i.e. that the OR in males is different to the OR in females). The calculations needed to

Table 18.6 Calculations required for the χ^2 test of heterogeneity.

Stratum (i)	$(d_{1i} \times h_{0i} - OR_{MH} \times d_{0i} \times h_{1i})^2$	$OR_{MH} \times V_i \times n_i^2$	$\dfrac{(d_{1i} \times h_{0i} - OR_{MH} \times d_{0i} \times h_{1i})^2}{OR_{MH} \times V_i \times n_i^2}$
Males (i = 1)	$(36 \times 50 - 2.13 \times 50 \times 14)^2$ $= 97056.2$	$2.13 \times 8.21 \times 150^2$ $= 392737$	$\dfrac{97056.2}{392737} = 0.247$
Females (i = 2)	$(24 \times 90 - 2.13 \times 10 \times 126)^2$ $= 269601$	$2.13 \times 7.08 \times 150^2$ $= 940728$	$\dfrac{269601}{940728} = 0.287$
Total			0.534

apply the formula above are given in Table 18.6. The resulting value of the χ^2 test of heterogeneity is:

$$\chi^2 = 0.534, \ \text{d.f.} = 1, \ P = 0.470$$

There is thus no evidence that gender modifies the association between rural/urban residence and leptospirosis antibodies.

When does effect modification matter?

As discussed above, Mantel–Haenszel methods assume that the true E–D odds ratio is the same in each stratum, and that the only reason for differences in the observed odds ratios between strata is sampling variation. We should therefore check this assumption, by applying the χ^2 test for heterogeneity, before reporting Mantel–Haenszel odds ratios, confidence intervals and P-values. This test has low *power* (see Chapter 35): it is unlikely to yield evidence for effect modification unless there are large differences between strata. A large P-value does not therefore establish the absence of effect modification. In fact, as the true odds ratios are never likely to be *exactly* the same in each stratum, effect modification is always present to some degree. Most researchers would accept, however, that minor effect modification should be ignored in order to simplify the presentation of the data.

The following box summarizes a practical approach to examining for effect modification, and recommends how analyses should be presented when evidence for effect modification is found. These issues are also discussed in Section 29.5 and Chapter 38, which describes strategies for data analysis.

> ## BOX 18.1   A PRACTICAL APPROACH TO EXAMINING FOR EFFECT MODIFICATION
>
> 1 Always examine the pattern of odds ratios in the different strata: how different do they look, and is there any trend across strata?
> 2 If there is clear evidence of effect modification, and substantial differences in the E–D association between strata, report this and report the E–D association separately in each stratum.
> 3 If there is moderate evidence of effect modification, use Mantel–Haenszel methods but in addition report stratum-specific estimates of the E–D association.
> 4 If there is no evidence of effect modification, report this and use Mantel–Haenszel methods.

18.6 STRATIFICATION ON MORE THAN ONE CONFOUNDING VARIABLE

It is possible to apply the Mantel–Haenszel methods to control simultaneously for the effects of two or more confounders. For example, we can control additionally for differences in age distribution between the urban and rural areas by grouping our population into four age groups and forming the $2 \times 4 = 8$ strata corresponding to all combinations of gender and age group. The drawback to this approach is that the number of strata increases rapidly as we attempt to control for the effects of more confounding variables, so that it becomes impossible to estimate the stratum-specific odds ratios (although the Mantel-Haenszel OR can still be derived).

The alternative is to use regression models. The use of logistic regression models to control for confounding is considered in detail in Chapter 20.

CHAPTER 19

Logistic regression: comparing two or more exposure groups

19.1 INTRODUCTION

In this chapter we introduce **logistic regression**, the method most commonly used for the analysis of *binary* outcome variables. We show how it can be used to examine the effect of a *single* exposure variable, and in particular, how it can be used to:

- Compare a binary outcome variable between two exposure (or treatment) groups.
- Compare more than two exposure groups.
- Examine the effect of an ordered or continuous exposure variable.

We will see that it gives *very similar results* to the methods for analysing *odds ratios* described in Chapters 16, 17 and 18, and is an alternative to them. We will also see how logistic regression provides a flexible means of analysing the association between a binary outcome and a *number* of exposure variables. In the next chapter, we will explain how it is used to control for confounding. We will also briefly describe the regression analysis of risk ratios, and methods for the analysis of categorical outcomes with more than two levels.

We will explain the principles of logistic regression modelling in detail in the next section, in the simple context of comparing two exposure groups. In particular, we will show how it is based on modelling odds ratios, and explain how to interpret the computer output from a logistic regression analysis. We will then introduce the general form of the logistic regression equation, and explain where the name 'logistic' comes from. Finally we will explain how to fit logistic regression models for categorical, ordered or continuous exposure variables.

Links between multiple regression models for the analysis of numerical outcomes, the logistic regression models introduced here, and other types of regression model introduced later in the book, are discussed in detail in Chapter 29.

19.2 LOGISTIC REGRESSION FOR COMPARING TWO EXPOSURE GROUPS

Introducing the logistic regression model

We will start by showing, in the simple case of two exposure groups, how logistic regression models the association between binary outcomes and exposure variables in terms of odds ratios. Recall from Chapter 16 that the *exposure odds ratio* (OR) is defined as:

$$\text{Exposure odds ratio} = \frac{\text{Odds in exposed group}}{\text{Odds in unexposed group}}$$

If we re-express this as:

$$\text{Odds in exposed} = \text{Odds in unexposed} \times \text{Exposure odds ratio}$$

then we have the basis for a simple model for the odds of the outcome, which expresses the odds in each group in terms of two **model parameters**. These are:

1 The **baseline** odds. We use the term **baseline** to refer to the exposure group against which all the other groups will be compared. When there are just two exposure groups as here, then the baseline odds are the odds in the unexposed group. We will use the parameter name 'Baseline' to refer to the odds in the baseline group.

2 The **exposure odds ratio**. This expresses the effect of the exposure on the odds of disease. We will use the parameter name 'Exposure' to refer to the exposure odds ratio.

Table 19.1 shows the odds in each of the two exposure groups, in terms of the parameters of the logistic regression model.

Table 19.1 Odds of the outcome in terms of the parameters of a logistic regression model comparing two exposure groups.

Exposure group	Odds of outcome	Odds of outcome, in terms of the parameter names
Exposed (group 1)	Baseline odds × exposure odds ratio	Baseline × Exposure
Unexposed (group 0)	Baseline odds	Baseline

The logistic regression model defined by the two equations for the odds of the outcome shown in Table 19.1 can be abbreviated to:

$$\text{Odds} = \text{Baseline} \times \text{Exposure}$$

Since the two parameters in this model *multiply* together, the model is said to be **multiplicative**. This is in contrast to the multiple regression models described in Chapter 11, in which the effects of different exposures were *additive*. If there were two exposures (A and B), the model would be:

$$\text{Odds} = \text{Baseline} \times \text{Exposure(A)} \times \text{Exposure(B)}$$

Thus if, for example, exposure A doubled the odds of disease and exposure B trebled it, a person exposed to both would have a six times greater odds of disease than a person in the baseline group exposed to neither. We describe such models in detail in the next chapter.

Example 19.1

All our examples of logistic regression models are based on data from a study of onchocerciasis ('river blindness') in Sierra Leone (McMahon *et al.* 1988, *Trans Roy Soc Trop Med Hyg* **82**; 595–600), in which subjects were classified according to whether they lived in villages in savannah (grassland) or rainforest areas. In addition, subjects were classified as infected if microfilariae (*mf*) of *Onchocerciasis volvulus* were found in skin snips taken from the iliac crest. The study included persons aged 5 years and above. Table 19.2 shows that the prevalence of micro-filarial infection appears to be greater for individuals living in rainforest areas compared to those living in the savannah; the associated odds ratio is $2.540/1.052 = 2.413$.

We will now show how to use logistic regression to examine the association between area of residence and microfilarial infection in these data. To use a **computer package to fit a logistic regression model**, it is necessary to specify just two items:

1 The *name of the outcome* variable, which in this case is *mf*. The **required convention for coding** is to code the outcome event (D) as 1, and the absence of the outcome event (H) as 0. The variable *mf* was therefore coded as 0 for uninfected subjects and 1 for infected subjects.

2 The *name of the exposure* variable(s). In this example, we have just one exposure variable, which is called *area*. The required *convention for coding* is that used throughout this book; thus *area* was coded as 0 for subjects living in savannah areas (the *baseline* or 'unexposed' group) and 1 for subjects living in rainforest areas (the 'exposed' group).

Table 19.2 Numbers and percentages of individuals infected with onchocerciasis according to their area of residence, in a study of 1302 individuals in Sierra Leone.

Area of residence	Microfilarial infection		Total	Odds of infection
	Yes	No		
Rainforest	$d_1 = 541$ (71.7%)	$h_1 = 213$ (28.3%)	754	$541/213 = 2.540$
Savannah (baseline group)	$d_0 = 281$ (51.3%)	$h_0 = 267$ (48.7%)	548	$281/267 = 1.052$
Total	822	480	1302	

Table 19.3 First ten lines of the computer dataset from the study of onchocerciasis.

id	mf	Area
1	1	0
2	1	1
3	1	0
4	0	1
5	0	0
6	0	1
7	1	0
8	1	1
9	1	1
10	1	1

The first ten lines of the dataset, when entered on the computer, are shown in Table 19.3. For example, subject number 1 lived in a savannah area and was infected, number 2 lived in a rainforest area and was also infected, whereas subject number 4 lived in a rainforest area but was not infected.

The **logistic regression model** that will be fitted is:

$$\text{Odds of } \textit{mf} \text{ infection} = \text{Baseline} \times \text{Area}$$

Its two parameters are:

1 baseline: the odds of infection in the baseline group (subjects living in savannah areas); and
2 area: the odds ratio comparing odds of infection among subjects living in rainforest areas with that among those living in savannah areas.

Table 19.4 shows the computer output obtained from fitting this model. The two *rows* in the output correspond to the two *parameters* of the logistic regression model; area is our exposure of interest, and the **constant** term refers to the baseline group. The same format is used for both parameters, and is based on what makes sense for interpretation of the effect of exposure. This means that some of the information presented for the constant (baseline) parameter is not of interest.

Table 19.4 Logistic regression output for the model relating odds of infection to area of residence, in 1302 subjects participating in a study of onchocerciasis in Sierra Leone.

	Odds ratio	z	$P > |z|$	95% CI
Area	2.413	7.487	0.000	1.916 to 3.039
Constant	1.052	0.598	0.550	0.890 to 1.244

The column labelled 'Odds ratio' contains the **parameter estimates**:

1 For the first row, labelled 'area', this is the *odds ratio* (2.413) comparing rainforest (area 1) with savannah (area 0). This is identical to the odds ratio which was calculated directly from the raw data (see Table 19.3).

2 For the second row, labelled 'constant', this is the *odds of infection in the baseline group* (1.052 = odds of infection in the savannah area, see Table 19.3). As we will see, this apparently inconsistent labelling is because output from regression models is labelled in a uniform way.

The remaining columns present *z* statistics, *P*-values and 95% confidence intervals corresponding to the model parameters. The values for *area* are exactly the same as those that would be obtained by following the procedures described in Section 16.7 for the calculation of a 95% confidence interval for an odds ratio, and the associated Wald test. They will be explained in more detail in the explanation of Table 19.5 below.

The logistic regression model on a log scale

As described in Chapter 16, confidence intervals for odds ratios are derived by using the standard error of the *log* odds ratio to calculate a confidence interval for the *log* odds ratio. The results are then *antilogged* to express them in terms of the original scale. The same is true for logistic regression models; they are *fitted on a log scale*. Table 19.5 shows the two equations that define the logistic regression model for the comparison of two exposure groups. The middle column shows the model for the odds of the outcome, as described above. Using the rules of logarithms (see p. 156, Section 16.5), it follows that corresponding equations on the log scale for the log of the odds of the outcome are as shown in the right-hand column. Note that as in the rest of the book all logs are to the base e (natural logarithms) unless they are explicitly denoted as logs to the base 10 by $\log_{10}$ (see Section 13.2).

Table 19.5 Equations defining the logistic regression model for the comparison of two exposure groups.

Exposure group	Odds of outcome	Log odds of outcome
Exposed (group 1)	Baseline odds × exposure OR	Log(baseline odds) + log(exposure OR)
Unexposed (group 0)	Baseline odds	Log(baseline odds)

Using the parameter names introduced earlier in this section, the logistic regression model on the log scale can be written:

$$\log(\text{Odds}) = \log(\text{Baseline}) + \log(\text{Exposure odds ratio})$$

In practice, we abbreviate it to:

$$\log(\text{Odds}) = \text{Baseline} + \text{Exposure}$$

since it is clear from the context that *output on the log scale refers to log odds and log odds ratios*. Note that whereas the exposure effect on the odds ratio scale is *multiplicative*, the exposure effect on the log scale is *additive*.

Example 19.1 (continued)
In this example, the model on the log scale is:

$$\log(\text{Odds of } \textit{mf} \text{ infection}) = \text{Baseline} + \text{Area}$$

where
1 *baseline* is the *log odds* of infection in the savannah areas; and
2 *area* is the *log odds ratio* comparing the odds of infection in rainforest areas with that in savannah areas.

Table 19.6 shows the results obtained on the log scale, for this model. We will explain each item in the table, and then discuss how the results relate to those on the odds ratio scale, shown in Table 19.4.

Table 19.6 Logistic regression output (log scale) for the association between microfilarial infection and area of residence.

	Coefficient	s.e.	z	$P > |z|$	95% CI
Area	0.881	0.118	7.487	0.000	0.650 to 1.112
Constant	0.0511	0.0854	0.598	0.550	−0.116 to 0.219

1 The two *rows* in the output correspond to the terms in the model; area is our exposure of interest, and as before the **constant term** corresponds to the baseline group.
2 The *first* column gives the results for the **regression coefficients** (corresponding to the parameter estimates on a log scale):
   (a) For the row labelled 'area', this is the **log odds ratio** comparing rainforest with savannah. It agrees with what would be obtained if it were calculated directly from Table 19.3, and with the value in Table 19.4:

$$\log \text{OR} = \log(2.540/1.052) = \log(2.413) = 0.881$$

   (b) For the row labelled 'constant', this is the **log odds in the baseline group** (the group with exposure level 0), i.e. the log odds of microfilarial infection in the savannah:

$$\log \text{odds} = \log(281/267) = \log(1.052) = 0.0511.$$

3 The *second* column gives the standard error(s) of the regression coefficient(s). In the simple example of a binary exposure variable, as we have here, the standard errors of the regression coefficients are exactly the same as those derived using the formulae given in Chapter 16. Thus:

    (a) s.e.(log OR comparing rainforest with savannah) is:

$$\sqrt{(1/d_1 + 1/h_1 + 1/d_0 + 1/h_0)} = \sqrt{(1/541 + 1/213 + 1/281 + 1/267)}$$
$$= 0.118$$

    (b) s.e.(log odds in savannah) is:

$$\sqrt{(1/d_0 + 1/h_0)} = \sqrt{(1/281 + 1/267)} = 0.0854$$

4 The 95% confidence intervals for the regression coefficients in the *last* column are derived in the usual way.

    (a) For the log OR comparing rainforest with savannah, the 95% CI is:

$$0.881 - (1.96 \times 0.118) \text{ to } 0.881 + (1.96 \times 0.118) = 0.650 \text{ to } 1.112$$

    (b) For the log odds in the savannah, the 95% CI is:

$$0.0511 - (1.96 \times 0.0854) \text{ to } 0.0511 + (1.96 \times 0.0854) = -0.116 \text{ to } 0.219$$

5 The z statistic in the *area* row of the third column is used to derive a **Wald test** (see Chapter 28) of the null hypothesis that the *area* coefficient $= 0$, i.e. that the exposure has no effect (since if log OR $= 0$, then OR must be equal to 1). This z statistic is simply the regression coefficient divided by its standard error:

$$z = 0.881/0.118 = 7.487$$

6 The *P*-value in the *fourth* column is derived from the z statistic in the usual manner (see Table A1 and Chapter 8), and can be used to assess the strength of the evidence against the null hypothesis that the true (population) exposure effect is zero. Thus, the *P*-value of 0.000 (which should be interpreted as < 0.001) for the log OR comparing rainforest with savannah indicates that there is strong evidence against the null hypothesis that the odds of microfilarial infection are the same in the two areas.

7 We are usually not interested in in the third and fourth columns (the z statistic and its *P*-value) for the *constant* row. However, for completeness, we will explain their meanings:

(a) The z statistic is the result of testing the null hypothesis that the log odds of infection in the savannah areas are 0 (or, equivalently, that the odds of infection are 1). This would happen if the risk of infection in the savannah areas was 0.5; in other words if people living in the savannah areas were equally likely to be infected as they were to be not infected.

(b) The P-value of 0.550 for the log odds in savannah areas indicates that there is no evidence against this null hypothesis.

Relation between outputs on the ratio and log scales

We will now explain the relationship between the two sets of outputs, since the results in Table 19.4 (output on the original, or ratio, scale) are derived from the results in Table 19.6 (output on the log scale). Once this is understood, it is rarely necessary to refer to the output displayed on the log scale: the most useful results are the odds ratios, confidence intervals and P-values displayed on the original scale, as in Table 19.4.

1 In Table 19.4, the column labelled 'Odds Ratio' contains the *exponentials* (antilogs) of the logistic regression coefficients shown in Table 19.6. Thus the OR comparing rainforest with savannah $= \exp(0.881) = 2.413$.

2 The z statistics and P-values are derived from the log odds ratio and its standard error, and so are identical in the two tables.

3 The 95% confidence intervals in Table 19.4 are derived by antilogging (exponentiating) the confidence intervals on the log scale presented in Table 19.6. Thus the 95% CI for the OR comparing rainforest with savannah is:

$$95\% \text{ CI} = \exp(0.650) \text{ to } \exp(1.112) = 1.916 \text{ to } 3.039$$

This is identical to the 95% CI calculated using the methods described in Section 16.7:

$$95\% \text{ CI (OR)} = \text{OR}/\text{EF to OR} \times \text{EF, where EF} = \exp[1.96 \times \text{s.e.}(\log \text{ OR})]$$

Note that since the calculations are multiplicative:

$$\frac{\text{Odds ratio}}{\text{Lower confidence limit}} = \frac{\text{Upper confidence limit}}{\text{Odds ratio}}$$

This can be a useful check on confidence limits presented in tables in published papers.

19.3 GENERAL FORM OF THE LOGISTIC REGRESSION EQUATION

We will now introduce the general form of the logistic regression model with several exposure variables, and explain how it corresponds to what we used above in the simple case when we are comparing two exposure groups, and therefore have a single exposure variable in our model. The general form of the logistic regression model is similar to that for multiple regression (see Chapter 11):

$$\text{log odds of outcome} = \beta_0 + \beta_1 x_1 + \beta_2 x_2 + \ldots + \beta_p x_p$$

The difference is that we are modelling a transformation of the outcome variable, namely the *log of the odds of the outcome*. The quantity on the right-hand side of the equation is known as the **linear predictor** of the log odds of the outcome, given the particular value of the p exposure variables x_1 to x_p. The β's are the **regression coefficients** associated with the p exposure variables.

The transformation of the probability, or risk, π of the outcome into the log odds is known as the **logit function**:

$$\text{logit}(\pi) = \log\left(\frac{\pi}{1 - \pi}\right)$$

and the name **logistic** is derived from this. Recall from Section 14.6 (Table 14.2) that while probabilities must lie between 0 and 1, odds can take any value between 0 and infinity (∞). The log odds are not constrained at all; they can take any value between $-\infty$ and ∞.

We will now show how the general form of the logistic regression model corresponds to the logistic regression model we used in Section 19.2 for comparing two exposure groups. The general form for comparing two exposure groups is:

$$\text{log odds of outcome} = \beta_0 + \beta_1 x_1$$

where x_1 (the exposure variable) equals 1 for those in the *exposed* group and 0 for those in the *unexposed* group. Table 19.7 shows the value of the log odds predicted

Table 19.7 Log odds of the outcome according to exposure group, as calculated from the linear predictor in the logistic regression equation.

Exposure group	Log odds of outcome, predicted from model	Log odds of outcome, in terms of the parameter names
Exposed ($x_1 = 1$)	$\beta_0 + \beta_1 \times 1 = \beta_0 + \beta_1$	log(Baseline odds) + log(Exposure odds ratio)
Unexposed ($x_1 = 0$)	$\beta_0 + \beta_1 \times 0 = \beta_0$	log(Baseline odds)

from this model in each of the two exposure groups, together with the log odds expressed in terms of the parameter names, as in Section 19.2.

We can see that the first regression coefficient, β_0, corresponds to the log odds in the unexposed (baseline) group. We will now show how the other regression coefficient, β_1, corresponds to the log of the exposure odds ratio. Since:

$$\text{Exposure OR} = \frac{\text{odds in exposed group}}{\text{odds in unexposed group}}$$

it follows from the rules of logarithms (see p. 156) that:

$$\log \text{OR} = \log(\text{odds in exposed group}) - \log(\text{odds in unexposed group})$$

Putting the values predicted from the logistic regression equation (shown in Table 19.7) into this equation gives:

$$\log \text{OR} = \beta_0 + \beta_1 - \beta_0 = \beta_1$$

The equivalent model on the ratio scale is:

$$\text{Odds of disease} = \exp(\beta_0 + \beta_1 x_1) = \exp(\beta_0) \times \exp(\beta_1 x_1)$$

In this *multiplicative model* $\exp(\beta_0)$ corresponds to the odds of disease in the baseline group, and $\exp(\beta_1)$ to the exposure odds ratio. Table 19.8 shows how this model corresponds to the model shown in Table 19.1.

Table 19.8 Odds of outcome according to exposure group, as calculated from the linear predictor in the logistic regression equation.

Exposure group	Odds of outcome, predicted from model	Odds of outcome, in terms of the parameter names
Exposed ($x_1 = 1$)	$\exp(\beta_0) \times \exp(\beta_1)$	Baseline odds $\times$ Exposure odds ratio
Unexposed ($x_1 = 0$)	$\exp(\beta_0)$	Baseline odds

19.4 LOGISTIC REGRESSION FOR COMPARING MORE THAN TWO EXPOSURE GROUPS

We now consider logistic regression models for **categorical exposure variables** with more than two levels. To examine the effect of categorical variables in logistic and other regression models, we look at the effect of each level compared to a **baseline** group. When the exposure is an *ordered* categorical variable, it may also be useful to examine the average change in the log odds per exposure group, as described in Section 19.5.

Table 19.9 Association between age group and microfilarial infection in the onchocerciasis study.

Age group (years)	Coded value in dataset	Microfilarial infection		Odds of infection	Odds ratio compared to the baseline group
		Yes	No		
5–9	0	46	156	$46/156 = 0.295$	1
10–19	1	99	119	$99/119 = 0.832$	$0.832/0.295 = 2.821$
20–39	2	299	125	$299/125 = 2.392$	$2.392/0.295 = 8.112$
≥ 40	3	378	80	$378/80 = 4.725$	$4.725/0.295 = 16.02$
Total		822	480		

Example 19.2

In the onchocerciasis study, introduced in Example 19.1, subjects were classified into four age groups: 5–9, 10–19, 20–39 and ≥ 40 years. Table 19.9 shows the association between age group and microfilarial infection. The odds of infection increased markedly with increasing age. A chi-squared test for association in this table gives $P < 0.001$, so there is clear evidence of an association between age group and infection. We chose the 5–9 year age group as the **baseline** exposure group, because its coded value in the dataset is zero, and calculated odds ratios for each non-baseline group relative to the baseline group.

The corresponding logistic regression model uses this same approach; the effect of each non-baseline age group is expressed in terms of the odds ratio comparing it with the baseline. The parameters of the model, on both the odds and log odds scales, are shown in Table 19.10.

Table 19.10 Odds and log odds of the outcome in terms of the parameters of a logistic regression model comparing four age groups.

Age group	Odds of infection	Log odds of infection
0 (5–9 years)	Baseline	Log(Baseline)
1 (10–19 years)	Baseline $\times$ Agegrp(1)	Log(Baseline) + Log(Agegrp(1))
2 (20–39 years)	Baseline $\times$ Agegrp(2)	Log(Baseline) + Log(Agegrp(2))
3 (≥ 40 years)	Baseline $\times$ Agegrp(3)	Log(Baseline) + Log(Agegrp(3))

Here, Agegrp(1) is the odds ratio (or, on the log scale, the log odds ratio) comparing group 1 (10–19 years) with group 0 (5–9 years, the baseline group), and so on. This regression model has four parameters:
1 the odds of infection in the 5–9 year group (the baseline group); and
2 the *three* odds ratios comparing the non-baseline groups with the baseline.
Using the notation introduced in Section 19.2, the four equations for the odds that define the model in Table 19.10 can be written in abbreviated form as:

$$\text{Odds} = \text{Baseline} \times \text{Agegrp}$$

or on a log scale, as:

$$\log(\text{Odds}) = \text{Baseline} + \text{Agegrp}$$

The effect of categorical variables is modelled in logistic and other regression models by using **indicator variables**, which are created automatically by most statistical packages when an exposure variable is defined as categorical. This is explained further in Box 19.1. Output from this model (expressed on the odds ratio scale, with the constant term omitted) is shown in Table 19.11.

Table 19.11 Logistic regression output (odds ratio scale) for the association between microfilarial infection and age group.

	Odds ratio	z	$P > |z|$	95% CI
agegrp(1)	2.821	4.802	0.000	1.848 to 4.308
agegrp(2)	8.112	10.534	0.000	5.495 to 11.98
agegrp(3)	16.024	13.332	0.000	10.658 to 24.09

BOX 19.1   USE OF INDICATOR VARIABLES IN REGRESSION MODELS

To model the effect of an exposure with more than two categories, we estimate the odds ratio for each non-baseline group compared to the base-line. In the logistic regression equation, we represent the exposure by a set of **indicator variables** (variables which take only the values 0 and 1) representing each non-baseline value of the exposure variable. The regression coefficients for these indicator variables are the corresponding (log) odds ratios. For example, to estimate the odds ratios comparing the 10–19, 20–39 and ≥ 40 year groups with the 5–9 year group, we create three indicator variables which we will call ageind_1, ageind_2 and ageind_3 (the name is not important). The table below shows the value of these indicator variables according to age group.

Value of indicator variables for use in logistic regression of the association between microfilarial infection and age group.

Age group	ageind_1	ageind_2	ageind_3
0 (5–9 years)	0	0	0
1 (10–19 years)	1	0	0
2 (20–29 years)	0	1	0
3 (≥ 40 years)	0	0	1

All three of these indicator variables (but not the original variable) are then included in a logistic regression model. Most statistical packages create the indicator variables automatically when the original variable is declared as categorical.

The *P*-values for the three indicator variables (corresponding to the non-baseline age groups) can be used to test the null hypotheses that there is no difference in odds of the outcome between the individual non-baseline exposure groups and the baseline group. However, these are not usually of interest: we need a test, analogous to the χ^2 test for a table with four rows and two columns, of the general null hypothesis that there is no association between age group and infection. We will see how to test such null hypotheses in regression models in Chapter 29, and in the next section we address the special case when the categorical variable is ordered, as is the case here. It is usually a mistake to conclude that there is a difference between one exposure group and the rest based on a particular (small) *P*-value corresponding to one of a set of indicator variables.

19.5 LOGISTIC REGRESSION FOR ORDERED AND CONTINUOUS EXPOSURE VARIABLES

Until now, we have considered logistic regression models for binary or categorical exposure variables. For binary variables, logistic regression estimates the odds ratio comparing the two exposure groups, while for categorical variables we have seen how to estimate odds ratios for each non-baseline group compared to the baseline. This approach does not take account of ordering of the exposure variable. For example, we did not use the fact that subjects aged ≥ 40 years are older than those aged 20–39 years, who in turn are older than those aged 10–19 years and so on.

Example 19.3

The odds of microfilarial infection in each age group in the onchocerciasis dataset are shown in Table 19.9 in Section 19.4, and are displayed in Figure 19.1. We do not have a straight line; the slope of the line increases with increasing age group. In other words, this increase in the odds of infection with increasing age does not appear to be constant.

However, Figure 19.2 shows that there *is* an approximately linear increase in the **log odds** of infection with increasing age group. This log-linear increase means that we are able to express the association between age and the log odds of microfilarial infection by a single linear term (as described below) rather than by a series of indicator variables representing the different groups.

Relation with linear regression models

Logistic regression models can be used to estimate the *most likely* value of the increase in log odds per age group, assuming that the increase is the same in each age group. (We will define the meaning of 'most likely' more precisely in Chapter

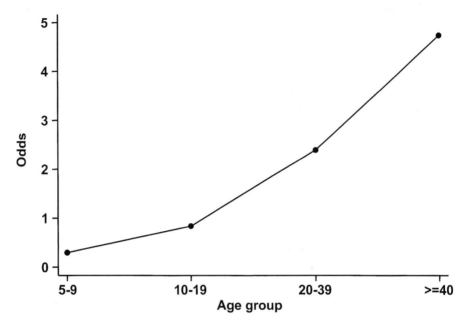

Fig. 19.1 Odds of microfilarial infection according to age group for the onchocerciasis data.

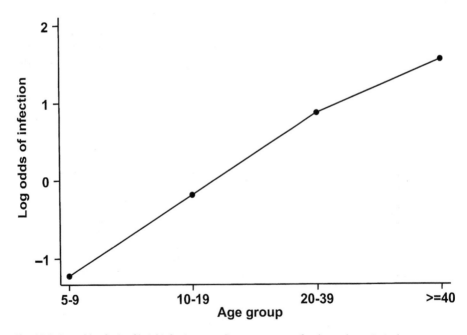

Fig. 19.2 Log odds of microfilarial infection according to age group for the onchocerciasis data.

28.) The model is analogous to the simple linear regression model described in Chapter 11. If we assume that:

$$y = \beta_0 + \beta_1 x$$

then the intercept β_0 is the value of y when $x = 0$, and the slope β_1 represents the increase in y when x increases by 1. Logistic regression models assume that:

$$\log \text{ odds} = \beta_0 + \beta_1 x$$

so that the intercept β_0 is the value of the log odds when $x = 0$, and the slope β_1 represents the increase in log odds when x increases by 1. We will use the notation

$$\log \text{ odds} = \text{Baseline} + [\text{X}]$$

where the square brackets indicate our assumption that variable X has a linear effect on the log odds of the outcome. For the onchocerciasis data, our model is

$$\log \text{ odds} = \text{Baseline} + [\text{Agegrp}]$$

Example 19.3 (continued)

Table 19.12(a) shows logistic regression output for the model assuming a linear effect of logistic regression on the log odds of microfilarial infection. The estimated increase in log odds for every unit increase in age group is 0.930 (95% CI = 0.805 to 1.055). This corresponds to an odds ratio per group of 2.534 (95% CI = 2.236 to 2.871; see output in Table 19.12b). The constant term corresponds to the estimated log odds of microfilarial infection in age group 0 (5–9 years, log odds = −1.115), *assuming a linear relation* between age group and the log odds of infection. It does not therefore numerically equal the baseline term in the

Table 19.12 Logistic regression output for the linear association between the log odds of microfilarial infection and age group (data in Table 19.9).

(a) Output on log scale.

	Coefficient	s.e.	z	$P > |z|$	95% CI
Age group	0.930	0.0638	14.587	0.000	0.805 to 1.055
Constant	−1.115	0.127	−8.782	0.000	−1.364 to −0.866

(b) Output on ratio scale.

	Odds ratio	z	$P > |z|$	95% CI
Age group	2.534	14.587	0.000	2.236 to 2.871

Table 19.13 Predicted log odds in each age group, derived from a logistic regression model assuming a linear relationship between the log odds of microfilarial infection and age group.

Age group	Logistic regression equation	Predicted log odds
0	log odds = constant + 0 × age group	$-1.115 + 0.930 \times 0 = -1.115$
1	log odds = constant + 1 × age group	$-1.115 + 0.930 \times 1 = -0.185$
2	log odds = constant + 2 × age group	$-1.115 + 0.930 \times 2 = 0.745$
3	log odds = constant + 3 × age group	$-1.115 + 0.930 \times 3 = 1.674$

regression equation when age is included as a categorical variable, as described in Section 19.4.

Substitution of the estimated regression coefficients into the logistic regression equation gives the **predicted log odds** in each age group. These are shown in Table 19.13. Figure 19.3 compares these predicted log odds from logistic regression with the observed log odds in each group. This shows that the linear assumption gives a good approximation to the observed log odds in each group. Section 29.6 describes how to test such linear assumptions.

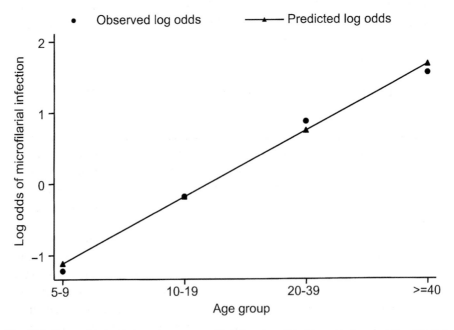

Fig. 19.3 Observed log odds in each age group (circles) and predicted log odds from logistic regression (triangles, connected by line).

CHAPTER 20

Logistic regression: controlling for confounding and other extensions

20.1 INTRODUCTION

In the last chapter we introduced the principles of logistic regression models, and described how to use logistic regression to examine the effect of a single exposure variable. We now describe how these models can be extended to control for the confounding effects of one or more additional variables. In addition, we briefly cover regression modelling for risk ratios, rather than odds ratios, and for outcomes with more than two levels.

20.2 CONTROLLING FOR CONFOUNDING USING LOGISTIC REGRESSION

In Chapter 18 we saw how to control for a **confounding** variable by dividing the sample into strata defined by levels of the confounder, and examining the effect of the exposure in each stratum. We then used the Mantel–Haenszel method to combine the odds ratios from each stratum into an overall summary odds ratio. We also explained how this approach assumes that effect modification (interaction) is not present, i.e. that the true odds ratio comparing exposed with unexposed individuals is the same in each stratum. We now see how making the same assumption allows us to control for confounding using logistic regression.

We will explain this in the context of the onchocerciasis dataset used throughout Chapter 19. Recall that we found strong associations of both area of residence and of age group with the odds of microfilarial (*mf*) infection. If the age distributions differ in the two types of area, then it is possible that age is a confounding variable for the association between area and *mf* infection. We will control for this possible confounding by fitting a logistic regression model, which includes the effects of both area and age group. We will start with *hypothetical* data, constructed so that it is easy to see how this logistic regression model works. We will then explain how to interpret the output when we apply the model to the real data.

Example 20.1 (hypothetical data)

Table 20.1 shows *hypothetical* data for the odds of *mf* infection according to area of residence (exposure) and age group. You can see that:

1 Table 20.1(a) shows that the exposure effect is *exactly* the same in each of the age groups; the age-specific odds ratios comparing exposed with unexposed individuals are all equal to 3.0. (Note also that when the age groups are combined, the crude odds ratio is $1.86/0.92 = 2.02$, which is considerably less than the individual age-specific odds ratios of 3, confirming that age group confounds the association between *mf* infection and area.)

2 Table 20.1(b) shows that the age group effect is *exactly* the same in each area of residence. For example, the odds ratio comparing age group 1 with age group 0 in the savannah areas is $0.5/0.2 = 2.5$, the same as the odds ratio in the forest areas ($1.5/0.6 = 2.5$). Similarly, the odds ratio comparing age group 2 with age group 0 are 10 in each area, and the odds ratios comparing age group 3 with age group 0 are 15 in each area.

Table 20.1 *Hypothetical* data for the odds of *mf* infection, according to area of residence and age group.

(a) Crude data, and odds of disease in each group (d = number infected and h = number uninfected), plus odds ratios for area in each age-group and overall.

Age group	Savannah areas (Unexposed)		Rainforest areas (Exposed)		Odds ratio for area effect
	d/h	Odds	d/h	Odds	
0	20/100	0.2	30/50	0.6	3.0
1	40/80	0.5	60/40	1.5	3.0
2	80/40	2.0	60/10	6.0	3.0
3	90/30	3.0	45/5	9.0	3.0
All age groups combined	230/250	0.92	195/105	1.86	2.02

(b) Age group odds ratios (comparing age groups 1, 2 and 3 with age group 0), in each type of area of residence.

Age group	Odds ratios for age group effects	
	Savannah areas	Rainforest areas
0	1.0	1.0
1	2.5 ($= 0.5/0.2$)	2.5 ($= 1.5/0.6$)
2	10.0 ($= 2.0/0.2$)	10.0 ($= 6.0/0.6$)
3	15.0 ($= 3.0/0.2$)	15.0 ($= 9.0/0.6$)

These two facts mean that we can *exactly* express the odds of *mf* infection in the eight area–age subgroups in terms of the following five *parameters*, as shown in Table 20.2(a):

1 0.2: the odds of mf infection at the *baseline* values of *both* area and age group;

2 3.0: the *area* odds ratio comparing the odds of infection in rainforest areas compared to savannah areas; and

3 2.5, 10.0 and 15.0: the three *age* odds ratios comparing age groups 1, 2 and 3 with age group 0 (respectively).

Table 20.2(b) shows the corresponding equations in terms of the parameter names; these follow the convention we introduced in Chapter 19. These equations define the *logistic regression model* for the effects of area and age group on the odds of *mf* infection. As described in Chapter 19, such a logistic regression model can be abbreviated to:

$$\text{Odds} = \text{Baseline} \times \text{Area} \times \text{Agegrp}$$

As explained in Section 19.2, it is a *multiplicative* model for the joint effects of area and age group. Note that the Baseline parameter now refers to the odds of the disease at the baseline of *both* variables. This model *assumes* that the odds ratio for area is the same in each age group and that the odds ratios for age group are the same in each area, i.e. that there is *no interaction* between the effects of area and age group.

Table 20.2 Odds of *mf* infection by area and age group, expressed in terms of the parameters of the logistic regression model: Odds = Baseline × Area × Age group.

(a) Expressed in terms of the parameter values.

	Odds of *mf* infection	
Age group	Savannah areas (Unexposed)	Rainforest areas (Exposed)
0	$0.2 = 0.2$	$0.6 = 0.2 \times 3.0$
1	$0.5 = 0.2 \times 2.5$	$1.5 = 0.2 \times 3.0 \times 2.5$
2	$2.0 = 0.2 \times 10.0$	$6.0 = 0.2 \times 3.0 \times 10.0$
3	$3.0 = 0.2 \times 15.0$	$9.0 = 0.2 \times 3.0 \times 15.0$

(b) Expressed in terms of the parameter names.

	Odds of *mf* infection	
Age group	Savannah areas (Unexposed)	Rainforest areas (Exposed)
0	Baseline	Baseline × Area
1	Baseline × Agegrp(1)	Baseline × Area × Agegrp(1)
2	Baseline × Agegrp(2)	Baseline × Area × Agegrp(2)
3	Baseline × Agegrp(3)	Baseline × Area × Agegrp(3)

(c) Expressed on a *log* scale, in terms of the parameter names.

	Log odds of *mf* infection	
Age group	Savannah areas (Unexposed)	Rainforest areas (Exposed)
0	log(Baseline)	log(Baseline) + log(Area)
1	log(Baseline) + log(Agegrp(1))	log(Baseline) + log(Area) + log(Agegrp(1))
2	log(Baseline) + log(Agegrp(2))	log(Baseline) + log(Area) + log(Agegrp(2))
3	log(Baseline) + log(Agegrp(3))	log(Baseline) + log(Area) + log(Agegrp(3))

As explained in Chapter 19, the calculations to derive confidence intervals and *P*-values for the parameters of logistic regression models are done on the log scale, in which case the baseline parameter refers to the *log odds* in the baseline group, and the other parameters refer to *log odds ratios*. The effects of the exposure variables are additive on the log scale (as described in Section 19.2). Table 20.2(c) shows the equations for the log odds in each of the area–age subgroups. The corresponding logistic regression model, defined by these eight equations, is:

$$\log(\text{Odds}) = \log(\text{Baseline}) + \log(\text{Exposure}) + \log(\text{Age})$$

Example 20.2 (real data)

In our hypothetical example, we were able to precisely express the odds in the *eight* sub-groups in the table in terms of *five* parameters, because we created the data so that the effect of area was exactly the same in each age group, and the effect of age exactly the same in savannah and rainforest areas. Of course, sampling variation means that real data is never this neat, even if the model proposed is correct. Table 20.3 shows the odds of *mf* infection in the eight area–age subgroups, using the data that were actually observed in the onchocerciasis study.

Table 20.3 Odds of microfilarial infection and odds ratios comparing individuals living in forest areas with those living in savannah areas, separately for each age group.

| | Area of residence | | |
Age group	Savannah	Rainforest	Odds ratio for area
0 (5–9 years)	16/77 = 0.208	30/79 = 0.380	1.828
1 (10–19 years)	22/50 = 0.440	77/69 = 1.116	2.536
2 (20–39 years)	123/85 = 1.447	176/40 = 4.400	3.041
3 (≥ 40 years)	120/55 = 2.182	258/25 = 10.32	4.730

From the previous chapter (Table 19.4) we know that the crude odds ratio for area is 2.413 (the odds ratio which does not take into account the effects of age group, or any other variables). We can see in Table 20.3 that in three out of the four age groups the stratum-specific odds ratios for the effect of area of residence are larger than this. If we use Mantel–Haenszel methods (*see* Chapter 18) to estimate the effect of area of residence controlling for age group, we obtain an estimated odds ratio of 3.039 (95% CI = 2.310 to 3.999). This is noticeably larger than the crude odds ratio of 2.413.

As in the hypothetical example above, we can express the odds of *mf* infection in the rainforest areas in terms of the odds ratios for the effect of area of residence in each age group (Table 20.4a). Alternatively, we can express the odds of *mf* infection in terms of the odds ratios for each of the three age groups compared to age group 0 (Table 20.4b). Note that (in contrast to the hypothetical example above) these sets of odds ratios are not exactly the same in each area. This means that we cannot calculate the parameter estimates directly from the raw data, as we

Table 20.4 Odds of *mf* infection, according to area of residence and age group, for the data observed in the onchocerciasis study.

(a) With the odds in the rainforest areas expressed in terms of the age-specific odds ratios for the association between area and infection.

	Area	
Age group	Savannah	Rainforest
0 (5–9 years)	0.208	0.208×1.828
1 (10–19 years)	0.440	0.440×2.536
2 (20–39 years)	1.447	1.447×3.041
3 ($\geq$ 40 years)	2.182	2.182×4.730

(b) With the odds of infection in age groups 2 to 4 expressed in terms of the area-specific odds ratios for the association between age group and infection.

	Area	
Age group	Savannah	Rainforest
0 (5–9 years)	0.208	0.380
1 (10–19 years)	0.208×2.118	0.380×2.939
2 (20–39 years)	0.208×6.964	0.380×11.59
3 ($\geq$ 40 years)	0.208×10.50	0.380×27.18

could for the simpler examples in Chapter 19. Instead we use a computer package to fit the model and to estimate the *most likely* values for the effect of area controlling for age group, and the effect of age group controlling for area, on the basis of the assumption that there is no interaction between the effects of the two variables. The meaning of 'most likely' is explained more precisely in Chapter 28.

The computer output from this model (on the odds ratio scale) is shown in Table 20.5. The estimated odds ratio of 3.083 (95% CI = 2.354 to 4.038) for area controlling for age group is very close to that derived using the Mantel–Haenszel method (OR 3.039, 95% CI = 2.310 to 3.999), and again is noticeably larger than

Table 20.5 Logistic regression output for the model for *mf* infection, including both area of residence and age group.

	Odds ratio	z	$P > |z|$	95% CI
Area	3.083	8.181	0.000	2.354 to 4.038
Agegrp(1)	2.599	4.301	0.000	1.682 to 4.016
Agegrp(2)	9.765	10.944	0.000	6.493 to 14.69
Agegrp(3)	17.64	13.295	0.000	11.56 to 26.93
Constant*	0.147	−9.741	0.000	0.100 to 0.217

*Constant (baseline odds) = estimated odds of *mf* infection for 5–9 year olds living in the savannah areas, assuming no interaction between the effects of area and age group.

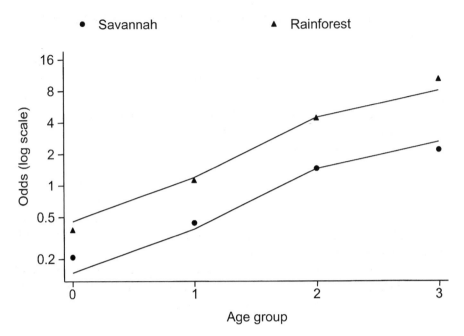

Fig. 20.1 Observed odds of *mf* infection in the eight area–age subgroups, together with lines showing the predicted odds from the logistic regression model defined in Table 20.2(b).

the crude odds ratio of 2.413. Thus the confounding effect of age meant that the crude odds ratio for area was too small.

We can use the parameter estimates shown in Table 20.5 to calculate the *predicted odds* in each group, using the equations for the odds in this logistic regression model, shown in Table 20.2(b). These calculations are shown in Table 20.6. Figure 20.1 compares the *observed* odds of *mf* infection in the eight area–age subgroups (shown in Table 20.3) with the *predicted* odds from the logistic regression model (shown by separate lines for the savannah and rainforest). The odds are plotted on a log scale; this means that, since the model *assumes* that the area odds ratios are the same in each age group, the two lines showing the predicted odds are *parallel*.

Table 20.6 Odds of *mf* infection by area and age group, as estimated from the logistic regression model.

	Odds of *mf* infection	
Age group	Savannah areas	Rainforest areas
0 (5–9 years)	0.147	$0.147 \times 3.083 = 0.453$
1 (10–19 years)	$0.147 \times 2.599 = 0.382$	$0.147 \times 3.083 \times 2.599 = 1.178$
2 (20–39 years)	$0.147 \times 9.765 = 1.435$	$0.147 \times 3.083 \times 9.765 = 4.426$
3 ($\geq$ 40 years)	$0.147 \times 17.64 = 2.593$	$0.147 \times 3.083 \times 17.64 = 7.993$

20.3 TESTING FOR INTERACTION, AND MORE COMPLEX LOGISTIC REGRESSION MODELS

We have explained the interpretation of logistic regression models for one and two variables in great detail. The extension to models for more than two variables is straightforward, and the interpretation of results follows the same principles. Regression modelling, including hypothesis testing, examining interaction between variables and modelling dose–response relationships, is described in more detail in Chapter 29. For now we note two important points:

1 In the logistic regression model for two variables (area and age group) described above, we assumed that the effect of each was the same regardless of the level of the other. In other words, we assumed that there was no **interaction** between the effects of the two variables. Interaction (also known as **effect modification**) was described in Chapter 18. It is straightforward to use regression modelling to examine this; see Section 29.5 for details.

2 Similarly, when we include three or more variables in a logistic regression model, we assume that there is no interaction between any of them. On the basis of this assumption, we estimate the effect of each, controlling for the effect of all the others.

More information about logistic regression models may be found in Hosmer and Lemeshow (2000).

20.4 REGRESSION ANALYSIS OF RISK RATIOS

Most regression analyses of binary outcomes are conducted using odds ratios: partly because of the mathematical advantages of analyses based on odds ratios (see Section 16.6) and partly because computer software to do logistic regression analyses is so widely available. However, it is straightforward to do regression analyses of risk ratios, if it is considered important to express exposure effects in that way.

This is carried out by relating the effect of the exposure variable(s) to the log of the risk of the outcome rather than the log of the odds, using a statistical software package that allows the user to fit **generalized linear models** (see Chapter 29) for a range of outcome distributions and a range of what are known as **link functions**. For logistic regression the outcome variable is assumed to have a binomial distribution (see Chapter 15) and the link function is the logit function $\text{logit}(\pi) = \log[\pi/(1 - \pi)]$ (see Section 19.3). To model exposure effects as risk ratios instead of odds ratios, we simply specify a log link function ($\log \pi$) instead of a logit link function. The outcome distribution is still binomial. The model is:

$$\log(\text{risk of outcome}) = \beta_0 + \beta_1 x_1 + \beta_2 x_2 + \ldots + \beta_p x_p$$

If the outcome is rare then odds ratios are approximately the same as risk ratios (see Section 16.6) and so the choice of odds ratio or risk ratio as the measure of exposure effect is unimportant. When the outcome is common, the two measures are different, and as stated in Section 16.6, it is important that odds ratios are not misinterpreted as risk ratios. The problem with the regression analysis of risk ratios is that when the outcome is common, it can prove difficult to fit models based on risk ratios, because they are constrained (see Section 16.6); this means that computer model-fitting routines often fail to produce results. Furthermore, exposure effects will differ depending on whether the presence *or* absence of the outcome event is considered as the outcome. For these reasons, it is likely that logistic regression will continue to be the method of choice for the regression analysis of binary outcome variables.

20.5 OUTCOMES WITH MORE THAN TWO LEVELS

Finally, we briefly describe extensions to logistic regression that may be used for categorical outcomes with more than two categories. In Chapter 2 we distinguished between categorical variables such as ethnic group, for which there is no natural ordering of the categories, and **ordered categorical** variables such as social class, in which the different categories, though non-numerical, have a natural ordering. We will briefly introduce the regression models appropriate for each of these types of outcome variable. We will denote the outcome variable by y, and assume that y has k possible categories.

Multinomial logistic regression

Multinomial logistic regression, also known as **polychotomous logistic regression**, extends logistic regression by estimating the effect of one or more exposure variables on the probability that the outcome is in a particular category. For example, in a study of risk factors for asthma the outcome might be defined as no asthma, allergic asthma and non-allergic asthma. One of the outcome levels is chosen as the comparison level, and $(k - 1)$ regression coefficients, corresponding to each other outcome level, are estimated for each exposure variable in the regression model. If there are only two outcome levels the model is identical to standard logistic regression. However, when the outcome has *more than* two levels, interpretation of the regression coefficients is less straightforward than for logistic regression, because the estimated effect of an exposure variable is measured by the combined effects of $(k - 1)$ regression coefficients.

Ordinal logistic regression

Ordinal logistic regression is an extension of logistic regression which is appropriate when the outcome variable is *ordered categorical*. For example, in a study of risk factors for malnutrition the outcome might be classified as severe, moderate, mild, or no malnutrition. The most commonly used type of model is the **proportional odds** model, whose parameters represent the exposure odds ratios for being in the highest j categories compared to the lowest $(k - j)$ categories. For example, if there were four outcome categories and a single exposure variable, then the exposure odds ratio would represent the combined comparison of outcome: category 4 with categories 3, 2 and 1, categories 4 and 3 with categories 2 and 1, and categories 4, 3 and 2 with category 1. It is assumed that the effect of exposure is the same for all such splits of the categories of the outcome variable. Some statistical software packages provide tests of this assumption, others do not.

Other, less commonly used models for ordered categorical outcome variables include the **continuation ratio model** and the **stereotype model**.

Further reading

Regression models for categorical variables with more than two levels are described by Agresti (1996). Models for ordered categorical outcome variables have been reviewed by Armstrong and Sloan (1989), and Ananth and Kleinbaum (1997).

CHAPTER 21

Matched studies

21.1 INTRODUCTION

In this chapter we introduce methods for studies in which we have binary outcome observations that are **matched** or **paired** in some way. The two main reasons why matching occurs are:

1 When the outcome is observed on the *same* individual on two separate occasions, under different exposure (or treatment) circumstances, or using two different methods.

2 The study has used a **matched design** in selecting individuals. This mainly occurs with **case–control studies**; each case (subjects with the disease) is matched with one or more controls (subjects without the disease), deliberately chosen to have the same values for major confounding variables. For example, controls might be selected because they are of similar age to a case, or because they live in the same neighbourhood as the case. We will discuss case–control studies in more detail in Chapter 34, where we will see that matched designs often have few advantages, and may have serious disadvantages, compared to unmatched designs. It is also *very occasionally* used in **clinical trials**, for example in a trial comparing two treatments for an eye condition, the two treatments may be randomly assigned to the left and right eyes of each patient.

It is essential that the matching be allowed for in the analysis of such studies.

21.2 COMPARISON OF TWO PROPORTIONS: PAIRED CASE

Example 21.1
Consider the results of an experiment to compare the Bell and Kato–Katz methods for detecting *Schistosoma mansoni* eggs in faeces in which two subsamples from each of 315 specimens were analysed, one by each method. Here, the exposure is the type of method, and the outcome is the test result. The correct way to analyse such data is to consider the results of each *pair* of subsamples. For any pair there are four

Table 21.1 Possible results when a pair of subsamples is tested using two methods for detecting *Schistosoma mansoni* eggs.

	Notation	Description
Both tests positive		Concordant pairs
Both tests negative		
Bell positive, Kato–Katz negative	*r*	Discordant pairs
Kato–Katz positive, Bell negative	*s*	

possible outcomes, as shown in Table 21.1. The results for each of the 315 specimens (pairs of subsamples) are shown in Table 21.2(a). Note that it would be incorrect to arrange the data as in Table 21.2(b) and to apply the standard chi-squared test, as this would take no account of the *paired* nature of the data, namely that it was the *same* 315 specimens examined with each method, and not 630 different ones.

One hundred and eighty-four specimens were positive with both methods and 63 were negative with both. These 247 specimens (the **concordant pairs**; see Table 21.1) therefore give us no information about which of the two methods is better at detecting *S. mansoni* eggs. The information we require is entirely contained in the 68 specimens for which the methods did not agree (the **discordant pairs**). Of these, 54 were positive with the Bell method only, compared to 14 positive with the Kato–Katz method only.

Table 21.2 Comparison of Bell and Kato–Katz methods for detecting *Schistosoma mansoni* eggs in faeces. The same 315 specimens were examined using each method. Data from Sleigh *et al.* (1982) *Transactions of the Royal Society of Tropical Medicine and Hygiene* **76**: 403–6 (with permission).

(a) Correct layout.

		Kato–Katz		
		+	−	Total
Bell	+	184	54(*r*)	238
	−	14(*s*)	63	77
Total		198	117	315

(b) Incorrect layout.

	Results		
	+	−	Total
Bell	238	77	315
Kato–Katz	198	117	315
Total	436	194	630

The proportions of specimens found positive with the two methods were 238/315 (0.756) using the Bell method and 198/315 (0.629) using the Kato–Katz method. The difference between the proportions was therefore 0.1270. This difference can also be calculated from the numbers of discordant pairs, *r* and *s*, and the total number of pairs, *n*:

$$\text{Difference between paired proportions} = \frac{r-s}{n},$$

$$\text{s.e.(difference)} = \frac{\sqrt{(r+s)}}{n}$$

In this example, the difference between the paired proportions is $(r - s)/n = (54 - 14)/315 = 0.1270$, the same as calculated above. Its standard error equals $[\sqrt{(r + s)}]/n = \sqrt{68}/315 = 0.0262$. An approximate **95% confidence interval** can be derived in the usual way:

$$95\% \text{ CI} = 0.1270 - (1.96 \times 0.0262) \text{ to } 0.1270 + (1.96 \times 0.0262)$$
$$= 0.0756 \text{ to } 0.1784$$

With 95% confidence, the positivity rate is between 7.6% and 17.8% higher if the Bell method is used to detect *S. mansoni* eggs than if the Kato–Katz method is used.

z-test for difference between proportions

If there was no difference in the abilities of the methods to detect *S. mansoni* eggs, we would not of course expect complete agreement since different subsamples were examined, but we would expect on average half the disagreements to be positive with the Bell method only and half to be positive with the Kato–Katz method only. Thus an appropriate test of the null hypothesis that there is no difference between the methods is to compare the proportion found positive with the Bell method only, namely 54/68, with the hypothetical value of 0.5. This may be done using the *z test*, as described in Section 15.6. As usual, we construct the test by dividing the difference by its standard error assuming the null hypothesis to be true, which gives:

$$z = \frac{54/68 - 0.5}{\sqrt{(0.5 \times 0.5/68)}} = 4.85, \; P < 0.001$$

There is strong evidence that the Bell method is more likely to detect *S. mansoni* eggs than the Kato–Katz method. (Note that other than for the sign of the z statistic exactly the same result would have been obtained had the proportion positive with the Kato–Katz method only, namely 14/68, been compared with 0.5.)

21.3 USING ODDS RATIOS FOR PAIRED DATA

An alternative approach to the analysis of matched pairs is to estimate the odds ratio comparing the Bell and Kato–Katz methods. Again, our analysis must take the pairing into account. This can be done using **Mantel–Haenszel** methods (see Section 18.4), with the data stratified into the individual pairs. Using the same notation as in Chapter 18, the notation for the *i*th pair is shown in Table 21.3. The Mantel–Haenszel estimate of the odds ratio (see Chapter 18) is given by:

$$OR_{MH} = \frac{\sum \dfrac{d_{1i} \times h_{0i}}{n_i}}{\sum \dfrac{d_{0i} \times h_{1i}}{n_i}}$$

Table 21.3 Notation for the 'stratified' 2×2 table giving the results for pair i.

	Outcome		Total
	+	−	
Bell method	d_{1i}	h_{1i}	1
Kato–Katz method	d_{0i}	h_{0i}	1
Total	d_i	h_i	2

As in the last section, the analysis can be simplified if we note that there are only four possible outcomes for each pair, and therefore only four possible types of 2×2 table. These are shown in Table 21.4, together with their contributions to the numerator and denominator in the formula for the Mantel–Haenszel OR. This shows that, again, only the discordant pairs contribute to the Mantel–Haenszel estimate of the odds ratio. The total for the numerator is $r/2$, while the total for the denominator is $s/2$. The estimated **odds ratio** is therefore:

$$\mathrm{OR}_{MH} = \frac{r/2}{s/2} = \frac{r}{s}, \text{ the ratio of the numbers of discordant pairs}$$

Table 21.4 Possible outcomes for each pair, together with their contributions to the numerator and denominator in the formula for the Mantel–Haenszel estimate of the odds ratio.

	Concordant pairs				Discordant pairs			
	+	−	+	−	+	−	+	−
Bell	1	0	0	1	1	0	0	1
Kato–Katz	1	0	0	1	0	1	1	0
Number of pairs					r		s	
$\dfrac{d_{1i} \times h_{0i}}{n_i}$	0		0		½		0	
$\dfrac{d_{0i} \times h_{1i}}{n_i}$	0		0		0		½	

An approximate **95% error factor** for the odds ratio is given by:

$$\mathrm{EF} = \exp[1.96 \times \sqrt{(1/r + 1/s)}]$$

In the example, the estimated odds ratio is given by $54/14 = 3.857$, while the error factor is $\exp[1.96 \times \sqrt{(1/54 + 1/14)}] = 1.193$. The approximate **95% confidence interval** is therefore given by:

95% CI = OR/EF to OR × EF = 3.857/1.193 to 3.857 × 1.193 = 3.234 to 4.601

McNemar's chi-squared test

A chi-squared test, based on the numbers of discordant pairs, can also be derived from the formula for the Mantel–Haenszel statistic presented in Chapter 18 and is given by:

$$\chi^2_{paired} = \frac{(r-s)^2}{r+s}, \text{d.f.} = 1$$

This is known as **McNemar's chi-squared test**. In the example $\chi^2 = (54 - 14)^2$ $/(54 + 14) = 40^2/68 = 23.53$, d.f. $= 1, P < 0.001$. Apart from rounding error, this χ^2 value is the same as the square of the z value obtained above $(4.85^2 = 23.52)$, the two tests being mathematically equivalent.

Validity

The use of McNemar's chi-squared test or the equivalent z test is valid provided that the total number of discordant pairs is at least 10. The approximate error factor for the 95% CI for the odds ratio is valid providing that the total number of pairs is greater than 50. If these conditions are not met then methods based on exact binomial probabilities should be used (these are described by Alman *et al.* 2000).

21.4 ANALYSING MATCHED CASE–CONTROL STUDIES

The methods described above can also be used for the analysis of case–control studies and clinical trials which have employed a matched design, as described in the introduction. The rationale for this and the design issues are discussed in more detail in Chapter 34.

Example 21.2
Table 21.5 shows data from a study to investigate the association between use of oral contraceptives and thromboembolism. The cases were 175 women aged 15–44 discharged alive from 43 hospitals after initial attacks of thromboembolism. For each case a female patient suffering from some other disease (thought to be unrelated to the use of oral contraceptives) was selected from the same hospital to act as a control. She was chosen to have the same residence, time of hospital-isation, race, age, marital status, parity, and income status as the case. Participants were questioned about their past contraceptive history, and in particular

Table 21.5 Results of a *matched* case–control study, showing the association between use of oral contraceptives (OC) and thromboembolism. With permission from Sartwell *et al.* (1969) *American Journal of Epidemiology* 90: 365–80.

		Controls		
		OC used	OC not used	Total
Cases	OC used	10	57	67
	OC not used	13	95	108
	Total	23	152	175
		OR = 57/13 = 4.38		

about whether they had used oral contraceptives during the month before they were admitted to hospital.

The pairing of the cases and controls is preserved in the analysis by comparing oral contraceptive use of each case against oral contraceptive use of their matched control. There were ten case–control pairs in which both case and control had used oral contraceptives and 95 pairs in which neither had. These 105 concordant pairs give no information about the association. This information is entirely contained in the 70 discordant pairs in which the case and control differed. There were 57 case–control pairs in which only the case had used oral contraceptives within the previous month compared to 13 in which only the control had done so. The odds ratio is measured by the ratio of these **discordant pairs** and equals 4.38, which suggests oral contraceptive use leads to a substantial increase in the risk of thromboembolism.

$$OR = \text{ratio of discordant pairs}$$
$$= \frac{\text{no. of pairs in which case exposed, control not exposed}}{\text{no. of pairs in which control exposed, case not exposed}}$$

The *error factor* is $\exp[1.96 \times \sqrt{(1/57 + 1/13)}] = 1.827$. The 95% CI for the odds ratio is therefore 4.38/1.827 to 4.38 × 1.827, which is 2.40 to 8.01. McNemar's χ^2 test gives: $\chi^2 = (95 - 10)^2/(95 + 10) = 26.4, P < 0.001$, corresponding to strong evidence against the null hypothesis that there is no association.

If *several* controls rather than a single matched control are selected for each case, the odds ratio can still be estimated by using Mantel–Haenszel methods. However, these methods are severely limited because they do not allow for further stratification on confounding variables which were not also matching variables. The solution to this problem is to use **conditional logistic regression**, which we describe next.

21.5 CONDITIONAL LOGISTIC REGRESSION

In general when analysing individually matched case–control studies we may wish to control for confounding variables, additional to those matched for in the design. This is done using **conditional logistic regression**, a variant of logistic regression in which cases are only compared to controls in the same matched set. In the simple case of individually-matched case–control studies with one control per case and no further confounders, conditional logistic regression will give identical results to the methods for paired data described earlier in the chapter. However, additional confounders may be included in the model, and there is no restriction on the numbers of cases and controls in each matched set.

Once the reader is familiar with the use of logistic regression, then conditional logistic regression should present no additional difficulties. The only difference is that in addition to the outcome and exposure variables, the computer software requires a variable that specifies which case (or cases) matches which control (or controls). Exposure effects are estimated by considering possible combinations of exposures, conditional on the observed exposures *within each matched set*. For example, if the set consists of one case and two controls, with only one of the set exposed and the other two unexposed, then the three possible combinations are:

	Case	Control 1	Control 2
1	Exposed	Unexposed	Unexposed
2	Unexposed	Exposed	Unexposed
3	Unexposed	Unexposed	Exposed

It is because the possible combinations are conditional on the total number of exposed and unexposed individuals in each matched set that the method is called *conditional* logistic regression. This argument extends in a straightforward manner to numeric exposure variables and to more than one exposure variable.

Example 21.3

Table 21.6 shows data from a matched case–control study of risk factors for infant death from diarrhoea in Brazil [Victora *et al.* (1987) *Lancet* **ii**: 319–322], in which an attempt was made to ascertain all infant deaths from diarrhoea occurring over a one-year period in two cities in southern Brazil, by means of weekly visits to all hospitals, coroners' services and death registries in the cities. Whenever the underlying cause of death was considered to be diarrhoea, a physician visited the parents or guardians to collect further information about the terminal illness, and data on possible risk factors. The same data were collected for two 'control' infants. Those chosen were the nearest neighbour aged less than 1 year, and the next nearest neighbour aged less than 6 months. This procedure was designed to provide a control group with a similar socio-economic distribution to that of the cases. The selection also ensures

Table 21.6 First 24 lines (eight case–control sets) of the dataset for the matched case–control study of risk factors for infant death from diarrhoea in southern Brazil. Reproduced with kind permission of C.G. Victora.

Observation number	case	set	water	agegp	bwtgp	social	income
1	1	1	0	2	3	1	3
2	0	1	1	3	4	2	2
3	0	1	1	2	3	1	3
4	1	2	1	1	2	1	2
5	0	2	1	3	4	2	3
6	0	2	1	2	4	1	2
7	1	3	1	2	3	2	2
8	0	3	1	5	3	2	4
9	0	3	1	1	3	2	4
10	1	4	1	3	3	1	2
11	0	4	1	4	3	1	3
12	0	4	1	2	4	1	2
13	1	5	1	2	2	2	2
14	0	5	1	4	2	2	2
15	0	5	1	1	2	2	3
16	1	6	1	2	3	2	2
17	0	6	1	4	4	1	2
18	0	6	1	2	3	1	2
19	1	7	1	2	1	1	2
20	0	7	1	4	3	1	2
21	0	7	1	2	4	1	2
22	1	8	1	3	3	1	3
23	0	8	1	5	2	1	2
24	0	8	1	2	4	1	1

that there are approximately twice as many controls less than 6 months old, as between 6–11 months; this matches what was known concerning the age distribution of the cases. During the one-year study period, data were collected on 170 cases together with their 340 controls. In addition to variable *case* (1 = case, 0 = control), the dataset contains a variable *set* which gives the number (from 1 to 170) of the set to which each case and its two matched controls belong. Table 21.6 contains the first 24 lines (eight case–control sets) of this dataset.

Variable *water* denotes whether the child's household had access to water in their house or plot (*water* = 1) or not (*water* = 0). Variable *agegp* (age group) is coded as 1 = 0–1 months, 2 = 2–3 months, 3 = 4–5 months, 4 = 6–8 months and 5 = 9–11 months. Variable *bwtgp* (birth weight group, kg) has values 1 = 1.50–2.49, 2 = 2.50–2.99, 3 = 3.00–3.49, 4 => 3.50 kg. The final two variables are *social* (household social group) from 1 (most deprived) to 3 (least deprived), and *income* (household income group) from 1 (least monthly income) to 4 (most monthly income).

Examining the effect of a single exposure variable

A total of 111 (65.3%) cases and 259 (76.2%) controls had access to water, suggesting that access to water might be protective against infant death from diarrhoea. Since this is a *matched* case–control study, the calculation of the odds ratio for this exposure and all other analyses must take into account the matching. Using Mantel–Haenszel methods stratified by set (170 strata, each containing 1 case and 2 controls) gives an estimated odds ratio of 0.275 (95% CI = 0.136 to 0.555). Access to water thus appears to be strongly protective against infant diarrhoea death. Table 21.7 shows corresponding output from a conditional logistic regression model (also stratifying on set for the effect of household water supply). The estimated odds ratio is similar to that derived using Mantel–Haenszel methods.

Table 21.7 Conditional logistic regression output (odds ratio scale) for the association between household water supply and infant diarrhoea death in southern Brazil.

	Odds ratio	z	$P > |z|$	95% CI
Water	0.2887	−3.67	0.000	0.1487 to 0.5606

A possible alternative approach to the analysis of such data is to fit a standard logistic regression model, incorporating an indicator variable in the model corresponding to each case–control set, as a way of controlling for the matching. It is important to note, however, that for finely matched data *this will give the wrong answer*, and that the odds ratios obtained will be further away from the null value of 1 than they should be. For data in which the sets consist of exactly one case and one control, the estimated odds ratio from such a model will be exactly the square of the odds ratio estimated using Mantel–Haenszel methods stratified by set, or using conditional logistic regression.

Controlling for confounders, additional to those used for matching

Since access to water may be associated with a household's social status, we may wish to control additionally for the effects of variables such as *social* and *income*. Because there are only three subjects in each stratum, further stratification using Mantel–Haenszel methods is not feasible. However, conditional logistic regression allows us to control for the effects of confounding variables in addition to those used in the matching. Table 21.8 shows output from a conditional logistic regression model, controlling for the effects of all the variables in Table 21.6. Here, *agegp*(2) is an indicator variable (see Section 19.4) which takes the value 1 for infants in age group 2 and 0 for infants in other age groups. However, the corresponding odds ratio of 2.6766 cannot be interpreted as the odds of death in age group 2 compared to age group 1, because age was used in the matching of cases to controls. The odds ratio for the effect of water is only slightly increased (closer to the null value of 1), so we would conclude that the additional variables

Table 21.8 Conditional logistic regression output (odds ratio scale) for the association between household water supply and infant diarrhoea death in southern Brazil, controlling for the effects of potentially confounding variables.

	Odds Ratio	z	$P > |z|$	95% CI
water	0.2991	−3.20	0.001	0.1427 to 0.6269
agegp(2)	2.6766	2.89	0.004	1.3719 to 5.2222
agegp(3)	2.4420	2.50	0.012	1.2121 to 4.9199
agegp(4)	3.2060	3.27	0.001	1.5940 to 6.4482
agegp(5)	0.8250	−0.43	0.666	0.3444 to 1.9758
bwtgp(2)	0.4814	−2.00	0.045	0.2354 to 0.9844
bwtgp(3)	0.4111	−2.52	0.012	0.2061 to 0.8199
bwtgp(4)	0.3031	−3.12	0.002	0.1431 to 0.6422
social(2)	0.9517	−0.21	0.830	0.6058 to 1.4951
social(3)	0.1527	−1.78	0.075	0.0192 to 1.2128
income(2)	0.7648	−0.85	0.394	0.4128 to 1.4170
income(3)	0.6970	−1.01	0.312	0.3459 to 1.4043
income(4)	0.6991	−0.86	0.389	0.3098 to 1.5774

included in the model had only a slight confounding effect, and that there is still a clear protective effect of having a water supply in a household.

PART D

LONGITUDINAL STUDIES: ANALYSIS OF RATES AND SURVIVAL TIMES

In this part of the book we describe methods for the analysis of **longitudinal studies**, that is studies in which subjects are followed over time. These may be subdivided into three main types:

- **cohort studies** in which a group of individuals is followed over time, and the incidence of one or more outcomes is recorded, together with exposure to one or more factors
- **survival studies** in which individuals are followed from the time they experience a particular event such as the diagnosis of disease, and the time to recurrence of the disease or death is recorded
- **intervention studies** in which subjects are randomized to two or more intervention or treatment groups (one of which is often a control group with no active intervention or treatment or with standard care); the occurrence of pre-specified outcomes is recorded

These different types of study are described in more detail in Chapter 34. Our focus is on methods for their analysis, where the *outcome of interest* is *binary*, and where:

1 individuals in the study *are followed over different lengths of time*, and/or

2 we are interested not only in whether or not the outcome occurs, but also the *time at which it occurs*.

Note that for longitudinal studies in which everyone is followed for *exactly* the same length of time, the methods described in Part C can be used if the outcome is defined as the *risk* or *odds* of the event of interest. The exception is studies when most subjects will experience the event of interest by the end of the follow-up. For example, in a trial of a new treatment approach for lung cancer, even if every patient were followed for 10 years, the focus would be on assessing whether the new treatment had extended the survival time, rather than comparing the proportion who survived in each group. This is because lung cancer has a very poor prognosis; the probability of anyone surviving for more than 10 years is close to zero.

In Chapter 22 we explain why variable follow-up times are common and the special issues that arise in their analysis, and we define **rates of disease and mortality** as the appropriate outcome measure. We then introduce the **Poisson distribution** for the *sampling distribution of a rate* and derive a standard error of a rate from it. In Chapter 23 we describe how to compare two rates, and how to control for the effects of *confounding* using **stratification** methods, and in Chapter

24 the use of **Poisson regression** methods. In Chapter 25 we describe the use of standardized rates to enable ready comparison between several groups. This part of the book concludes with the group of methods known as **survival analysis**; Chapter 26 covers the use of life tables, Kaplan–Meier estimates of survival curves and log rank tests, and Chapter 27 describes Cox (proportional hazards) regression for the analysis of survival data. In contrast to the other methods for the analysis of longitudinal studies presented earlier in this part, survival analysis methods do not require the rate(s) to be constant during specified time periods.

We will assume throughout this part of the book that individuals can only experience one occurrence of the outcome of interest. This is not the case where the outcome of interest is a **disease or condition that can recur**. Examples are episodes of diarrhoea, acute respiratory infection, malaria, asthma and myocardial infarction, which individuals may experience more than once during the course of the study. Although we can apply the methods described in this part of the book by defining the outcome as the occurrence of one or more events, and using the time until the *first* occurrence of the event, a more appropriate approach is to use the methods presented in Chapter 31, which describes the analysis of **clustered data**. The methods in Chapter 31 also apply to the analysis of longitudinal studies in which we take **repeated measures of a quantitative outcome variable**, such as blood pressure or lung function, on the same individual.

CHAPTER 22

Longitudinal studies, rates and the Poisson distribution

22.1 INTRODUCTION

In this chapter we introduce the **rate** of event occurrence, as the outcome measure for the analysis of longitudinal studies. We explain why variable follow-up times happen, show how rates are estimated and discuss what they mean and how they relate to the measure of event occurrence described in Part C. We then describe the **Poisson distribution** for the *sampling distribution of a rate*, and use its properties to derive confidence intervals for rates. In the next chapter we introduce two measures used to compare rates in different exposure groups; the **rate ratio** and the **rate difference**.

22.2 CALCULATING PERIODS OF OBSERVATION (FOLLOW-UP TIMES)

In the majority of longitudinal studies, individuals are followed for different lengths of time. Methods that take this into account are the focus of this part of the book. Variable follow-up times occur for a variety of reasons:

- for logistic reasons, individuals may be recruited over a period of time but followed to the same end date
- in an intervention or cohort study, new individuals may be enrolled during the study because they have moved into the study area
- in a survival study, there may be a delay between the diagnosis of the event and recruitment into the study
- some individuals may be lost to follow up, for example because of emigration out of the study area or because they choose to withdraw from the study
- some individuals may die from causes other than the one that is the focus of interest
- in studies where the population of interest is defined by their age, for example women of child bearing age (ie. 15–44 years), individuals may move into or out of the group during the study as they age.

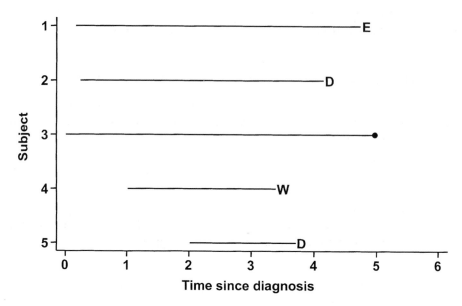

Fig. 22.1 Follow-up histories for 5 subjects in a study of mortality after a diagnosis of prostate cancer (D = died, E = emigrated, W = withdrew, • = reached the end of follow-up without experiencing the disease event).

Figure 22.1 depicts an example from a study of prostate cancer, which shows that subjects were recruited to the study at varying times after diagnosis and exited at different points in time. Only subject 3 was followed for the full 5 years: subjects 2 and 5 died, subject 1 emigrated and subject 4 withdrew from the study. Survival times for subjects who are known to have survived up to a certain point in time, such as subjects 1 and 4, but whose survival status past that point is not known, are said to be **censored**.

An individual's **period of observation** (or **follow-up time**) starts when they join the study and stops when they experience the outcome, are lost to follow-up, or the follow-up period ends, whichever happens first. This is the time during which, were they to experience an event, the event would be recorded in the study. This period is also called the **period at risk**. It is often measured in years, when it is called **person-years-at-risk** or **pyar**.

The occurrence and timings of outcome events, losses to follow-up, and recruitment of new participants are most accurately determined through regular surveillance of the study population. In some countries this may be possible using national databases, for example of deaths or cancer events, by 'flagging' the subjects under surveillance in the study so that the occurrence of events of interest can be routinely detected. In other settings it may be necessary to carry out community-based surveillance. For logistic simplicity, and cost considerations, this is sometimes carried out by conducting just two cross-sectional surveys, one at the beginning and one at the end of the study period, and enquiring about changes in the intervening period. If the exact date of an outcome event, loss to follow-up, or new recruitment cannot be determined through questioning, it is usually assumed to have occurred half-way through the interval between the surveys.

Using statistical computer packages to calculate periods of follow-up

When analysing longitudinal studies, it is important to choose a statistical computer package that allows easy manipulation of dates. Many packages provide a facility for automatic recoding of dates as the total number of days that have elapsed since the start of the Julian calendar, or from a chosen reference date such as 1/Jan/1960. Thus, for example, 15/Jan/1960 would be coded as 14, 2/Feb/1960 as 32, 1/Jan/1959 as −365 and so on. It is then easy to calculate the time that has elapsed between two dates. If the recoded variables are *startdate* and *exitdate*, and since (taking leap years into account) there are on average 365.25 days in a year, the follow-up time in years is given by:

$$\text{Follow-up time in years} = (exitdate - startdate)/365.25$$

22.3 RATES

The **rate** of occurrence of an outcome event measures the number of new events that occur per person per unit time, and is denoted by the Greek letter λ (lambda). Some examples of rates are:

- In the UK, the *incidence rate* of prostate cancer is 74.3/100 000 men/year. In other words, 74.3 new cases of prostate cancer are detected among every 100 000 men each year
- In the UK, the *mortality rate* from prostate cancer is 32.5/100 000 men/year. In other words 32.5 out of every 100 000 men die from prostate cancer each year
- In the UK, the incidence rate of abortions among teenage girls aged 16–19 years rose from 6.1/1000 girls/year in 1969 to 26.0/1000 girls/year in 1999

The rate is estimated from study data by dividing the total number (d) of events observed by the total (T) of the individual person-years of observation.

$$\text{Rate, } \lambda = \frac{\text{number of events}}{\text{total person-years of observation}} = \frac{d}{T}$$

Note that the sum, T, of the individual person-years is equivalent to the average number of persons under observation multiplied by the length of the study.

The rate is also known as the **incidence rate** (or **incidence density**) of the outcome event, except when the outcome of interest is death, in which case it is called the **mortality rate**. For rare events, the rate is often multiplied by 1000 (or even 10 000 or 100 000) and expressed per 1000 (or 10 000 or 100 000) person-years-at-risk. For a **common disease** such as diarrhoea or asthma, which may occur more than once in the same person, the incidence rate measures the average number of attacks per person per year (at risk). However, the standard methods for the analysis of rates (described in this part of the book) are not valid when individuals may experience multiple episodes of disease. We explain how to deal with this situation in Chapter 31.

Example 22.1

Five hundred children aged less than 5 years living in a community in rural Guatemala were enrolled in a study of acute lower respiratory infections. Fifty-seven were hospitalized for an acute lower respiratory infection, after which they were no longer followed in the study. The study lasted for 2 years, but because of migration, the occurrence of infections, passing the age of 5, and losses to follow-up, the number under surveillance declined with time and the total child-years at risk was $T = 873$ (i.e. an average population size of 436 over the 2 years). The rate of acute lower respiratory infections was therefore estimated to be:

$$\lambda = 57/873 = 0.0653 \text{ per child-year}$$

This can also be expressed per 1000 child-years at risk, as:

$$\lambda = 57/873 \times 1000 = 65.3 \text{ per 1000 child-years}$$

Note that the estimated rate will be the same whether the child-years of follow-up arise from following (for example) 1000 children for 1 year, 500 children for 2 years or 250 children for 4 years (and so on).

Understanding rates and their relationship with risks

The rate relates the number of new events to total observation time. This is in contrast to the **risk**, or **cumulative incidence** (see Chapter 15), in which the number of new events is related to the number at risk at the beginning of the observation period; the longer the period of observation the greater the risk will be, since there will be more time for events to occur. Measures of risk therefore contain an implicit but not explicit time element.

Figure 22.2 illustrates the accumulation of new cases of a disease over a 5 year period in a population *initially disease free*, for two somewhat different incidence rates: (a) $\lambda = 0.3$/person/year, and (b) $\lambda = 0.03$/person/year. For ease of understanding, we are illustrating this assuming that the population remains constant over the 5 years, and that there is complete surveillance; that is that there are no losses to follow-up, and no migration either in or out.

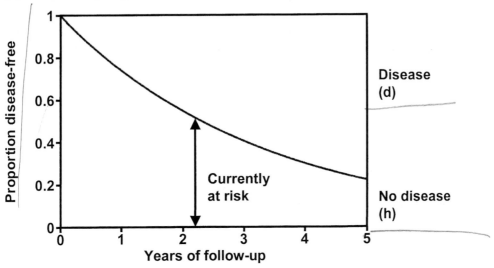

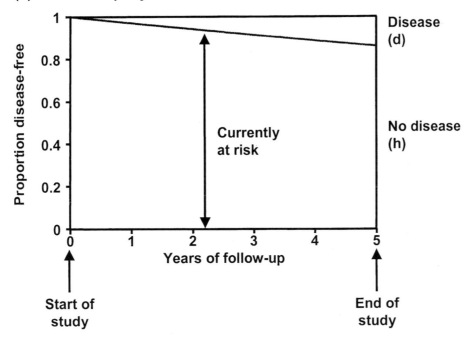

Fig. 22.2 A graphical representation of two follow-up studies which lasted for 5 years. In the top graph (a) the rate of disease is 0.3/person/year, and the disease-free population declines exponentially with time. In the bottom graph (b) the rate is 0.03/person/year, and the decline in the disease-free population is approximately linear over the period of the study.

The disease rate applies to the number of people disease-free at a particular point in time. Understanding the effect of this is a bit like understanding the calculation of compound interest rates. In Figure 22.2(a), the incidence rate is high, and so the proportion of the population remaining disease free is changing rapidly over time. The disease rate is therefore operating on an ever-diminishing proportion of the population as time goes on. This means that the number of new cases per unit time will be steadily decreasing.

In other words, although the disease rate is constant over time, the cumulative incidence and risk do not increase at a constant pace; their increase slows down over time. This is reflected by a steadily decreasing gradient of the graph showing how the disease-free population is diminishing over time (or equivalently how the number who have experienced the disease, that is the cumulative incidence, is accumulating). It can be shown mathematically that when the rate is constant over time, this graph is described by an *exponential* function, and that:

$$\text{Proportion disease free at time } t = e^{-\lambda t}$$

$$\text{Risk up to time } t = 1 - e^{-\lambda t}$$

$$\text{Average time to contracting the disease} = 1/\lambda$$

In Figure 22.2(b), the incidence rate is low and so the proportion of the population remaining disease-free decreases slowly over time. It remains sufficiently close to one over the 5 years that the exponential curve is approximately linear, corresponding to a constant increase of new cases (and therefore of risk) over time. In fact when the value of λ is very *small*, the risk is approximately equal to the rate multiplied by the time:

$$\text{When } \lambda \text{ is very small, risk up to time } t \approx \lambda t, \text{ so that}$$

$$\lambda \approx \frac{\text{risk}}{t}$$

Table 22.1 shows the values of the risks (up to 1, 2 and 5 years) that result from these two very different rates. This confirms what we can see visually in Figure 22.2. For the high rate ($\lambda = 0.3$/person/year), the number of new cases per unit time is steadily decreasing; the increase is always less than the rate because the size of the 'at risk' population is decreasing rapidly. Thus at 1 year, the cumulative risk is a bit less than the rate (0.26 compared to 0.3), at 2 years it is considerably less than twice the rate (0.45 compared to 0.6), and so on. In contrast, for the low rate ($\lambda = 0.03$/person/year), the number of new cases is increasing steadily, and the risk increases by approximately 0.03/year.

Table 22.1 Risks of disease up to 1, 2 and 5 years corresponding to rates of $\lambda = 0.3$/person/year, and $\lambda = 0.03$/person/year.

	Risk of disease		
Rate of disease	Over 1 year	Over 2 years	Over 5 years
0.3/person/year	$1 - e^{-0.3} = 0.26$	$1 - e^{-0.3 \times 2} = 0.45$	$1 - e^{-0.3 \times 5} = 0.78$
0.03/person/year	$1 - e^{-0.03} = 0.03$	$1 - e^{-0.03 \times 2} = 0.06$	$1 - e^{-0.03 \times 5} = 0.14$

We have demonstrated that when λ is very small, the risk up to time t approximately equals λt. This is equivalent to the rate, λ, being approximately equal to the value of the risk per unit time (risk/t). We will now show that the value of risk/t also gets close to the rate as the length of the time interval gets very small. This is true whatever the size of the rate, and is the basis of the **formal definition of a rate**, as the value of risk/t when t is very small.

$$\lambda = \frac{\text{risk}}{t}, \text{ when } t \text{ is very small}$$

Table 22.2 illustrates this for the fairly high rate of $\lambda = 0.3$/person/year. Over 5 years, the risk per year equals 0.1554, just over half the value of the rate. If the length of time is decreased to 1 year, the risk per year is considerably higher at 0.2592, but still somewhat less than the rate of 0.3 per year. As the length of time decreases further, the risk per year increases; by one month it is very close to the rate, and by one day almost equal to it.

Table 22.2 Risk of disease, and risk/t, for different lengths of time interval t, when the rate, $\lambda = 0.3$/person/year.

	Length of time interval, t						
	5 years	1 year	1 month (30 days)	1 week	1 day	1 hour	1 minute
t (years)	5	1	0.08219	0.01918	0.002740	0.0001142	0.000001900
risk $= 1 - e^{-0.3t}$	0.7769	0.2592	0.02436	0.005737	0.0008216	0.00003420	0.0000005710
risk/t	0.1554	0.2592	0.2963	0.2992	0.2999	0.3000	0.3000

22.4 THE POISSON DISTRIBUTION

We have already met the normal distribution for means and the binomial distribution for proportions. We now introduce the **Poisson distribution**, named after the French mathematician, which is appropriate for describing the *number* of occurrences of an event during a period of time, provided that these events occur independently of each other and at random. An example would be the number of congenital malformations of a given type occurring in a particular district each year, provided that that there are no epidemics or specific environmental hazards and that the population is constant from year to year (also see Example 22.2).

The Poisson distribution is also appropriate for the *number* of particles found in a unit of space, such as the number of malaria parasites seen in a microscope field of a blood slide, provided that the particles are distributed *randomly* and *independently* over the total space. The two properties of randomness and independence must both be fulfilled for the Poisson distribution to hold. For example, the number of *Schistosoma mansoni* eggs in a stool slide will not be Poisson, since the eggs tend to cluster in clumps rather than to be distributed independently.

After introducing the Poisson distribution in general for the number of events, we will explain its application to the analysis of rates.

Definition of the Poisson distribution

The Poisson distribution describes the sampling distribution of the number of occurrences, d, of an event during a period of time (or region of space). It depends upon just one parameter, which is the mean number of occurrences, μ, in periods of the same length (or in equal regions of space).

$$\text{Probability } (d \text{ occurrences}) = \frac{e^{-\mu} \mu^d}{d!}$$

Note that, by definition, both 0! and μ^0 equal 1. The probability of zero occurrences is therefore $e^{-\mu}$ (e is the mathematical constant 2.71828...).

$$\text{Mean number of occurrences} = \mu$$
$$\text{s.e. of number of occurrences} = \sqrt{\mu}$$

The standard error for the number of occurrences equals the square root of the mean, which is estimated by the square root of the observed number of events, $\sqrt{d}$.

Example 22.2
A district health authority which plans to close the smaller of two maternity units is assessing the extra demand this will place on the remaining unit. One factor being considered is the risk that on any given day the demand for admissions will

exceed the unit's capacity. At present the larger unit averages 4.2 admissions per day and can cope with a maximum of 10 admissions per day. This results in the unit's capacity being exceeded only on about one day per year. After the closure of the smaller unit the average number of admissions is expected to increase to 6.1 per day. The Poisson distribution can be used to estimate the proportion of days on which the unit's capacity is then likely to be exceeded. For this we need to determine the probability of getting 11 or more admissions on any given day. This is most easily calculated by working out the probabilities of 0, 1, 2 . . . or 10 admissions and subtracting the total of these from 1, as shown in Table 22.3. For example:

$$\text{Probability (three admissions)} = \frac{e^{-6.1}\, 6.1^3}{3!}$$

The calculation shows that the probability of 11 or more admissions in a day is 0.0470. The unit's capacity is therefore likely to be exceeded 4.7% of the time, or on about 17 days per year.

Table 22.3 The probabilities of the number of admissions made during a day in a maternity unit, based on a Poisson distribution with a mean of 6.1 admissions per day.

No. of admissions	Probability
0	0.0022
1	0.0137
2	0.0417
3	0.0848
4	0.1294
5	0.1579
6	0.1605
7	0.1399
8	0.1066
9	0.0723
10	0.0440
Total (0 − 10)	0.9530
11+ (by subtraction, 1 − 0.9530)	0.0470

Shape of the Poisson distribution

Figure 22.3 shows the shape of the Poisson distribution for various values of its mean, μ. The distribution is very skewed for small means, when there is a sizeable probability that zero events will be observed. It is symmetrical for large means and is adequately approximated by the normal distribution for values of $\mu = 10$ or more.

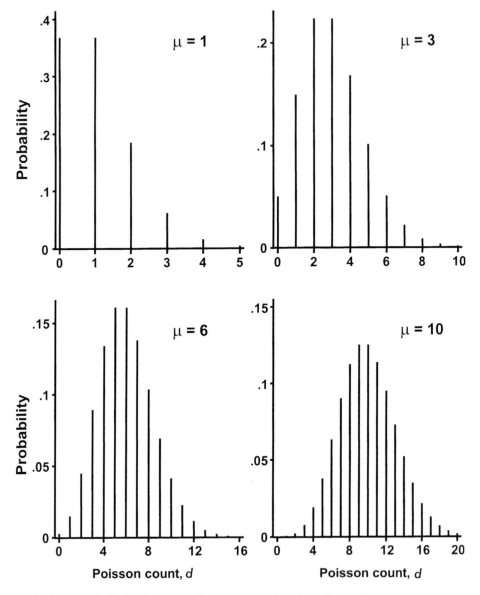

Fig. 22.3 Poisson distribution for various values of μ. The horizontal scale in each diagram shows values of the number of events, d.

Use of the Poisson distribution

The Poisson distribution (and its normal approximation) can be used whenever it is reasonable to assume that the outcome events are occurring independently of each other and randomly in time. This assumption is, of course, less likely to be true for infectious than for non-communicable diseases but, provided there is no strong evidence of disease clustering, the use is still justified. Specific techniques exist to detect disease clustering in time and/or space (see Elliott *et al.*, 2000), such as the possible clustering of cases of leukaemia or variant Creutzfeldt–Jakob disease in a particular area. Such clusters violate what might otherwise be a Poisson distribution.

22.5 STANDARD ERROR OF A RATE

We now discuss the use of the Poisson distribution for the analysis of rates. Recall that:

$$\text{Rate, } \lambda = \frac{\text{number of events}}{\text{total person-years of observation}} = \frac{d}{T}$$

Although the value of the total person-years of observation (T) is affected by the number of events, and the time at which they occur (since an individual's period of observation only contributes until they experience an event, as then they are no longer at risk), it can be shown that we do not need to explicitly consider this variation in T. We can therefore calculate the standard error of a rate as follows:

$$\text{s.e. (rate)} = \frac{\text{s.e. (number of events)}}{T} = \frac{\sqrt{d}}{T} = \sqrt{\frac{\lambda}{T}}$$

The right hand version of the formula (derived by replacing $\sqrt{d}$ with $\sqrt{(\lambda T)}$) makes it clear that the standard error of the rate will be smaller the larger the total person-years of observation, as λ will be the same, on average, whatever the value of this.

Example 22.1 (continued)
We showed earlier that in the 2-year morbidity study in rural Guatemala the rate of acute lower respiratory infections, expressed per 1000 child-years at risk, was estimated to be 65.3 per 1000 child-years. The standard error of the rate is:

$$\text{s.e.} = \frac{\sqrt{d}}{T} \times 1000 = \frac{\sqrt{57}}{873} \times 1000 = 8.6$$

22.6 CONFIDENCE INTERVAL FOR A RATE

A confidence interval for a rate can be derived from its standard error, in the usual way. However, it is preferable to work on the log scale and to derive a confidence interval for the log rate, and then to antilog this to give a confidence interval for a rate, since this takes account of the constraint that the rate must be greater than or equal to zero. We now show how to do this.

The formula for the standard error of the log rate is derived using the **delta method** (see Box 16.1 on p. 157), and is:

$$\text{s.e. } (\log \text{ rate}) = \frac{1}{\sqrt{d}}$$

Thus, perhaps surprisingly, the standard error of the log rate depends only on the number of events, and not on the length of follow-up time. In the same way as shown in Chapter 16, the steps of calculating the confidence interval on the log scale and then converting it to give a confidence interval for the rate can be combined into the following formulae:

$$95\% \text{ CI (rate)} = \text{rate/EF to rate} \times \text{EF}$$

$$\text{Error factor (EF)} = \exp(1.96/\sqrt{d})$$

Example 22.1 (continued)
For the Guatemala morbidity study there were 57 lower respiratory infections in 873 child-years at risk. The log rate per 1000 child-years at risk, is $\log(\lambda) = \log(1000 \times 57/873) = \log(65.3) = 4.179$. The standard error of this log rate is:

$$\text{s.e. } (\log \text{ rate}) = 1/\sqrt{d} = 1/\sqrt{57} = 0.132$$

1 The 95% confidence interval for the log rate is therefore:

$$95\% \text{ CI} = 4.179 - (1.96 \times 0.132) \text{ to } 4.179 + (1.96 \times 0.132) = 3.919 \text{ to } 4.438$$

The 95% confidence interval for the rate is:

$$95\% \text{ CI} = \exp(3.919) \text{ to } \exp(4.438) = 50.36 \text{ to } 84.65 \text{ infections per}$$

$$1000 \text{ child-years}$$

2 Alternatively, we may calculate the 95% CI using the 95% error factor (EF) for the rate:

$$EF = \exp(1.96/\sqrt{d}) = \exp(1.96/\sqrt{57}) = 1.296$$

The 95% confidence interval for the rate is:

$$95\% \text{ CI} = \frac{\lambda}{EF} \text{ to } \lambda \times EF = 65.3/1.296 \text{ to } 65.3 \times 1.296$$
$$= 50.36 \text{ to } 84.65 \text{ infections per 1000 child-years}$$

CHAPTER 23

Comparing rates

23.1 INTRODUCTION

In this chapter we describe the two measures used to compare rates in different exposure groups: the **rate difference** and the **rate ratio**. We then show how to use Mantel–Haenszel methods to estimate rate ratios controlling for confounding factors. In Part C we emphasized the similarity between Mantel–Haenszel methods, which use stratification to estimate odds ratios for the effect of exposure controlled for the effects of confounding variables, and logistic regression models. Mantel–Haenszel methods for rate ratios are closely related to the corresponding regression model for rates, Poisson regression, which is introduced in Chapter 24.

23.2 COMPARING TWO RATES

We now see how the rates of disease in two exposure groups may be compared, using two different measures: the **rate difference** and the **rate ratio**.

Rate differences

Example 23.1
The children in the Guatemala morbidity study analysed in Example 22.1 were subdivided according to the quality of their housing conditions. The data are shown in Table 23.1, together with the notation we will use. We will consider children living in poor housing conditions to be the exposed group and, as in Part C, denote exposed and unexposed groups by the subscripts 1 and 0 respectively. The **rate difference** comparing poor with good housing is $93.0 - 46.3 = 46.7$ infections per 1000 child-years.

Table 23.1 Incidence of lower respiratory infection among children aged less than 5 years, according to their housing conditions.

Housing condition	Number of acute lower respiratory infections	Child-years at risk	Rate/1000 child-years
Poor (exposed)	$d_1 = 33$	$T_1 = 355$	$\lambda_1 = 93.0$
Good (unexposed)	$d_0 = 24$	$T_0 = 518$	$\lambda_0 = 46.3$
Total	$d = 57$	$T = 873$	$\lambda = 65.3$

The **standard error of a rate difference** is:

$$\text{s.e. (rate difference)} = \sqrt{\left(\frac{d_1}{T_1^2} + \frac{d_0}{T_0^2}\right)}$$

This can be used in the usual way to derive a 95% confidence interval. In this example,

$$\text{s.e.} = \sqrt{\left(\frac{d_1}{T_1^2} + \frac{d_0}{T_0^2}\right)} = \sqrt{\left(\frac{33}{355^2} + \frac{24}{518^2}\right)} \times 1000$$
$$= 18.7 \text{ infections per } 1000 \text{ child-years}$$

and the 95% confidence interval is:

$$46.7 - 1.96 \times 18.7 \text{ to } 46.7 + 1.96 \times 18.7$$
$$= 10.0 \text{ to } 83.4 \text{ infections per } 1000 \text{ child-years}$$

With 95% confidence, the rate of lower respiratory infections among children living in poor housing exceeds the rate among children living in good housing by between 10.0 and 83.4 infections per 1000 child-years.

Rate ratios

As explained in more detail in the next chapter, the analysis of rates is usually done using **rate ratios** rather than rate differences. The rate ratio is defined as:

$$\text{Rate ratio} = \frac{\text{rate in exposed}}{\text{rate in unexposed}} = \frac{\lambda_1}{\lambda_0} = \frac{d_1/T_1}{d_0/T_0} = \frac{d_1 \times T_0}{d_0 \times T_1}$$

As for risk ratios and odds ratios, we use the **standard error of the log rate ratio** to derive confidence intervals, and tests of the null hypothesis of no difference between the rates in the two groups. This (again derived using the **delta method**) is given by:

$$\text{s.e. of log(rate ratio)} = \sqrt{(1/d_1 + 1/d_0)}$$

The **95 % confidence interval for the rate ratio** is:

$$95\% \text{ CI} = \text{rate ratio}/\text{EF to rate ratio} \times \text{EF, where}$$

$$\text{EF} = \exp[1.96 \times \text{s.e. of log(rate ratio)}]$$

z-test for the rate ratio

A *z*-**test** (Wald test, see Chapter 28) of the null hypothesis that the rates in the two groups are equal is given by:

$$z = \frac{\text{log(rate ratio)}}{\text{s.e. of log(rate ratio)}}$$

Example 23.1 (continued)
The rate ratio comparing children living in poor housing with those living in good housing is:

$$\text{rate ratio} = \frac{33/355}{24/518} = 2.01$$

The standard error of the log(rate ratio) is $\sqrt{(1/33 + 1/24)} = 0.268$, and the 95 % error factor is:

$$95\% \text{ EF} = \exp(1.96 \times 0.268) = 1.69$$

A 95 % confidence interval for the rate ratio is thus:

$$95\% \text{ CI} = 2.01/1.69 \text{ to } 2.01 \times 1.69 = 1.19 \text{ to } 3.39$$

With 95% confidence, the rate of acute lower respiratory infections among children living in poor housing is between 1.19 and 3.39 times the rate among children living in good housing. The z statistic is $\log(2.01)/0.268 = 2.60$; the corresponding P value is 0.009. There is therefore good evidence against the null hypothesis that infection rates are the same among children living in good and poor quality housing.

Relationship between rate ratio, risk ratio and odds ratio

From Chapter 16, we know that for a rare event the risk ratio is approximately equal to the odds ratio. And in the last chapter we saw that for a rare event, risk up to time t approximately equals λt. It therefore follows that for a rare event the risk ratio and rate ratio are also approximately equal:

$$\text{Risk ratio} \approx \frac{\lambda_1 t}{\lambda_0 t} = \frac{\lambda_1}{\lambda_0} = \text{Rate ratio} \approx \text{Odds ratio}$$

However when the event is not rare the three measures will all be different. These different measures of the association between exposure and outcome event, and of the impact of exposure, are discussed in more detail in Chapter 37.

23.3 MANTEL–HAENSZEL METHODS FOR RATE RATIOS

Recall from Chapter 18 that a **confounding** variable is one that is related both to the outcome variable and to the exposure of interest (see Figure 18.1), and that is not a part of the causal pathway between them. Ignoring the effects of confounding variables may lead to bias in our estimate of the exposure–outcome association. We saw that we may allow for confounding in the analysis via **stratification**: restricting estimation of the exposure–outcome association to individuals with the same value of the confounder. We then used **Mantel–Haenszel** methods to combine the stratum-specific estimates, leading to an estimate of the *summary odds ratio*, controlled for the confounding.

We now present Mantel–Haenszel methods for rate ratios. Table 23.2 shows the notation we will use for the number of events and person-years in each group, in stratum i. The notation is exactly the same as that in Table 23.1, but with the subscript i added, to refer to the stratum i.

Table 23.2 Notation for the table for stratum i.

	Number of events	Person-years at risk
Group 1 (Exposed)	d_{1i}	T_{1i}
Group 0 (Unexposed)	d_{0i}	T_{0i}
Total	$d_i = d_{0i} + d_{1i}$	$T_i = T_{0i} + T_{1i}$

The data consist of c such tables, where c is the number of different values the confounding variable can take. The estimate of the rate ratio for stratum i is

$$RR_i = \frac{d_{1i}/T_{1i}}{d_{0i}/T_{0i}} = \frac{d_{1i} \times T_{0i}}{d_{0i} \times T_{1i}}$$

Mantel–Haenszel estimate of the rate ratio controlled for confounding

As for the odds ratio, the **Mantel–Haenszel estimate of the rate ratio** is a *weighted average* (see Section 18.3) of the rate ratios in each stratum. The weight for each rate ratio is:

$$w_i = \frac{d_{0i} \times T_{1i}}{T_i}$$

Since the numerator of the weight is the same as the denominator of the rate ratio in stratum i, $w_i \times RR_i = (d_{1i} \times T_{0i})/T_i$. These weights therefore lead to the following formula for the **Mantel–Haenszel estimate of the rate ratio**:

$$RR_{MH} = \frac{\Sigma(w_i \times RR_i)}{\Sigma w_i} = \frac{\Sigma \dfrac{d_{1i} \times T_{0i}}{T_i}}{\Sigma \dfrac{d_{0i} \times T_{1i}}{T_i}}$$

Following the notation of Clayton and Hills (1993), this can alternatively be written as:

$$RR_{MH} = Q/R, \text{ where}$$
$$Q = \Sigma \frac{d_{1i} \times T_{0i}}{T_i} \text{ and } R = \Sigma \frac{d_{0i} \times T_{1i}}{T_i}$$

Example 23.2

Data on incidence of acute lower respiratory infections from a study in Guatemala were presented in Example 23.1 and Table 23.1. The rate ratio comparing children living in poor with good housing conditions is 2.01 (95% CI 1.19 to 3.39). Table 23.3 shows the same information, stratified additionally by the type of cooking stove used in the household.

Table 23.3 Association between incidence of acute lower respiratory infection and housing conditions, stratified by type of cooking stove.

(a) Wood burning stove (stratum 1)

Housing condition	Number of infections	Child-years at risk	Rate/1000 child-years
Poor (exposed)	$d_{11} = 28$	$T_{11} = 251$	$\lambda_{11} = 111.6$
Good (unexposed)	$d_{01} = 5$	$T_{01} = 52$	$\lambda_{01} = 96.2$
Total	$d_1 = 33$	$T_1 = 303$	$\lambda_1 = 108.9$

Rate ratio $= 1.16$ (95% CI 0.45 to 3.00), $P = 0.76$

(b) Kerosene or gas stove (stratum 2)

Housing condition	Number of infections	Child-years at risk	Rate/1000 child-years
Poor (exposed)	$d_{12} = 5$	$T_{12} = 104$	$\lambda_{12} = 48.1$
Good (unexposed)	$d_{02} = 19$	$T_{02} = 466$	$\lambda_{02} = 40.8$
Overall	$d_2 = 24$	$T_2 = 570$	$\lambda_2 = 42.1$

Rate ratio $= 1.18$ (95% CI 0.44 to 3.16), $P = 0.74$

Table 23.4 Person-years of observation according to housing conditions and type of cooking stove.

	Type of stove	
Housing condition	Wood burning stove	Gas or kerosene stove
Poor (exposed)	$T_{11} = 251$	$T_{21} = 104$
Good (unexposed)	$T_{10} = 52$	$T_{20} = 466$

Examination of the association between quality of housing and infection rates in the two strata defined by type of cooking stove shows that there is little evidence of an association in either stratum. Type of cooking stove is a strong confounder of the relationship between housing quality and infection rates, because most poor quality houses have wood burning stoves while most good quality houses have kerosene or gas stoves. This can be seen by tabulating the person-years of observation according to housing condition and cooking stove, as shown in Table 23.4.

Table 23.5 shows the calculations needed to derive the Mantel–Haenszel rate ratio combining the stratified data, presented in Table 23.3, on the association between housing conditions (the exposure variable) and the incidence of acute lower respiratory infection (the outcome), controlling for type of stove.

The Mantel–Haenszel estimate of the rate ratio equals:

$$RR_{MH} = Q/R = 8.89/7.61 = 1.17$$

Table 23.5 Calculations required to derive the Mantel–Haenszel summary rate ratio, with associated confidence interval and P value.

Stratum i	RR_i	$w_i = \frac{d_{0i} \times T_{1i}}{T_i}$	$w_i \times RR_i$	V_i	d_{1i}	E_{1i}
Wood stove ($i = 1$)	1.16	4.14	4.81	4.69	28	27.34
Kerosene/gas ($i = 2$)	1.18	3.47	4.09	3.58	5	4.38
Total		$R = 7.61$	$Q = 8.89$	$V = 8.27$	$O = 33$	$E = 31.72$

After controlling for the confounding effect of type of stove, the rate of infection is only slightly (17%) greater among children living in poor housing conditions compared to children living in good housing conditions.

Standard error and confidence interval for the Mantel–Haenszel RR

As is usual for ratio measures, the **95% confidence interval for RR_{MH}** is derived using the standard error of $\log(RR_{MH})$, denoted by s.e.$_{MH}$.

$$95\% \text{ CI} = RR_{MH}/EF \text{ to } RR_{MH} \times EF, \text{ where}$$

$$\text{the error factor EF} = \exp(1.96 \times \text{s.e.}_{MH})$$

The simplest formula for the **standard error of $\log RR_{MH}$** (Clayton and Hills 1993) is:

$$\text{s.e.}_{MH} = \sqrt{\left(\frac{V}{Q \times R}\right)}, \text{ where}$$

$$V = \Sigma V_i, \text{ and } V_i = \frac{d_i \times T_{1i} \times T_{0i}}{T_i^2}$$

V is the sum across the strata of the variances V_i for the number of exposed individuals experiencing the outcome event, i.e. the variances of the d_{1i}'s. Note that the formula for the variance V_i of d_{1i} for stratum i gives the same value regardless of which group is considered as exposed and which is considered as unexposed.

Example 23.2 (continued)
Using the results of the calculations for Q, R and V shown in Table 23.5, we find that:

$$\text{s.e.}_{\text{MH}} = \sqrt{\left(\frac{V}{Q \times R}\right)} = \sqrt{\left(\frac{8.27}{8.89 \times 7.61}\right)} = 0.35$$

so that $EF = \exp(1.96 \times 0.35) = 1.98$, $RR_{\text{MH}}/EF = 1.17/1.98 = 0.59$, and $RR_{\text{MH}} \times EF = 1.17 \times 1.98 = 2.32$. The 95% confidence interval is therefore:

$$95\% \text{ CI for } RR_{\text{MH}} = 0.59 \text{ to } 2.32$$

Mantel–Haenszel χ^2 test of the null hypothesis

Finally, we test the null hypothesis that $RR_{\text{MH}} = 1$ by calculating the **Mantel–Haenszel χ^2 test statistic**:

$$\chi^2_{\text{MH}} = \frac{(\Sigma d_{1i} - \Sigma E_{1i})^2}{\Sigma V_i} = \frac{(O - E)^2}{V} = \frac{U^2}{V}; \text{ d.f.} = 1$$

This is based on a comparison in each stratum of the number of exposed individuals observed to have experienced the disease event (d_{1i}) with the expected number in this category (E_{1i}) if there were no difference in the rates between the exposed and unexposed. The expected numbers are calculated in the same way as for the standard χ^2 test described in Chapter 17.

$$E_{1i} = \frac{d_i \times Y_{1i}}{Y_i}$$

The formula has been simplified by writing O for the sum of the observed numbers, E for the sum of the expected numbers and U for the difference between them:

$$O = \Sigma d_{1i}, \; E = \Sigma E_{1i} \text{ and } U = D - E$$

Note that χ^2_{MH} *has just 1 degree of freedom irrespective of how many strata are summarized.*

Example 23.2 (continued)

From the data presented in Table 23.5, a total of $O = 33$ children living in poor housing experienced acute lower respiratory infections, compared with an expected number of 31.72, based on assuming no difference in rates between poor and good housing. Thus the Mantel–Haenszel χ^2 statistic is:

$$\chi^2_{MH} = \frac{U^2}{V} = \frac{(33 - 31.72)^2}{8.27} = 0.20 \text{ (1 d.f., } P = 0.655)$$

After controlling for type of cooking stove, there is no evidence of an association between quality of housing and incidence of lower respiratory infections.

Test for effect modification (interaction)

Use of Mantel–Haenszel methods to control for confounding assumes that the exposure–outcome association is the same in each of the strata defined by the levels of the confounder, in other words that the confounder does not modify the effect of the exposure on the outcome event. If this is true, $RR_i = RR_{MH}$, and it follows that:

$$(d_{1i} \times T_{0i} - RR_{MH} \times d_{0i} \times T_{1i}) = 0$$

The χ^2 **test for heterogeneity** is based on a *weighted* sum of the squares of these differences:

$$\chi^2 = \Sigma \frac{(d_{1i} \times T_{0i} - RR_{MH} \times d_{0i} \times T_{1i})^2}{RR_{MH} \times V_i \times T_i^2}, \text{ d.f.} = c - 1$$

where V_i is as defined above, and c is the number of strata. The greater the differences between the stratum-specific rate ratios and RR_{MH}, the larger will be the heterogeneity statistic.

Example 23.2 (continued)
The rate ratios in the two strata were very similar (1.16 in houses with wood-burning stoves and 1.18 in houses with kerosene or gas stoves). We do not, therefore, expect to find evidence of effect modification. Application of the formula for the test for heterogeneity gives $\chi^2 = 0.0005$ (1 d.f.), $P = 0.98$. There is thus no evidence that type of cooking stove modifies the association between quality of housing and rates of respiratory infections.

CHAPTER 24

Poisson regression

24.1 INTRODUCTION

In this chapter we introduce **Poisson regression** for the analysis of rates. This is used to estimate **rate ratios** comparing different exposure groups in the same way that logistic regression is used to estimate *odds ratios* comparing different exposure groups. We will show how it can be used to:

- compare the rates between two exposure (or treatment) groups
- compare more than two exposure groups
- examine the effect of an ordered or continuous exposure variable
- control for the confounding effects of one or more variables
- estimate and control for the effects of **exposures that change over time**

We will see that Poisson regression models comparing two exposure groups give identical rate ratios, confidence intervals and *P*-values to those derived using the methods described in Section 23.2. We will also see that Poisson regression to control for confounding is closely related to the Mantel–Haenszel methods for rate ratios, described in Section 23.3. Finally, we will show how to estimate and control for the effects of variables that change over time, by splitting the follow-up time for each subject.

Like logistic regression models, Poisson regression models are fitted on a *log scale*. The results are then antilogged to give rate ratios and confidence intervals. Since the principles and the approach are exactly the same as those outlined for logistic regression in Part B, a more concise treatment will be given here; readers are referred to Chapters 19 and 20 for more detail. More general issues in regression modelling are discussed in Chapter 29.

24.2 POISSON REGRESSION FOR COMPARING TWO EXPOSURE GROUPS

Introducing the Poisson regression model

The *exposure rate ratio* is defined as:

$$\text{Exposure rate ratio} = \frac{\text{rate in exposed group}}{\text{rate in unexposed group}}$$

If we re-express this as:

$$\text{Rate in exposed group} = \text{Rate in unexposed group} \times \text{Exposure rate ratio}$$

then we have the basis for a model which expresses the rate in each group in terms of two **model parameters**. These are:

1 The **baseline rate**. As in Chapters 19 and 20, we use the term **baseline** to refer to the exposure group against which all the other groups are compared. When there are just two exposure groups, then the baseline rate is the rate in the unexposed group. We use the parameter name Baseline to refer to the rate in the baseline group.

2 The **exposure rate ratio**. This expresses the effect of the exposure on the rate of disease. We use the parameter name Exposure to refer to the exposure rate ratio.

As with logistic regression, Poisson regression models are fitted on a log scale. The two equations that define this model for the *rate* of an outcome event are shown in Table 24.1, together with the corresponding equations for the *log rate*. The equations for the rate can be abbreviated to:

$$\text{Rate} = \text{Baseline} \times \text{Exposure}$$

The two equations that define the Poisson regression model on the log scale can be written:

$$\log(\text{Rate}) = \log(\text{Baseline}) + \log(\text{Exposure rate ratio})$$

Table 24.1 Equations defining the Poisson regression model for the comparison of two exposure groups.

Exposure group	Rate	Log rate
Exposed (*group 1*)	Baseline rate × exposure rate ratio	Log(baseline rate) + log(exposure rate ratio)
Unexposed (*group 0*)	Baseline rate	Log(baseline rate)

In practice, we abbreviate it to:

$$\log(\text{Rate}) = \text{Baseline} + \text{Exposure}$$

since it is clear from the context that output on the log scale refers to log rate and log rate ratios. Note that whereas the exposure effect on the rate ratio scale is *multiplicative*, the exposure effect on the log scale is *additive*.

Example 24.1

All the examples in this chapter are based on a sample of 1786 men who took part in the Caerphilly study, a study of risk factors for cardiovascular disease. Participants were aged between 43 and 61 when they were first examined, and were followed for up to 19 years. The first examinations took place between July 1979 and October 1983, and the follow-up for the outcome (myocardial infarction or death from heart disease) ended in February 1999. Further information about the study can be found at www.epi.bris.ac.uk/mrc-caerphilly.

The first ten lines of the dataset are shown in Table 24.2. Variable '*cursmoke*', short for *current smoker* at recruitment, was coded as 1 for subjects who were smokers and 0 for subjects who were non-smokers, and variable 'MI' was coded as 1 for subjects who experienced a myocardial infarction or died from heart disease during the follow-up period and 0 for subjects who did not. Variable '*years*' is the years of follow-up for each subject (the time from *examdate* to *exitdate*); it was derived using a statistical computer package, as described in Section 22.2.

There were 990 men who were current smokers at the time they were recruited into the study, and 796 men who had never smoked or who were ex-smokers. Table 24.3 shows rates of myocardial infarction in these two groups. The *rate ratio* comparing smokers with never/ex-smokers is $16.98/9.68 = 1.700$.

Table 24.2 First ten lines of the computer dataset from the Caerphilly study. Analyses of the Caerphilly study are by kind permission of the MRC Steering Committee for the Management of MRC Epidemiological Resources from the MRC Epidemiology Unit (South Wales).

id	dob	examdate	exitdate	years	MI	cursmoke
1	20/May/1929	17/Jun/1982	31/Dec/1998	16.54	0	1
2	9/Jul/1930	10/Jan/1983	24/Dec/1998	15.95	0	0
3	6/Feb/1929	23/Dec/1982	26/Nov/1998	15.93	0	1
4	24/May/1931	7/Jul/1983	22/Nov/1984	1.38	1	0
5	9/Feb/1934	3/Sep/1980	19/Dec/1998	18.29	0	0
6	14/Mar/1930	17/Nov/1981	31/Dec/1998	17.12	0	0
7	13/May/1933	30/Oct/1980	27/Dec/1998	18.16	0	1
8	23/May/1924	24/Apr/1980	24/Jan/1986	5.75	1	1
9	20/Jun/1931	11/Jun/1980	12/Dec/1998	18.50	0	1
10	12/May/1929	17/Nov/1979	20/Jan/1995	15.18	1	0

Table 24.3 Rates of myocardial infarction among men who were and were not current smokers at the time they were recruited to the Caerphilly study.

Current smoker at entry to the study	Number of myocardial infarctions	Person-years at risk	Rate per 1000 person-years
Yes (exposed)	$d_1 = 230$	$T_1 = 13\,978$	$\lambda_1 = 230/13.978 = 16.98$
No (unexposed)	$d_0 = 118$	$T_0 = 12\,183$	$\lambda_0 = 118/12.183 = 9.68$
Overall	$d = 348$	$T = 26\,161$	$\lambda = 348/26.161 = 13.30$

We will now show how to use Poisson regression to examine the association between smoking and rates of myocardial infarction in these data. To use a **computer package to fit a Poisson regression model**, it is necessary to specify three items:

1 The *name of the outcome* variable, which in this case is MI. If each line of the dataset represents an individual (as is the case here) then the outcome variable is coded as 1 for individuals who experienced the event and 0 for individuals who did not experience the event. If *data have been grouped according to the values of different exposure variables* then the outcome contains the total number of events in each group.

2 The *total exposure time*, for the individual or the group (depending on whether each line in the dataset represents an individual or a group). As will be explained in Section 24.3, this is used as an **offset** in the Poisson regression model.

3 The *name of the exposure* variable(s). In this example, we have just one exposure variable, which is called *cursmoke*. The *required convention for coding* is that used throughout this book; thus *cursmoke* was coded as 0 for men who were never/ex-smokers at the start of the study (the *unexposed* or *baseline* group) and 1 for men who were current smokers at the start of the study (the *exposed* group).

The **Poisson regression model** that will be fitted is:

$$\text{Rate of myocardial infarction} = \text{Baseline} \times \text{Cursmoke}$$

Its two parameters are:

1 Baseline: the rate of myocardial infarction in the baseline group (never/ex-smokers), and

2 Cursmoke: the rate ratio comparing current smokers with never/ex-smokers.

Output on the ratio scale

Table 24.4 shows the computer output obtained from fitting this model. The two *rows* in the output correspond to the two *parameters* of the logistic regression model; cursmoke is our exposure of interest and the **constant** term refers to the

Table 24.4 Poisson regression output for the model relating rates of myocardial infarction with smoking at the time of recruitment to the Caerphilly study.

	Rate ratio	z	P > |z|	95% CI
Cursmoke	1.700	4.680	0.000	1.361 to 2.121
Constant	0.00969	−50.37	0.000	0.00809 to 0.0116

baseline group. The same format is used for both parameters, and is based on what makes sense for interpretation of the effect of exposure. This means that some of the information presented for the constant (baseline) parameter is not of interest.

The column labelled 'Rate Ratio' contains the **parameter estimates**:

1 For the first row, labelled 'cursmoke', this is the *rate ratio* (1.700) comparing smokers at recruitment with never/ex-smokers. This is identical to the rate ratio that was calculated directly from the raw data (see Table 24.3).

2 For the second row, labelled 'constant', this is the *rate of myocardial infarction in the baseline group* (0.00969 = 118/12 183, see Table 24.3). As we explained in the context of logistic regression, this apparently inconsistent labelling is because output from regression models is labelled in a uniform way.

The remaining columns present z statistics, P-values and 95 % confidence intervals corresponding to the model parameters. They will be explained in more detail after the explanation of Table 24.5 below.

Output on the log scale

Table 24.5 shows Poisson regression output, on the log scale, for the association between smoking and rates of myocardial infarction. The model is:

$$\text{Log(Rate)} = \text{Baseline} + \text{Cursmoke}$$

where
- Baseline is the log rate of myocardial infarction in never/ex-smokers, and
- Cursmoke is the log rate ratio comparing the rate of myocardial infarction in smokers with that in never/ex-smokers.

Table 24.5 Poisson regression output (log scale) for the association between smoking and rates of myocardial infarction.

	Coefficient	s.e.	z	P > |z|	95% CI
Cursmoke	0.530	0.113	4.680	0.000	0.308 to 0.752
Constant	−4.64	0.092	−50.37	0.000	−4.82 to −4.45

The interpretation of this output is very similar to that described for logistic regression in Chapter 19; readers are referred there for a more detailed discussion of all components of the output.

1 The *first* column gives the results for the **regression coefficients** (corresponding to the parameter estimates on a log scale). For the row labelled 'cursmoke' this is the *log rate ratio* comparing smokers with non-smokers. It agrees with what would be obtained if it were calculated directly from Table 24.3:

$$\text{log rate ratio} = \log(16.98/9.68) = \log(1.70) = 0.530$$

For the row labelled 'constant', the regression coefficient is the *log rate in the baseline group*, i.e. the log rate of myocardial infarction among non-smokers:

$$\text{log rate} = \log(118/12\,183) = \log(0.00969) = -4.637$$

2 The *second* column gives the *standard errors* of the regression coefficients. For a binary exposure variable, these are exactly the same as those derived using the formulae given in Section 23.2. Thus:

$$\text{s.e.(log rate ratio)} = \sqrt{(1/d_1 + 1/d_0)} = \sqrt{(1/118 + 1/230)} = 0.113$$

$$\text{s.e.(log rate in never/ex-smokers)} = \sqrt{(1/d_0)} = \sqrt{(1/118)} = 0.092$$

3 The *95% confidence intervals* for the regression coefficients in the *last* column are derived in the usual way. For the log rate ratio comparing smokers with never/ex-smokers, the 95% CI is:

$$95\% \text{ CI} = (0.530 - (1.96 \times 0.113)) \text{ to } (0.530 + (1.96 \times 0.113))$$
$$= 0.308 \text{ to } 0.752$$

4 Each *z statistic* in the *third* column is the regression coefficient divided by its standard error. They can be used to derive a Wald test of the null hypothesis that the corresponding regression coefficient = 0.

5 The *P-values* in the *fourth* column are derived from the *z* statistics in the usual manner (see Table A1 in the Appendix) and can be used to test the null hypothesis that the true (population) value for the corresponding population parameter is zero. For example the *P*-value of 0.000 (i.e. < 0.001) for the log rate ratio comparing smokers with never/ex-smokers indicates that there is strong evidence against the null hypothesis that rates of myocardial infarction are the same in smokers as in non-smokers.

As previously explained in the context of logistic regression, we are usually not interested in the *z* statistic and corresponding *P*-value for the *constant* parameter.

Relation between outputs on the ratio and log scales

As with logistic regression, the results in Table 24.4 (output on the original, or ratio, scale) are derived from the results in Table 24.5 (output on the log scale). Once the derivation of the ratio scale output is understood, it is rarely necessary to refer to the log scale output: the most useful results are the rate ratios, confidence intervals and *P*-values displayed on the ratio scale, as in Table 24.4. Note that the output corresponding to the constant term (baseline group) is often omitted from computer output, since the focus of interest is on the parameter estimates (rate ratios) comparing the different groups.

1 In Table 24.4, the column labelled 'Rate Ratio' contains the *exponentials* (antilogs) of the Poisson regression coefficients shown in Table 24.5. Thus the rate ratio comparing smokers with never/ex-smokers $= \exp(0.530) = 1.700$.

2 The *z* statistics and *P*-values are derived from the regression coefficients and their standard errors, and so are identical in the two tables.

3 The 95% confidence intervals in Table 24.4 are derived by antilogging (exponentiating) the confidence intervals on the log scale presented in Table 24.5. Thus the 95% CI for the rate ratio comparing smokers with never/ex-smokers is:

$$95\% \text{ CI} = \exp(0.308) \text{ to } \exp(0.752) = 1.361 \text{ to } 2.121$$

This is identical to the 95% CI calculated using the methods described in Section 23.2.

$$95\% \text{ CI for rate ratio} = \text{rate ratio}/\text{EF to rate ratio} \times \text{EF}$$

where the *error factor* $\text{EF} = \exp(1.96 \times \text{s.e.}(\log \text{ rate ratio}))$. Note that since the calculations are multiplicative:

$$\frac{\text{Rate ratio}}{\text{Lower confidence limit}} = \frac{\text{Upper confidence limit}}{\text{Rate ratio}}$$

This can be a useful check on confidence limits presented in tables in published papers.

24.3 GENERAL FORM OF THE POISSON REGRESSION MODEL

The general form of the Poisson regression model is similar to that for logistic regression (Section 19.3) and that for multiple regression (Section 11.4). It relates the **log rate** to the values of one or more exposure variables:

$$\log(\text{rate}) = \beta_0 + \beta_1 x_1 + \beta_2 x_2 + \ldots + \beta_p x_p$$

The quantity on the right hand side of the equation is known as the **linear predictor** of the log rate, given the particular value of the p exposure variables x_1 to x_p. The β's are the **regression coefficients** associated with the p exposure variables.

Since $\log(\text{rate}) = \log(d/T) = \log(d) - \log(T)$, the general form of the Poisson regression model can also be expressed as:

$$\log(d) = \log(T) + \beta_0 + \beta_1 x_1 + \beta_2 x_2 + \ldots + \beta_p x_p$$

The term $\log(T)$ is known as an **offset** in the regression model. To use statistical packages to fit Poisson regression models we must specify the outcome as the *number* of events and give the exposure time T, which is then included in the offset term, $\log(T)$.

We now show how this general form corresponds to the model we used in Section 24.2 for comparing two exposure groups. The general form for comparing two groups is:

$$\text{Log rate} = \beta_0 + \beta_1 x_1$$

where x_1 (the exposure variable) equals 1 for those in the *exposed* group and 0 for those in the *unexposed* (*baseline*) group.

Using a similar argument to that given in Section 19.3 in the context of logistic regression models, it is straightforward to show that:

1 β_0 (the *intercept*) corresponds to the log rate in the unexposed (baseline) group, and

2 β_1 corresponds to the log of the rate ratio comparing exposed and unexposed groups (the exposure rate ratio).

The equivalent model on the ratio scale is:

$$\text{Rate of disease} = \exp(\beta_0) \times \exp(\beta_1 x_1)$$

In this *multiplicative model* $\exp(\beta_0)$ corresponds to the rate of disease in the baseline group, and $\exp(\beta_1)$ to the exposure rate ratio.

24.4 POISSON REGRESSION FOR CATEGORICAL AND CONTINUOUS EXPOSURE VARIABLES

We now consider Poisson regression models for categorical exposure variables with more than two levels, and for ordered or continuous exposure variables. The principles have already been outlined in detail in Chapter 19, in the context of logistic regression. The application to Poisson regression will be illustrated by examining the association between social class and rates of myocardial infarction in the Caerphilly study.

Poisson regression to compare more than two exposure groups

To examine the effect of **categorical exposure variables** in Poisson and other regression models, we look at the effect of each level compared to a *baseline* group. This is done using *indicator variables*, which are created automatically by most statistical packages, as explained in more detail in Box 19.1 on page 200.

Example 24.2

In the Caerphilly study, a Poisson regression model was fitted to investigate the evidence that rates of myocardial infarction were higher among men in less privileged social classes. Table 24.6 shows the output, with the social class variable, *socclass*, coded from 1 = social class I (most affluent) to 6 = social class V (most deprived). The model was fitted with social class group III non-manual as the baseline group, since this was the largest group in the study, comprising 925 (51.8%) of the men. The regression confirms that there is a pattern of increasing rates of myocardial infarction in more deprived social classes. This trend is investigated further in Table 24.7 below.

Note that some statistical computer packages will allow the user to specify which exposure group is to be treated as the baseline group. In other packages, it may be necessary to recode the values of the variable so that the group chosen to be the baseline group has the lowest coded value.

Table 24.6 Poisson regression output for the effect of social class on the rate of myocardial infarction. The model has six parameters: the rate in the baseline group (rate not shown in the table) and the five rate ratios comparing the other groups with this one. It can be written in abbreviated form as: Rate $=$ Baseline $\times$ Socclass.

	Rate ratio	z	$P > |z|$	95% CI
Socclass(1), I	0.403	−2.36	0.018	0.190 to 0.857
Socclass(2), II	0.759	−1.75	0.080	0.557 to 1.034
Socclass(3), III non-manual	1 (baseline group)			
Socclass(4), III manual	0.956	−0.25	0.802	0.675 to 1.355
Socclass(5), IV	0.965	−0.21	0.836	0.693 to 1.344
Socclass(6), V	1.316	1.14	0.253	0.821 to 2.109

Poisson regression for ordered and continuous exposure variables

Example 24.2 (continued)

To investigate further the tendency for increasing rates of myocardial infarction with increasing deprivation, we can perform a **test for trend** by fitting a Poisson regression model for the linear effect of social class. This will assume a constant

Table 24.7 Poisson regression output for the model for the linear effect of social class on rates of myocardial infarction: Rate = Baseline × [Socclass], where [Socclass] is the rate ratio per unit increase in social class.

	Rate ratio	z	$P > |z|$	95% CI
Socclass	1.117	2.411	0.016	1.021 to 1.223

increase in the log rate ratio for each unit increase in social class, and correspondingly a constant rate ratio per increase in social class. The results are shown in Table 24.7. The estimated rate ratio per unit increase in social class is 1.117 (95% CI 1.021 to 1.223, $P = 0.016$). There is some evidence of an association between increasing social deprivation and increasing rates of myocardial infarction.

24.5 POISSON REGRESSION: CONTROLLING FOR CONFOUNDING

Readers are referred to Chapter 20 for a detailed discussion of how regression models control for confounding in a manner that is analogous to the stratification procedure used in Mantel–Haenszel methods. Both methods assume that the true exposure effect comparing exposed with unexposed individuals is the same in each of the strata defined by the levels of the confounding variable.

Example 24.3
In Section 24.4 we found evidence that rates of myocardial infarction in the Caerphilly study increased with increasing social deprivation. There was also a clear association (not shown here) between social class and the prevalence of smoking at the time of recruitment, with higher smoking rates among men of less privileged social classes. It is therefore possible that social class confounds the association between smoking and rates of myocardial infarction. We will examine this using both Mantel–Haenszel and Poisson regression analyses to estimate the rate ratio for smoking after controlling for social class. We will then compare the results.

Table 24.8 shows the rate ratios for smokers compared to non-smokers in strata defined by social class, together with the Mantel–Haenszel estimate of the rate ratio for smoking controlling for social class. This equals 1.65 (95% CI 1.32 to 2.06), only slightly less than the crude rate ratio of 1.70 (see Table 24.4). It appears therefore that social class is not an important confounder of the association between smoking and rates of myocardial infarction.

Table 24.9 shows the output (on the rate ratio scale) from the corresponding Poisson regression. This model *assumes* that the rate ratio for smoking is the same regardless of social class, and (correspondingly) that the rate ratios for social class are the same regardless of smoking. The estimated rate ratio for smoking controlled for social class is 1.645, almost identical to the Mantel–Haenszel estimate (see Table 24.8). There is also little difference between the crude effect of social class (Table 24.6) and the effect of social class controlling for smoking.

Table 24.8 Rate ratios for the association of smoking with rates of myocardial infarction in the Caerphilly study, separately in social class strata, together with the Mantel–Haenszel estimate of the rate ratio for smoking controlling for social class.

Social class stratum	Rate ratio (95% CI) for smokers compared to non-smokers
I (most affluent)	2.07 (0.46 to 9.23)
II	1.49 (0.86 to 2.58)
III non-manual	1.68 (1.23 to 2.30)
III manual	1.38 (0.73 to 2.62)
IV	1.75 (0.91 to 3.35)
V (least affluent)	2.15 (0.77 to 5.96)
Mantel–Haenszel estimate of the rate ratio for smokers compared to non-smokers, controlling for social class	1.65 (1.32 to 2.06)

$$\chi^2 \text{ for heterogeneity of rate ratios} = 0.82 \text{ (d.f.} = 5, \ P = 0.98)$$

Table 24.9 Poisson regression output for the model including both current smoking and social class. The model can be written in abbreviated form as Rate = Baseline × Cursmoke × Socclass, where the baseline group are non-smokers in Socclass (3).

	Rate ratio	z	$P > |z|$	95% CI
Cursmoke	1.645	4.351	0.000	1.315 to 2.058
Socclass(1)	0.445	−2.103	0.035	0.209 to 0.946
Socclass(2)	0.830	−1.176	0.240	0.608 to 1.133
Socclass(4)	1.014	0.075	0.940	0.715 to 1.437
Socclass(5)	0.976	−0.142	0.887	0.701 to 1.359
Socclass(6)	1.333	1.194	0.232	0.832 to 2.136

Note the different forms of the output for the Mantel–Haenszel and Poisson regression approaches. The Mantel–Haenszel output shows us stratum-specific effects of the exposure variable, which draws our attention to differences between strata and reminds us that when we control for smoking we assume that the effect of smoking is the same in different social classes. The Poisson regression output shows us the effect of smoking controlled for social class, and the effect of social class controlled for smoking. However, we should be aware of the need to test the underlying assumption that the effect of each variable is the same regardless of the value of the other: that is that there is no **effect modification**, also known as **interaction**. For Mantel–Haenszel methods this was described in Section 23.3. We see how to examine interaction in regression models in Chapter 29.

24.6 SPLITTING FOLLOW-UP TO ALLOW FOR VARIABLES WHICH CHANGE OVER TIME

In any long-term study the values of one or more of the exposure variables may change over time. The most important such change is in the **age** of subjects in the study. Since rates of most disease outcomes are strongly associated with age, we will usually wish to control for age in our analysis.

To allow for changes in age, or for any exposure variable whose value changes during the study, we simply divide the follow-up time for each person into distinct periods, during which the variable does not change. Since age, of course, changes constantly we divide the follow-up time into **age groups**. For example, in the Caerphilly study we might use five-year age groups: 40–44, 45–49, 50–54 and so on. Note that age 50–54 means 'from the date of the 50th birthday to the day before the 55th birthday'. The underlying assumption is that rates do not differ much *within* an age group, so that for example it assumes that the rate of myocardial infarction will be similar for a 54-year-old and a 50-year-old. Narrower age bands will be appropriate when rates vary rapidly with age; for example in a study of infant mortality.

Table 24.10 and Figure 24.1 illustrate the division of the follow-up period into 5-year age bands for subject numbers 1 and 2 in the Caerphilly dataset. Subject 1 was aged 58.52 years when he was recruited, and therefore started in the 55–59 age group. He passed through the 60–64, 65–69 and 70–74 age groups, and was in the 75–79 age group at the end of the study (at which time he was aged 75.36). Subject 2 was also in the 55–59 age group when he was recruited. He was in the 60–64 age group when he experienced a myocardial infarction on 27 Feb 1985, at which time he was aged 61.81.

It is important to note that the value of MI (myocardial infarction, the outcome variable) is equal to 0 for every interval unless the subject experienced an MI at the end of the interval, in which case it is 1. Thus for subject 1, the value of MI is 0 for every interval, and for subject 2 it is 0 for the first interval and 1 for the second interval. In general, the value of the outcome variable for a subject who experienced the outcome will be zero for every interval except the last.

Having divided the follow-up time in this way, we may now use **Mantel–Haenszel** or **Poisson regression** methods to examine the way in which disease rates change with age group, or to examine the effects of other exposures having

Table 24.10 Follow-up time split into 5-year age bands for the first two subjects in the Caerphilly study.

Date at start of interval	Date at end of interval	Age group	Age at start of interval	Age at end of interval	Years in interval	MI
Subject 1, born 22 Aug 1923, recruited 1 Mar 1982, exit (at end of follow-up) 31 Dec 1998						
1 Mar 1982	21 Aug 1983	55–59	58.52	60	1.48	0
22 Aug 1983	21 Aug 1988	60–64	60	65	5	0
22 Aug 1988	21 Aug 1993	65–69	65	70	5	0
22 Aug 1993	21 Aug 1998	70–74	70	75	5	0
22 Aug 1998	31 Dec 1998	75–79	75	75.36	0.36	0
Subject 2, born 8 May 1923, recruited 30 May 1982, exit (on date of MI) 27 Feb 1985						
30 May 1982	7 May 1983	55–59	59.06	60	0.94	0
8 May 1983	27 Feb 1985	60–64	60	61.81	1.81	1

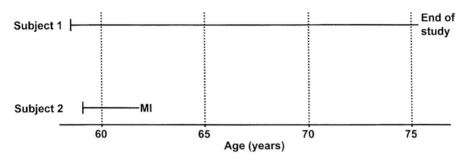

Fig. 24.1 Age of subjects 1 and 2 during the Caerphilly study. The dotted vertical lines denote 5-year age bands.

controlled for the effects of age group. Perhaps surprisingly, we analyse the contributions from the different time periods from the same individual in exactly the same way as if they were from different individuals. See Clayton and Hills (1993) for the reasons why this is justified. Also, note that if we analyse this expanded data set (with follow-up split into age groups) but omit age group from the analysis we will get exactly the same answer as in the analysis using the original intervals. This is because the number of events and the total follow-up time are exactly the same in the original and expanded datasets.

Table 24.11 shows the total number of events (d) and person-years (T) in the different age groups in the Caerphilly study, together with the rates per 1000 person-years and corresponding 95% confidence intervals. Rates of myocardial infarction generally increased with increasing age.

Table 24.11 Rates of myocardial infarction in different age groups in the Caerphilly study.

Age group	d	T	Rate per 1000 person-years	95% CI
45–49	12	1 627	7.376	4.189 to 12.989
50–54	42	4 271	9.833	7.267 to 13.305
55–59	73	6 723	10.858	8.632 to 13.657
60–64	102	7 115	14.336	11.807 to 17.406
65–69	76	4 287	17.726	14.157 to 22.195
70–74	30	1 872	16.029	11.207 to 22.926
75–79	13	266	48.958	28.428 to 84.315

This same approach may be used to examine any effect that may change over time. For example:

- if **repeat measurements of exposures** are made on different occasions after baseline, we may divide the follow-up time into the periods following each measurement, with *time-updated* values of the exposure measured at the beginning of each period.
- **secular changes** can be analysed by dividing time into different **time periods** (for example, 1970 to 1974, 1975 to 1979, etc.).

Joint effects may be investigated by dividing the period of follow-up according to the values of two variables. Note that the way in which individuals move through different categories of age group and time period may be displayed in a **Lexis diagram** (see Clayton and Hills, 1993 or Szklo and Nieto, 2000).

In Section 27.5, we explain how Poisson regression with follow-up time split into intervals is related to **Cox regression** analysis of survival data, and in Section 27.4 we discuss the criteria for choice of the time axis.

CHAPTER 25

Standardization

25.1 INTRODUCTION

Death rates and disease incidence rates are usually strongly related to age, and often differ for the two sexes. Population mortality and incidence rates therefore depend critically on the age–sex composition of the population. For example, a relatively older population would have a higher crude mortality rate than a younger population even if, age-for-age, the rates were the same. It is therefore misleading to use overall rates when comparing two different populations unless they have the same age–sex structure. We saw in Chapter 23 how to use Mantel–Haenszel methods and in Chapter 24 how to use Poisson regression to compare rates between different groups after controlling for variables such as age and sex.

We now describe the use of **standardization** and **standardized rates** to produce comparable measures between populations or sub-groups, adjusted for major confounders, such as any age–sex differences in the composition of the different populations or subgroups. **Mantel–Haenszel** or **regression methods** should be used to make formal comparisons between them.

There are two methods of standardization: *direct* and *indirect*, as summarized in Table 25.1. Both use a **standard population**.

Table 25.1 Comparison of direct and indirect methods of standardization.

	Direct standardization	Indirect standardization
Method	Study rates applied to standard population	Standard rates applied to study population
Data required		
Study population(s)	Age–sex specific rates	Age–sex composition + total deaths (or cases)
Standard population	Age–sex composition	Age–sex specific rates (+ overall rate)
Result	Age–sex adjusted rate	Standardized mortality (morbidity) ratio (+ age–sex adjusted rate)

- In **direct standardization**, the age–sex specific rates from each of the populations under study are applied to a *standard* population. The result is a set of **standardized rates**.
- In **indirect standardization**, the age–sex specific rates from a *standard* population are applied to each of the study populations. The result is a set of **standardized mortality (or morbidity) ratios (SMRs)**.

The choice of method is usually governed by the availability of data and by their (relative) accuracy. Thus, direct standardization gives more accurate results when there are small numbers of events in any of the age–sex groups of the study populations. The indirect method will be preferable if it is difficult to obtain national data on age–sex specific rates.

Both methods can be extended to adjust for other factors besides age and sex, such as different ethnic compositions of the study groups. The direct method can also be used to calculate **standardized means**, such as age–sex adjusted mean blood pressure levels for different occupational groups.

25.2 DIRECT STANDARDIZATION

Example 25.1

Table 25.2 shows the number of cases of prostate cancer and number of person-years among men aged ≥ 65 living in France between 1979 and 1996. The data are shown separately for six 3-year time periods. Corresponding rates of prostate cancer per 1000 person-years at risk (pyar) are shown in Table 25.3

Table 25.3 shows that the crude rates (those derived from the total number of cases and person-years, ignoring age group) increased to a peak of 2.64/1000 pyar in 1988–90 and then declined. However Table 25.2 shows that the age-distribution of the population was also changing during this time: the number of person-years in the oldest (≥ 85 year) age group more than doubled between 1979–81 and 1994–96, while increases in other age groups were more modest. The oldest age group also experienced the highest rate of prostate cancer, in all time periods.

Table 25.2 Cases of prostate cancer/1000 person-years among men aged ≥ 65 living in France between 1979 and 1996.

	Time period					
Age group	1979–81	1982–84	1985–87	1988–90	1991–93	1994–96
65–69	2021/2970	1555/2197	1930/2686	2651/3589	2551/3666	2442/3764
70–74	3924/2640	3946/2674	3634/2272	2842/1860	3863/2703	4158/3177
75–79	5297/1886	5638/1946	6018/1980	6211/2028	4640/1598	4253/1659
80–84	4611/985	5400/1134	6199/1189	6844/1294	6926/1393	6412/1347
≥ 85	3273/478	3812/539	4946/616	6581/764	7680/878	8819/1003
Total	19126/8959	20351/8490	22727/8743	25129/9535	25660/10238	26084/10950

Table 25.3 Rates of prostate cancer (per 1000 person-years) in men aged ≥ 65 living in France between 1979 and 1996.

	Time period					
Age group	1979–81	1982–84	1985–87	1988–90	1991–93	1994–96
65–69	0.68	0.71	0.72	0.74	0.70	0.65
70–74	1.49	1.48	1.60	1.53	1.43	1.31
75–79	2.81	2.90	3.04	3.06	2.90	2.56
80–84	4.68	4.76	5.21	5.29	4.97	4.76
≥ 85	6.85	7.07	8.03	8.61	8.75	8.79
Crude rate	2.13	2.40	2.60	2.64	2.51	2.38
Standardized rate	2.35	2.40	2.60	2.64	2.64	2.39

This means that the overall rates in each time period need to be adjusted for the age distribution of the corresponding population before they can meaningfully be compared. We will do this using the method of direct standardization.

1 The first step in direct standardization is to identify a standard population. This is usually one of the following:
   - one of the study populations
   - the total of the study populations
   - the census population from the local area or country

The choice is to some extent arbitrary. Different choices lead to different summary rates but this is unlikely to affect the interpretation of the results unless the patterns of change are different in the different age group strata (see point 5). Here we will use the number of person-years for the period 1985–87.

2 Second, for *each of the time periods of interest*, we calculate what would be the overall rate of prostate cancer in our standard population if the age-specific rates equalled those of the time period of interest. This is called the *age standardized survival rate* for that time period.

$$\text{Age standardized rate} = \begin{array}{c}\text{Overall rate in standard population}\\\text{if the age-specific rates were the same}\\\text{as those of the population of interest}\end{array} = \frac{\Sigma(w_i \times \lambda_i)}{\Sigma w_i}$$

In the above definition, w_i is the person-years at risk in age group i in the standard population, $\lambda_i = d_i/pyar_i$ is the rate in age group i in the time period of interest and the summation is over all age groups. Note that this is simply a **weighted average** (see Section 18.3) of the rates in the different age groups in the time period of interest, weighted by the person-years at risk in each age group in the standard population.

Table 25.4 Calculating the age standardized rate of prostate cancer for 1979–81, using direct standardization with the person-years during 1985–87 as the standard population.

Age group	Standard population: thousands of person-years in 1985–87, w_i	Study population: Rates in 1979–81, λ_i	Estimated number of cases in standard population, $w_i \times \lambda_i$
65–69	2686	0.68	1827.7
70–74	2272	1.49	3377.0
75–79	1980	2.81	5561.0
80–84	1189	4.68	5566.0
≥ 85	616	6.85	4217.9
All ages	$\Sigma w_i = 8743$		$\Sigma(w_i \times \lambda_i) = 20549.6$
		Age adjusted rate $= 2.35$	

For example, Table 25.4 shows the details of the calculations for the age-standardized rate for 1979–81, using the person-years in 1985–87 as the standard population. In the 65 to 69-year age group, applying the rate of 0.68 per 1000 person-years to the 2686 person-years in that age group in the standard population gives an estimated number of cases in this age group of $0.68 \times 2686 = 1827.7$. Repeating the same procedure for each age group, and then summing the numbers obtained, gives an overall estimate of 20549.6 cases out of the total of 8743 thousand person-years in the *standard* population: an age-standardized rate for the *study* population of 2.35 per 1000 person-years.

3 The results for all the time periods are shown in the bottom row of Table 25.3. The crude and standardized rates of prostate cancer in the different time periods are plotted in Figure 25.1(a). This shows that the crude rate was lower than the directly standardized rate in the 1979–81 period, but similar thereafter. This is because, as can be seen in Table 25.2, in the 1979–81 period there were proportionally fewer person-years in the oldest age groups, in which prostate cancer death rates were highest.

4 The standard error for the standardized rate is calculated as:

Standard error of standardized rate	Standard error of standardized proportion
$\dfrac{1}{\Sigma w_i}\sqrt{\left(\Sigma \dfrac{w_i^2 d_i}{(pyar_i)^2}\right)}$	$\dfrac{1}{\Sigma w_i}\sqrt{\left(\Sigma \dfrac{w_i^2 p_i(1-p_i)}{n_i}\right)}$

where the left hand formula is used for standardized rates and the right hand formula for standardized proportions. In these formulae the weights w_i are the person-years or number of individuals in the standard population. Using this formula, the standard error of the standardized rate in 1979–81 is 0.017 per 1000 person-years, so that the 95% confidence interval for the standardized rate in 1979–81 is:

$$95\% \ \mathrm{CI} = 2.35 - 1.96 \times 0.017 \ \text{to} \ 2.35 + 1.96 \times 0.017$$
$$= 2.32 \ \text{to} \ 2.38 \ \text{per} \ 1000 \ \text{person-years}$$

5 Finally, it is important to inspect the patterns of rates in the individual strata before standardizing, because when we standardize we assume *that the patterns of change in the rates are similar in each stratum*. If this is not the case then the choice of standard population will influence the observed pattern of change in the standardized rates. For example, in Figure 25.1(b) it can be seen that the rate in the ≥85 year age group increased more sharply than the rates in the other age groups. This means that the greater the proportion of individuals in the ≥85 year age group in the standard population, the sharper will be the increase in the standardized rate over time.

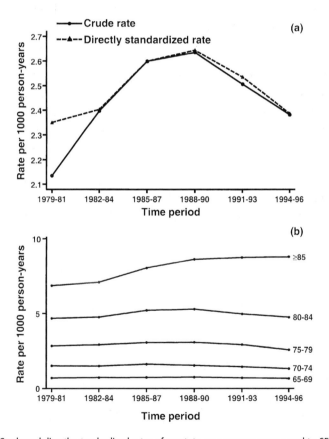

Fig. 25.1 (a) Crude and directly standardized rates of prostate cancer among men aged ≥ 65 years living in France between 1979 and 1986, with the population in 1985–87 chosen as the standard population. (b) Time trends in age-specific rates of prostate cancer, among men aged ≥ 65 years living in France between 1979 and 1986.

25.3 INDIRECT STANDARDIZATION

Example 25.2

Table 25.5 shows mortality rates from a large one-year study in an area endemic for onchocerciasis. One feature of interest was to assess whether blindness, the severest consequence of onchocerciasis, leads to increased death rates. From the results presented in Table 25.5 it can be seen that:

- not only does mortality increase with age and differ slightly between males and females, but
- the prevalence of blindness also increases with age and is higher for males than for females.

The blind sub-population is therefore on average older, with a higher proportion of males, than the non-blind sub-population. This means that it would have a higher crude mortality rate than the non-blind sub-population, even if the individual age–sex specific rates were the same. An overall comparison between the blind and non-blind will be obtained using the method of indirect standardization.

1 As for direct standardization, the *first* step is to identify a standard population. The usual choices are as before, with the restrictions that age–sex specific mortality rates are needed for the standard population and that the population chosen for this should therefore be large enough to have reliable estimates of these rates. In this example the rates among the non-blind will be used.

2 These standard rates are then applied to the population of interest to calculate the *number of deaths* that would have been *expected* in this population if the mortality experience were the same as that in the standard population.

   For example, in stratum 1 (males aged 30–39 years) one would expect a proportion of 19/2400 of the 120 blind to die, if their risk of dying was the same as that of the non-blind males of similar age. This gives an expected 0.95 deaths for this age group. In total, 22.55 deaths would have been expected among the blind compared to a total observed number of 69.

3 The ratio of the observed to the expected number of deaths is called the **standardized mortality ratio (SMR)**. It equals 3.1 (69/22.55) in this case. Overall, blind persons were 3.1 times more likely to die during the year than non-blind persons.

$$
\text{Standardized mortality ratio (SMR)} = \frac{\text{observed number of deaths}}{\substack{\text{expected number of deaths if the} \\ \text{age–sex specific rates were the same} \\ \text{as those of the } \textit{standard} \text{ population}}} = \frac{\Sigma d_i}{\Sigma E_i}
$$

The SMR measures how much more (or less) likely a person is to die in the study population compared to someone of the same age and sex in the standard population. A value of 1 means that they are equally likely to die, a value larger

Table 25.5 Use of indirect standardization to compare mortality rates between the blind and non-blind, collected as part of a one-year study in an area endemic for onchocerciasis. The mortality rates among the non-blind have been used as the standard rates.

Age (yrs)	Stratum (i)	Non-blind persons			% blind	Blind persons			Expected number of deaths among blind if rates were the same as those of the non-blind ($E_i = \lambda_i \times T_i$)
		Number of person-years	Number of deaths	Deaths/1000/ yr (λ_i)		Number of person-years (T_i)	Number of deaths (d_i)	Deaths/1000/yr	
Males									
30–39	1	2400	19	7.9	4.8	120	3	25.0	0.95
40–49	2	1590	21	13.2	9.7	171	7	40.9	2.26
50–59	3	1120	20	17.9	17.9	244	13	53.3	4.36
60+	4	610	20	32.8	28.0	237	24	101.3	7.77
Females									
30–39	5	3100	23	7.4	2.6	84	2	23.8	0.62
40–49	6	1610	22	13.7	4.1	69	3	43.5	0.94
50–59	7	930	16	17.2	15.3	168	8	47.6	2.89
60+	8	270	8	29.6	25.6	93	9	96.8	2.76
Total		11630	149	12.8	9.3		69	58.2	22.55
SMR				1.0				3.1 (69/22.5)	
Age-sex adjusted mortality rate				12.8				39.7 (3.1 × 12.8)	

than 1 that they are more likely to die, and a value smaller than 1 that they are less likely to do so. The SMR is sometimes multiplied by 100 and expressed as a percentage. Since the non-blind population was used as the standard, its expected and observed numbers of deaths are equal, resulting in an SMR of 1.

4 The 95% confidence interval for the SMR is derived using an error factor (EF) in the same way as that for a rate ratio (see Section 23.2):

$$95\% \text{ CI} = \text{SMR}/\text{EF to SMR} \times \text{EF}, \text{ where}$$
$$\text{EF} = \exp(1.96/\sqrt{d_i})$$

In this example, $\text{EF} = \exp(1.96/\sqrt{69}) = 1.266$, and the 95% confidence interval for the SMR is:

$$95\% \text{ CI} = \frac{\text{SMR}}{\text{EF}} \text{ to SMR} \times \text{EF} = 3.06/1.266 \text{ to } 3.06 \times 1.266 = 2.42 \text{ to } 3.87$$

5 Age–sex adjusted mortality rates may be obtained by multiplying the SMRs by the crude mortality rate of the standard population, when this is known. This gives age–sex adjusted mortality rates of 12.8 and 39.7/1000/year for the non-blind and blind populations respectively.

$$\begin{array}{ccc}\text{Age–sex adjusted} \\ \text{mortality rate}\end{array} = \text{SMR} \times \begin{array}{c}\text{crude mortality rate of} \\ \text{standard population}\end{array}$$

25.4 USE OF POISSON REGRESSION FOR INDIRECT STANDARDIZATION

We may use Poisson regression to derive the SMR, by fitting a model with:
- each row of data corresponding to the strata in the study population;
- the number of events in the study population as the outcome. In Example 25.2 this would be the number of deaths in the blind population;
- *no* exposure variables (a 'constant-only' model);
- specifying the *expected number* of events in each stratum (each row of the data), instead of the number of person-years, as the offset in the model. In Example 25.2, these are the expected number of deaths given in the right hand column of Table 25.5.

Table 25.6 shows the output from fitting such a model to the data in Example 25.2. The output is on the log scale, so the SMR is calculated by antilogging the

Table 25.6 Poisson regression output (log scale), using the expected number of deaths in the blind population as the offset.

	Coefficient	s.e.	z	$P > \lvert z \rvert$	95% CI
Constant	1.1185	0.1204	9.29	0.000	0.8825 to 1.3544

coefficient for the constant term. It equals $\exp(1.1185) = 3.1$, the same as the value calculated above.

$$SMR = \exp(\text{regression coefficient for constant term})$$

The 95% CI for the SMR is derived by antilogging the confidence interval for the constant term. It is $\exp(0.8825)$ to $\exp(1.3544) = 2.42$ to 3.87. It should be noted that indirect standardization assumes that the age–sex specific rates in the standard population are known without error. Clearly this is not true in the example we have used: the consequence of this is that confidence intervals for the SMR derived in this way will be somewhat too narrow. For comparison, a standard Poisson regression analysis of the association between blindness and death rates for the data in Table 25.5 gives a rate ratio of 3.05, and a 95% CI of 2.24 to 4.15.

Extension to several SMRs

It is fairly straightforward to extend this procedure to estimate, for example, the SMRs for each area in a geographical region by calculating the observed and expected number of deaths in each age–sex stratum in each area, and fitting a Poisson regression model including indicator variables for each area, and *omitting* the constant term. The SMRs would then be the antilogs of the coefficients for the different area indicator variables.

CHAPTER 26

Survival analysis: displaying and comparing survival patterns

26.1 INTRODUCTION

The methods described so far in this part of the book assume that rates are constant over the period of study, or within time periods such as age groups defined by splitting follow-up time as described in Section 24.6. However, in longitudinal studies in which there is a clear event from which subjects are followed, such as diagnosis of a condition or initiation of treatment, it may not be reasonable to assume that rates are constant, even over short periods of time. For example:

- the risk of death is very high immediately after heart surgery, falls as the patient recovers, then rises again over time;
- the recurrence rate of tumours, following diagnosis and treatment of breast cancer, varies considerably with time.

Methods for **survival analysis** allow analysis of such rates without making the assumption that they are constant. They focus on:

1 the **hazard** $h(t)$: the instantaneous rate at time t. They do not assume that the hazard is constant within time periods;

2 the **survivor function** $S(t)$, illustrated by the **survival curve**. This is the probability that an individual will survive (i.e. has not experienced the event of interest) up to and including time t.

We start by describing two ways of estimating the survival curve; life tables and the Kaplan–Meier method. We will then explain the proportional hazards assumption, and discuss how to compare the survival of two groups using Mantel–Cox methods. In the next chapter we will discuss regression analysis of survival data. We will see that these methods are closely related to, and often give similar results to, the Mantel–Haenszel and Poisson regression methods for the analysis of rates.

In Chapter 22 we stated that survival times for subjects who are known to have survived up to a certain point in time, but whose survival status past that point is not known, are said to be **censored**. Throughout this and the next chapter we will assume that the probability of being censored (either through loss to follow-up or because of death from causes other than the one being studied) is unrelated to the probability that the event of interest occurs. If this assumption is violated then we say that there is **informative censoring**, and special methods must be used.

26.2 LIFE TABLES

Life tables are used to display the survival pattern of a community when we do not know the exact survival time of each individual, but we do know the number of individuals who survive at a succession of time points. They may take one of two different forms. The first, a *cohort life table*, shows the actual survival of a group of individuals through time. The starting point from which the survival time is measured may be birth, or it may be some other event. For example, a cohort life table may be used to show the mortality experience of an occupational group according to length of employment in the occupation, or the survival pattern of patients following a treatment, such as radiotherapy for small-cell carcinoma of bronchus (Table 26.1). The second type of life table, a *current life table*, shows the expected survivorship through time of a hypothetical population to which current age-specific death rates have been applied. Historically, this was more often used for actuarial purposes and was less common in medical research. In recent times, this approach has been used to model the burden of disease due to different causes and conditions (Murray & Lopez, 1996).

Example 26.1
Table 26.1 shows the survival of patients with small-cell carcinoma of bronchus, month by month following treatment with radiotherapy. This table is based on data collected from a total of 240 patients over a 5 year period. The data themselves are summarized in columns 1–4 of the life table; the construction of a **cohort life table** is shown in columns 5–8.

Column 1 shows the number of months since treatment with radiotherapy began. Columns 2 and 3 contain the number of patients alive at the beginning of each month and the number who died during the month. For example, 12 of the 240 patients died during the first month of treatment, leaving 228 still alive at the start of the second month. The number of patients who were censored during each month (known to have survived up to month i but lost to follow-up after that time) is shown in column 4. The total number of persons at risk of dying during the month, adjusting for these losses, is shown in column 5. This equals the

Table 26.1 Life table showing the survival pattern of 240 patients with small-cell carcinoma of bronchus treated with radiotherapy.

(1) Interval (months) since start of treatment i	(2) Number alive at beginning of interval a_i	(3) Deaths during interval d_i	(4) Number censored (lost to follow-up) during interval c_i	(5) Number of persons at risk $n_i = a_i - c_i/2$	(6) Risk of dying during interval $r_i = d_i/n_i$	(7) Chance of surviving interval $s_i = 1 - r_i$	(8) Cumulative chance of survival from start of treatment $S(i) = S(i-1) \times s_i$
1	240	12	0	240.0	0.0500	0.9500	0.9500
2	228	9	0	228.0	0.0395	0.9605	0.9125
3	219	17	1	218.5	0.0778	0.9222	0.8415
4	201	36	4	199.0	0.1809	0.8191	0.6893
5	161	6	2	160.0	0.0375	0.9625	0.6634
6	153	18	7	149.5	0.1204	0.8796	0.5835
7	128	13	5	125.5	0.1036	0.8964	0.5231
8	110	11	3	108.5	0.1014	0.8986	0.4700
9	96	14	3	94.5	0.1481	0.8519	0.4004
10	79	13	0	79.0	0.1646	0.8354	0.3345
11	66	15	4	64.0	0.2344	0.7656	0.2561
12	47	6	1	46.5	0.1290	0.8710	0.2231
13	40	6	0	40.0	0.1500	0.8500	0.1896
14	34	4	2	33.0	0.1212	0.8788	0.1666
15	28	5	0	28.0	0.1786	0.8214	0.1369
16	23	7	1	22.5	0.3111	0.6889	0.0943
17	15	12	0	15.0	0.8000	0.2000	0.0189
18	3	3	0	3.0	1.0000	0.0000	0.0000

number alive at the beginning of the month minus half the number lost to follow-up, assuming that on average these losses occur half-way through the month.

Column 6 shows the risk of dying during a month, calculated as the number of deaths during the month divided by the number of persons at risk. Column 7 contains the complementary chance of surviving the month.

Column 8 shows the cumulative chance of surviving. This is calculated by applying the rules of conditional probability (see Chapter 14). It equals the chance of surviving up to the end of the previous month, multiplied by the chance of surviving the month. For example, the chance of surviving the first month was 0.9500. During the second month the chance of surviving was 0.9605. The overall chance of surviving two months from the start of treatment was therefore $0.9500 \times 0.9605 = 0.9125$. In this study all the patients had died by the end of 18 months.

More generally, the cumulative chance of surviving to the end of month i is given by:

$$S(i) = \text{chance of surviving to month } (i-1) \times \text{chance of surviving month } i$$
$$= S(i-1) \times s_i \text{ or } s_1 \times s_2 \times \ldots \times s_i$$

These are the **probabilities $S(i)$ of the survivor function**. The survival curve is illustrated in Figure 26.1.

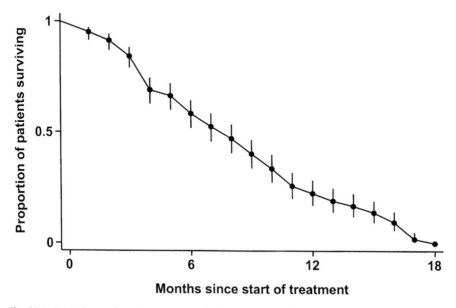

Fig. 26.1 Survival curve for patients with small-cell carcinoma of the bronchus treated with radiotherapy, drawn from life table calculations presented in Table 26.1.

Confidence interval for the survival curve

The 95% confidence interval for each $S(i)$ is derived using an error factor (see Kalbfleisch & Prentice, 1980, pp. 14, 15 for details) as follows:

$$95\% \text{ CI} = S(t)^{(1/\text{EF})} \text{ to } S(t)^{\text{EF}}, \text{ where}$$

$$\text{EF} = \exp\left[1.96 \times \frac{\sqrt{[\Sigma d/(n(n-d))]}}{[\Sigma \log((n-d)/n)]^2}\right]$$

In this formula, the summations are over all the values of d and n, up to and including time interval i. Figure 26.1 includes the 95% confidence intervals calculated in this way, using the data in columns 3 and 5 of Table 26.1. Because derivation of such confidence intervals involves a substantial amount of calculation, it is usually done using a statistical computer package.

Life expectancy

Also of interest is the average length of survival, or **life expectancy**, following the start of treatment. This may be crudely estimated from the survival curve as the time corresponding to a cumulative probability of survival of 0.5, or it may be calculated using columns 1 and 8 of the life table. For each interval, the length of the interval is multiplied by the cumulative chance of surviving. The total of these values plus a half gives the life expectancy. (The addition of a half is to allow for the effect of grouping the life table in whole months and is similar to the continuity corrections we have encountered in earlier chapters.)

$$\text{Life expectancy} = 0.5 + \sum \left(\begin{array}{c} \text{length of} \\ \text{interval} \end{array} \times \begin{array}{c} \text{cumulative chance} \\ \text{of survival} \end{array} \right)$$

In Table 26.1 all the intervals are of 1 month and so the life expectancy is simply the sum of the values in column 8 plus a half, which equals 7.95 months.

26.3 KAPLAN–MEIER ESTIMATE OF THE SURVIVAL CURVE

In many studies we know the exact follow up time (for example, to within 1 day) for each individual in the study, and may therefore wish to estimate the survivor function $S(t)$ using this information rather than by dividing the survival time into discrete periods, as is done in the life table method. This avoids the assumption that individuals lost to follow-up are censored half way through the interval. The difference between the approaches is likely to be minimal if the periods in the life table are short, such as 1 month, but for longer periods (such as 1 year) information is likely to be lost by grouping.

The estimate using exact failure and censoring times is known as the **Kaplan–Meier** estimate, and is based on a similar argument to that used in deriving life tables. To derive the Kaplan–Meier estimate, we consider the **risk sets** of individuals still being studied at *each time, t, at which an event occurs*. If there are n_t individuals in the risk set at time t, and d_t events occur at that precise time then the estimated *risk*, r_t, of an event at time t is d_t/n_t, and so the estimated **survival probability at time t** is:

$$s_t = 1 - r_t = \frac{n_t - d_t}{n_t}$$

At *all* times at which no event occurs, the estimated survival probability is 1.

To estimate the survivor function, we use a similar conditional probability argument to that used in deriving life tables. We number the times at which disease events occur as t_1, t_2, t_3 and so on. Since the estimated survival probability until just before t_1 is 1:

$$S(t_1) = 1 \times s_{t_1} = s_{t_1}$$

The survival probability remains unchanged until the next disease event, at time t_2. The survivor function at this time t_2 is:

$$S(t_2) = S(t_1) \times s_{t_2} = s_{t_1} \times s_{t_2}$$

In general, the survival probability up to and including event j is:

$$S(t_j) = S(t_{(j-1)}) \times s_{t_j} = s_{t_1} \times s_{t_2} \times \ldots \times s_{t_j}$$

This is known as the **product-limit formula**. Note that loss to follow-up does not affect the estimate of survival probability: the next survival probability is calculated on the basis of the new denominator, reduced by the number of subjects lost to follow-up since the last event.

Example 26.2
The examples for the rest of this chapter are based on data from a randomized trial (see Chapter 34) of Azathioprine for primary biliary cirrhosis, a chronic and eventually fatal liver disease (Christensen *et al.*, 1985). The trial was designed to

compare an active treatment, Azathioprine, against placebo. Between October 1971 and December 1977, 248 patients were entered into the trial and followed for up to 12 years. A total of 184 patients had the values of all prognostic variables measured at baseline. Of these, 31 had central cholestasis (a marker of disease severity) at entry. Among these 31 patients there were 24 deaths, and 7 losses to follow-up, as shown in Table 26.2.

The first death was at 19 days, so the risk of death at 19 days was $r_{19} = 1/31 = 0.0323$. The survival probability at 19 days is therefore $s_{19} = 1 - 0.0323 = 0.9677$, and the survivor function $S(19) = s_{19} = 0.9677$. The next death was at 48 days; at this point 30 patients were still at risk. The risk of death at 48 days was $r_{48} = 1/30 = 0.0333$. The survival probability at 48 days is therefore $s_{48} = 1 - 0.0333 = 0.9667$, and the survivor function $S(48) = s_{19} \times s_{48} = 0.9355$. Similarly, the estimate of the survivor function at 96 days is $s_{19} \times s_{48} \times s_{96} = 0.9677 \times 0.9667 \times 0.9655 = 0.9032$, and so on.

Displaying the Kaplan–Meier estimate of S(t)

The conventional display of the Kaplan–Meier estimate of the survival curve for the 31 patients with central cholestasis is shown in Figure 26.2. The survival curve is shown as a **step function**; the curve is horizontal at all times at which there is no outcome event, with a vertical drop corresponding to the change in the survivor function at each time when an event occurs. At the right-hand end of the curve, when there are very few patients still at risk, the times between events and the drops in the survivor function become large, because the estimated risk ($r_t = d_t/n_t$) is large at each time t at which an event occurs, as n_t is small. The survivor function should be interpreted cautiously when few patients remain at risk.

Confidence interval for the survival curve

Confidence intervals for $S(t)$ are derived in the same way as described earlier for life tables.

26.4 COMPARISON OF HAZARDS: THE PROPORTIONAL HAZARDS ASSUMPTION

The main focus of interest in survival analysis is in comparing the survival patterns of different groups. For example, Figure 26.3 shows the Kaplan–Meier estimates of the survivor functions for the two groups of patients with and without central cholestasis at baseline. It seems clear that survival times for patients without central cholestasis at baseline were much longer, but how should we quantify the difference in survival? The differences between the survival curves are obviously not constant. For example both curves start at 1, but never come together

Table 26.2 Derivation of the Kaplan–Meier estimate of the survivor function $S(t)$, for 31 patients with primary biliary cirrhosis complicated by central cholestasis. Analyses of this study are by kind permission of Dr E. Christensen.

Time (days) t	Number at risk at time of event(s) n_t	Number of deaths at time t d_t	Number lost to follow-up at time t c_t	Risk of death $r_t = d_t/n_t$	Probability of survival $s_t = 1 - r_t$	Survivor function $S(t) = S(t_{previous}) \times s_t$
19	31	1	0	0.0323	0.9677	0.9677
48	30	1	0	0.0333	0.9667	0.9355
96	29	1	0	0.0345	0.9655	0.9032
150	28	1	0	0.0357	0.9643	0.8710
177	27	1	0	0.0370	0.9630	0.8387
193	26	1	0	0.0385	0.9615	0.8065
201	25	1	0	0.0400	0.9600	0.7742
245	24	1	0	0.0417	0.9583	0.7419
251	23	1	0	0.0435	0.9565	0.7097
256	22	1	0	0.0455	0.9545	0.6774
302	21	0	1	0	1	0.6774
341	20	1	0	0.0500	0.9500	0.6435
395	19	1	0	0.0526	0.9474	0.6097
421	18	1	0	0.0556	0.9444	0.5758
464	17	1	0	0.0588	0.9412	0.5419
578	16	1	0	0.0625	0.9375	0.5081
582	15	0	1	0	1	0.5081
586	14	0	1	0	1	0.5081
688	13	1	0	0.0769	0.9231	0.4690
828	12	0	1	0	1	0.4690
947	11	1	0	0.0909	0.9091	0.4263
1159	10	0	1	0	1	0.4263
1219	9	1	0	0.1111	0.8889	0.3790
1268	8	1	0	0.1250	0.8750	0.3316
1292	7	0	1	0	1	0.3316
1693	6	1	0	0.1667	0.8333	0.2763
1881	5	1	0	0.2000	0.8000	0.2211
1940	4	1	0	0.2500	0.7500	0.1658
1975	3	1	0	0.3333	0.6667	0.1105
2338	2	0	1	0	1	0.1105
2343	1	1	0	1	0	0

$$\log(H_1(t)) - \log(H_0(t)) = \log(\text{constant})$$

Therefore, if the proportional hazards assumption is correct then graphs of the log of the cumulative hazard function in the exposed and unexposed groups will be parallel.

Figure 26.4 shows the log cumulative hazard against time since start of treatment for primary biliary cirrhosis patients with and without central cholestasis at baseline. It suggests that there is no major violation of the proportional hazards assumption, since the lines appear to be reasonably parallel. In this example time has been plotted on a log scale to stretch out the early part of the time scale, compared to the later, because more events occur at the beginning of the study than near the end. Note, however, that this does not affect the relative positioning of the lines; they should be parallel whether time is plotted on a log scale or on the original scale.

It can be shown mathematically that that the cumulative hazard is related to the survival function by the following formulae:

$$H(t) = -\log(S(t)), \text{ or equivalently}$$

$$S(t) = e^{-H(t)}$$

Because of this, graphs of $\log(-\log(S(t)))$ are also used to examine the proportional hazards assumption.

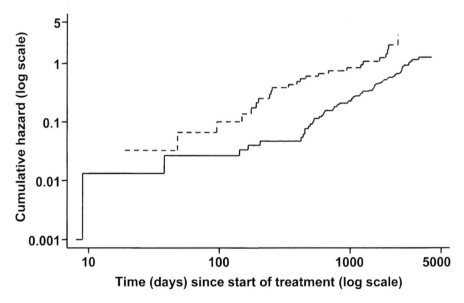

Fig. 26.4 Cumulative hazard (log scale) against time (log scale) for primary biliary cirrhosis patients with and without central cholestasis at baseline, in order to check the proportional hazards assumption.

Links between hazards, survival and risks when rates are constant

In Section 22.3 we described the relationship between risks and rates, and noted that when the event rate, λ, is constant over time then the proportion of the population event-free decreases exponentially over time. This proportion is exactly the same as the survivor function, $S(t)$. In the box below we extend the set of relationships to include the hazard, and cumulative hazard. Note that the hazard is constant over time, and that the cumulative hazard increases linearly over time. This is in contrast to the risk which does not increase at a steady pace; its rate of increase decreases with time.

> *When the event rate, λ, is constant over time:*
>
> $h(t) = \lambda$
>
> $H(t) = \lambda t$
>
> $S(t) = e^{-\lambda t}$
>
> Risk up to time $t = 1 - e^{-\lambda t}$
>
> Average survival time $= 1/\lambda$

26.5 COMPARISON OF HAZARDS USING MANTEL–COX METHODS: THE LOG RANK TEST

Mantel–Cox estimate of the hazard ratio

The Mantel–Cox method is a special application of the Mantel–Haenszel procedure, in which we construct a separate 2×2 table for each time at which an event occurs. It combines the contributions from each table, assuming that the hazard ratio is constant over the period of follow-up. We will use the same notation as that given in Table 18.3. Usually, there is only one event at a particular time, so in each table either d_{1i} is 0 and d_{0i} is 1 or vice-versa, but the procedure also works if there are ties (more than one event at a particular time). The **Mantel–Cox estimate of the hazard ratio** is given by:

> $\mathrm{HR_{MC}} = Q/R$, where
>
> $Q = \Sigma \dfrac{d_{1i} \times h_{0i}}{n_i}$ and $R = \Sigma \dfrac{d_{0i} \times h_{1i}}{n_i}$

Standard error and confidence interval of the Mantel–Cox HR

The standard error of log HR_{MC} is:

$$s.e._{MC} = \sqrt{(V/(Q \times R))}, \quad \text{where}$$
$$V = \Sigma V_i = \Sigma \frac{d_i \times n_{0i} \times n_{1i}}{n_i^2}$$

V is the sum across the strata of the variances V_i for the number of exposed individuals experiencing the outcome event.

This may be used to derive a 95% confidence interval for HR_{MC} in the usual way:

$$95\% \ CI = HR_{MC}/EF \ \text{to} \ HR_{MC} \times EF, \quad \text{where}$$
$$EF = \exp(1.96 \times s.e._{MC})$$

Mantel–Cox χ^2 (or log rank) test

Finally, we test the null hypothesis that $HR_{MC} = 1$ by calculating the **Mantel–Cox χ^2 statistic**, which is based on comparisons in each stratum of the number of exposed individuals *observed* to have experienced the event (d_{1i}), with the *expected* number in this category (E_{1i}) if there were no difference in the hazards between exposed and unexposed. Note that χ^2_{MC} *has just 1 degree of freedom irrespective of how many events occur.*

$$\chi^2_{MC} = \frac{U^2}{V}; \ d.f. = 1, \quad \text{where}$$
$$U = \Sigma(d_{1i} - E_{1i}), \ \text{and} \ E_{1i} = \frac{d_i \times n_{1i}}{n_i}$$

This χ^2 test is also known as the **log rank test**; the rather obscure name comes from an alternative derivation of the test.

Example 26.3

In the trial of survival in primary biliary cirrhosis patients, there were 72 deaths among the 153 patients without central cholestasis at baseline, and 24 deaths among the 31 patients with central cholestasis at baseline. Table 26.3

Table 26.3 Calculations needed to derive the Mantel–Cox estimate of the hazard ratio and the corresponding (log rank) test statistic for survival in primary biliary cirrhosis patients, with and without central cholestasis at baseline.

Day, i	n_{0i}	d_{0i}	n_{1i}	d_{1i}	$Q_i = \dfrac{d_{1i} \times h_{0i}}{n_i}$	$R_i = \dfrac{d_{0i} \times h_{1i}}{n_i}$	$U_i = d_i - \dfrac{d_i \times n_{1i}}{n_i}$	$V_i = \dfrac{d_i \times n_{1i} \times n_{0i}}{n_i^2}$
9	152	2	31	0	0	0.3388	−0.3388	0.2814
19	150	0	31	1	0.8287	0	0.8287	0.1419
38	150	2	30	0	0	0.3333	−0.3333	0.2778
48	148	0	30	1	0.8315	0	0.8315	0.1401
96	148	0	29	1	0.8362	0	0.8362	0.1370
144	148	1	28	0	0	0.1591	−0.1591	0.1338
150	147	0	28	1	0.8400	0	0.8400	0.1344
167	147	1	27	0	0	0.1552	−0.1552	0.1311
177	145	0	27	1	0.8430	0	0.8430	0.1323
193	144	0	26	1	0.8471	0	0.8471	0.1296
201	144	0	25	1	0.8521	0	0.8521	0.1260
207	144	1	24	0	0	0.1429	−0.1429	0.1224
245	143	0	24	1	0.8563	0	0.8563	0.1231
251	143	0	23	1	0.8614	0	0.8614	0.1194
256	143	0	22	1	0.8667	0	0.8667	0.1156
…	…	…	…	…	…	…	…	…
Totals					21.224	5.538	15.686	7.387

shows the calculations needed to derive the Mantel–Cox hazard ratio and associated log rank test statistic for the first 15 days on which one or more deaths
occurred, together with the total values of U, V, Q and R for the whole dataset.

The estimated hazard ratio is $Q/R = 21.224/5.538 = 3.833$. The interpretation
is that, on average, the hazard in patients with central cholestasis at baseline was
3.833 times the hazard in patients without central cholestasis.

The standard error of the log hazard ratio is

$$\sqrt{[V/(Q \times R)]} = \sqrt{[7.387/(21.224 \times 5.538)]} = 0.2507$$

The error factor is therefore $\exp(1.96 \times 0.2507) = 1.635$, so that the 95% CI for
the hazard ratio is 2.345 to 6.264. The (log rank) χ^2 statistic is:

$$\chi^2_{MC} = \frac{15.686^2}{7.387} = 33.31, \ P < 0.001$$

There is thus strong evidence that the hazard rates, and hence survival rates,
differed between the two groups.

These methods can also be extended to adjust for different compositions of the
different groups, such as different sex ratios or different age distributions. For
instance, we could stratify additionally on sex, and apply the method in the same
way.

CHAPTER 27

Regression analysis of survival data

27.1 INTRODUCTION

We now describe **Cox regression**, also known as **proportional hazards regression**. This is the most commonly used approach to the regression analysis of survival data. It uses the same approach as the Mantel–Cox method described in Section 26.5:

- it assumes that the ratio of the hazards comparing different exposure groups remains constant over time. This is known as the **proportional hazards** assumption;

- it is based on considering the **risk sets** of subjects still being followed up at each time that an event occurred. At the time of each event, the values of the exposure variables for the subject who experienced the disease event are compared to the values of the exposure variables for all the other subjects still being followed and who did not experience the disease event.

After introducing Cox regression, we then consider:

- what to do when the proportional hazards assumption does not appear to hold;
- the way in which the choice of time axis influences the nature of the risk sets;
- the link between Cox and Poisson regression;
- the use of parametric survival models as an alternative approach.

General issues in regression modelling, including fitting linear effects and testing hypotheses, are discussed in more detail in Chapter 29.

27.2 COX REGRESSION

The mathematical form of the **Cox proportional hazards model** is:

$$\text{Log}(h(t)) = \log(h_0(t)) + \beta_1 x_1 + \beta_2 x_2 + \ldots + \beta_p x_p$$

where $h(t)$ is the hazard at time t, $h_0(t)$ is the **baseline hazard** (the hazard for an individual in whom all exposure variables $= 0$) at time t, and x_1 to x_p are the p exposure variables.

On the *ratio scale* the model is:

$$h(t) = h_0(t) \times \exp(\beta_1 x_1 + \beta_2 x_2 + \ldots + \beta_p x_p)$$

When there is a single exposure variable (x_1) and just two exposure groups ($x_1 = 1$ for exposed individuals and 0 for unexposed individuals) the model is described by two equations, as shown in Table 27.1.

The **hazard ratio** comparing exposed with unexposed individuals at time t is therefore:

$$HR(t) = \frac{h_0(t) \exp(\beta_1)}{h_0(t)} = \exp(\beta_1)$$

The model thus assumes that the hazard ratio remains constant over time; it equals $\exp(\beta_1)$. It is this assumption that is highlighted in the name 'proportional hazards' regression. The regression coefficient β_1 is the estimated *log hazard ratio* comparing exposed with unexposed individuals.

Table 27.1 Equations defining the Cox regression model for the comparison of two exposure groups, at time t.

Exposure group	Log(Hazard at time t)	Hazard at time t
Exposed ($x_1 = 1$)	$\log(h_0(t)) + \beta_1$	$h_0(t) \times \exp(\beta_1)$
Unexposed ($x_1 = 0$)	$\log(h_0(t))$	$h_0(t)$

Example 27.1
Table 27.2 shows the output from a Cox regression analysis of the effect of central cholestatis at baseline (variable name *cencho0*) in primary biliary cirrhosis patients. There is clear evidence that this increased the hazard rate. The results are very similar to the Mantel–Cox estimate of the hazard ratio (3.833, 95% CI $= 2.345$ to 6.264), derived in Section 26.5. The square of the Wald z-test statistic is $5.387^2 = 29.02$, similar to but a little smaller than the log rank χ^2 statistic of 33.31, derived in Section 26.5. Three points should be noted:

1 Cox regression analysis is based on a **conditional likelihood** estimation procedure, in which the values of the exposure variables are compared between individuals *within* the risk sets of individuals being followed at each time at which

Table 27.2 Cox regression output for the model for the effect of central cholestasis at baseline in the study of survival in patients with primary biliary cirrhosis, introduced in Example 26.2.

	Hazard ratio	z	$P > |z|$	95% CI
cencho0	3.751	5.387	0.000	2.319 to 6.067

an event occurs. *The baseline hazard (which can vary over time) is therefore not estimated and is not displayed.*

2 As explained earlier, the model is based on the proportional hazards assumption. This assumption may be investigated graphically, as described in Section 26.4. Alternatively, statistical tests of the proportional hazards assumption are available, as discussed below.

3 As with all regression models, it is straightforward to estimate the effect of more than one exposure variable. As usual, we assume that the effects of different exposures combine in a *multiplicative* manner: this was explained in detail in Section 20.2, in the context of logistic regression. On the basis of this assumption, we may interpret the estimated effect of each exposure variable as the effect after controlling for the confounding effects of other exposure variables in the model. This assumption may be examined by fitting interaction terms (see Section 29.4).

27.3 NON-PROPORTIONAL HAZARDS

Non-proportional hazards correspond to an interaction between the exposure variable and time: in other words the exposure effect (hazard ratio) changes over time. In addition to the graphical examination of proportional hazards described in Section 26.4, many software packages provide statistical tests of the proportional hazards assumption. Three analysis options when evidence of non-proportional hazards is found are:

1 Extend the model to include an exposure-time interaction term. For example, for a single binary exposure variable, the model could assume:

$$\text{hazard ratio} = \exp(\beta_1 + \beta_2 t)$$

In theory, there is no reason that complex changes of the exposure hazard ratios over time should not be modelled. However, not all statistical software will allow this.

2 If the variable for which there is evidence of non-proportional hazards is a confounder, rather than the main exposure of interest, then the regression may be *stratified* according to the values of this confounding variable. This modifies the risk sets, so that they include only individuals with the same value of the confounding variable. The effect of the confounder is not estimated, but its effects are controlled for without assuming proportional hazards.

3 Split the follow-up time into different periods, as described in Section 24.6. It is then straightforward to fit models that allow the exposure effect to differ between time periods. Splitting follow-up time can also be used to derive tests of the proportional hazards assumption, by looking for interactions between exposure and time period (see Section 29.4 for a description of tests for interaction in regression models).

27.4 CHOICE OF TIME AXIS IN SURVIVAL ANALYSES

When following subjects after diagnosis or treatment of a disease, it may be reasonable to suppose that the major determinant of variation in the hazard will be the time since diagnosis or treatment. This was the assumption we made in the study of primary biliary cirrhosis, when we examined patients from the time they were treated. Our **risk sets** were constructed by considering all subjects who were at risk at the times after the start of treatment at which events occurred.

However, there are different options for the choice of time axis which may be more suitable in other situations. For example, consider the Caerphilly study of risk factors for cardiovascular disease, in which the dates of the first examinations took place between July 1979 and October 1983, and participants were aged between 43 and 61 when they were first examined. There are three possible choices for the time scale for construction of risk sets:

1 time since recruitment to the study;
2 time since birth (i.e. age);
3 year of the study (i.e. date).

Each of these choices will lead to different risk sets (sets of subjects at risk when an event occurred) at the times at which events occur. We illustrate the differences between these time scales using ten patients randomly chosen from the Caerphilly study. Their dates of birth, entry to, and exit from, the study, together with the corresponding ages and time in the study are shown in Table 27.3.

Table 27.3 Dates and ages of entry to, and exit from, the Caerphilly study for ten randomly selected subjects.

Subject number	Date of birth	Date of first examination	Date of exit	Age at entry	Age at exit	Years in study (T)	MI
151	20 Oct 1931	30 May 1980	18 Dec 1998	48.61	67.16	18.55	0
158	21 Mar 1933	2 Dec 1981	9 May 1984	48.70	51.13	2.43	1
658	12 Aug 1925	22 Oct 1981	18 Jul 1996	56.19	70.93	14.74	1
941	28 Oct 1933	29 May 1982	19 Dec 1998	48.58	65.14	16.56	0
1376	19 Sep 1935	21 Mar 1982	25 Nov 1998	46.50	63.18	16.68	0
1467	9 Jan 1930	6 Jul 1982	3 Aug 1993	52.49	63.56	11.08	0
1650	19 Nov 1927	24 Nov 1982	31 Dec 1998	55.01	71.12	16.10	0
1673	14 Feb 1926	3 Jul 1983	31 Dec 1998	57.38	72.88	15.50	0
1754	21 Jul 1921	1 Oct 1980	31 Dec 1998	59.20	77.45	18.25	0
1765	27 Mar 1924	30 Dec 1982	13 Dec 1998	58.76	74.71	15.95	0

The risk sets corresponding to the three different choices of time axis are illustrated in Figure 27.1. The horizontal lines represent the follow-up time for each subject. The follow-up line ends in a closed circle for subjects who experienced an MI (numbers 158 and 658). It ends in an open circle for subjects who were censored, either because they were lost to follow-up (subject 1467 on 3 August 1993), or because they were still healthy at the time of their end of study follow-up in November or December 1998 (the other seven subjects). Subjects whose follow-up is intersected by the dotted vertical lines, at the times of the MIs, are members of the risk set for that MI, i.e. those with whom the covariates of the patient who experienced the MI are compared.

1 *Risk sets* corresponding to *time from entry to the study*, Figure 27.1(a): at the time of the first MI all subjects were still being followed and are therefore in the risk set, while at the time of the second MI all subjects except 158 and 1467 are in the risk set.

    The majority of published applications of Cox regression use this choice, in which all subjects start at time 0. This is partly because Cox regression was originally developed for data on survival following a defined event, and also because until recently most computer programs for Cox regression insisted that all subjects enter at time 0. However, there is no reason why risk sets should not be constructed on the basis of delayed entry, and some statistical packages now allow flexible choices of time axis in Cox regression. In contrast, choices (2) and (3) both imply that subjects enter the study at different times, as well as having different periods of follow-up.

2 *Risk sets* corresponding to choosing *age as the time axis*, Figure 27.1(b): these consist of all subjects who were still being followed at a time when they were the same age as that of the subject who experienced the MI. Since subject 158 was relatively young when he experienced his MI, only three other subjects are members of this risk set. Similarly only four other subjects are members of the risk set for subject 658.

3 *Risk sets* corresponding to choosing *calendar time as the time axis*, Figure 27.1(c): in this example, because subjects were recruited over a relatively short period, the risk sets are the same as for (a), but in general this need not be the case.

Criteria for choice of time axis

In general, the best choice of time axis in survival analysis will be the scale over which we expect the hazard to change most dramatically. In studies of survival following diagnosis of a disease such as cancer, the best time axis is usually time since recruitment (start of study). Calendar time would be a sensible choice in studies of survival following an environmental disaster, such as the leak of poisonous fumes from a factory, which occurred at a particular time. In contrast, recruitment to the Caerphilly study did not depend on the participant experiencing

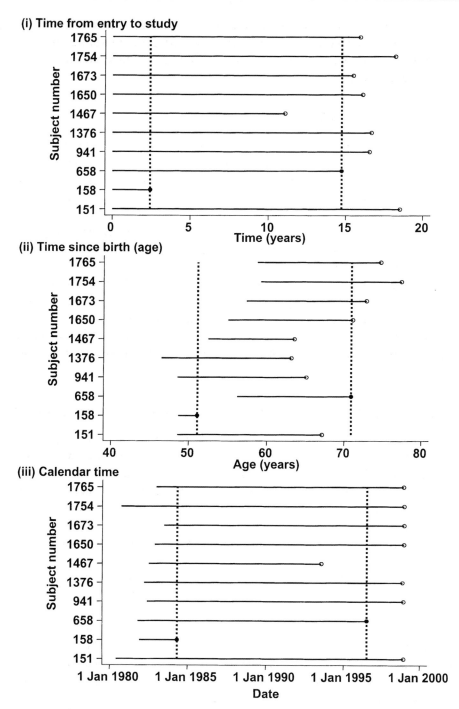

Fig. 27.1 Risk sets corresponding to three different choices of time axis, for ten patients randomly chosen from the Caerphilly study. The follow-up line ends in a closed circle for subjects who experienced an MI and an open circle for subjects who were censored. The dotted vertical lines show the risk sets at the time of each MI for the different choices of time axis.

a particular event: simply on the person living in Caerphilly and being in later middle age at the time the study was established. Therefore measuring time from recruitment to the study does not seem a sensible choice of time axis: in this case age is a better choice.

More than one time axis

Finally, we may wish to do a Cox regression that allows for the effect of more than one variable to change over time. There are two main reasons for doing this:

1 we may want to allow for changing rates of disease according to, say, age group, while keeping time since an event such as diagnosis of disease as the time axis used to define the risk sets;

2 we may want to allow for the effect of exposures which are measured more than once, and estimate the association of the most recent exposure measurement with rates of disease.

The procedure is the same in each case. We simply split the follow-up time for each subject into periods defined by (1) age group, or (2) the time between exposure measurements, in the same way as described at the end of Section 24.6. Providing that the software being used for Cox regression will allow for delayed entry, we then fit a standard Cox regression model, controlling for the effects of the time-varying exposures.

27.5 LINKS BETWEEN POISSON REGRESSION AND COX REGRESSION

We have described two different regression models for the analysis of longitudinal studies. In Poisson regression we assume that rates are constant within time periods, and estimate rate ratios comparing exposed with unexposed groups. In Cox regression we make no assumptions about how the hazard changes over time; instead we estimate hazard ratios comparing different exposure groups. This is done by constructing *risk sets*, which consist of all subjects being followed at the time at which each event occurs, and assuming that the hazard ratio is the same across risk sets.

At the end of Chapter 24 we saw that we may allow for variables which change over time in Poisson regression by splitting the follow-up time, for example into 5-year age groups, and estimating the rate ratio separately in each time period, compared to a baseline period. This is illustrated in Figure 27.2, using 5-year age groups, for the ten subjects from the Caerphilly study. We consider the total number of events, and total length of follow-up, in each age group. Now suppose that we make the age groups smaller (1-year, say). Only age groups in which an event occurs will contribute to the analysis, and the follow-up time within each of these groups will be approximately equal. As we make the time intervals progressively shorter, we will be left with the risk sets analysed in Cox regression.

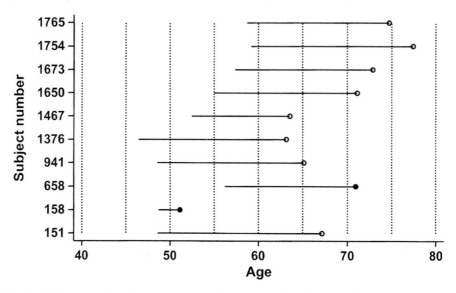

Fig. 27.2 Follow-up split into 5-year age groups, for ten subjects from the Caerphilly study.

27.6 PARAMETRIC SURVIVAL MODELS

Parametric survival models are an alternative regression approach to the analysis of survival data in which, instead of ignoring the hazard function, as in Cox proportional hazards models, we model the survivor function in the baseline group using one of a choice of mathematical functions. For example, we have already seen in Sections 22.3 and 26.4 that if the rate (hazard) is constant over time then the survivor function is exponential. This is exactly the assumption of Poisson regression, which means that it is therefore identical to a parametric survival model assuming an exponential survivor function. Other commonly used survivor function distributions are the Weibull, Gompertz, gamma, lognormal and log-logistic functions. **Weibull models** assume proportional hazards and usually give very similar estimated hazard ratios to those from Cox models. Because parametric survival models explicitly estimate the survivor function they may be of particular use when the aim of a study is to predict survival probabilities in different groups. For more details, see Cox and Oakes (1984) or Collett (2003).

PART E

STATISTICAL MODELLING

Previous parts of the book have discussed methods of analysis according to the different types of outcome (and exposure) variables. An understanding of what statistical method is appropriate given the type of data that have been collected is obviously crucial, but it is also important to realize that different statistical methods have much in common, so that an understanding of one method helps in understanding others. For example, the interpretation of confidence intervals and P-values follows the same logic, regardless of the particular situation in which they are derived. We have seen that computer output from different regression models is presented in a similar way, and issues such as testing hypotheses, examining interactions between exposure effects and selection of the most appropriate model also apply to all regression models.

In this part of the book we present statistical methods that apply to many types of exposure and outcome variables. We begin, in Chapter 28, by introducing likelihood: the concept that underlies most commonly used statistical methods. In Chapter 29 we consider general issues in regression modelling, including the use of likelihood ratio tests of hypotheses about the parameters of regression models.

Chapter 30 introduces methods that can be used when the usual model assumptions are violated: these provide a means of checking the robustness of results derived using standard methods. A common situation in which standard assumptions are violated is when data are clustered; that is when observations on individuals within a cluster tend to be *more similar* to each other than to individuals in other clusters. Failure to take account of clustering can lead to confidence intervals that are too narrow, and P-values that are too small. Chapter 31 introduces methods that are appropriate for the analysis of such data.

Chapter 32 focuses on how evidence can be summarized on a particular subject in order to make it accessible to medical practitioners and inform the practice of **evidence-based medicine**. In particular it covers systematic reviews of the medical literature, the statistical methods which are used to combine effect estimates from different studies (meta-analysis), and sources of bias in meta-analysis and how these may be detected.

Finally, in Chapter 33 we briefly describe the Bayesian approach to statistical inference.

Likelihood

28.1 INTRODUCTION

In this chapter, we introduce the concept of **likelihood** and explain how **likelihood theory** provides the basis for a general approach to using data to yield estimates of **parameters** of interest. The idea that we use data to estimate parameters of interest using an underlying probability model is fundamental to statistics. This ranges from:

- simple models to estimate a single parameter of interest, based on assuming a normal, binomial or Poisson distribution for the outcome of interest. For example, estimating the risk of vertical transmission of HIV during pregnancy or childbirth, in HIV-infected mothers given antiretroviral therapy during pregnancy, is based on assuming a binomial distribution for the occurrence (or not) of vertical transmission, or a normal approximation to this binomial distribution;
- to multivariable regression models assuming a particular distribution for the outcome based on the values of a number of exposure variables. Such models relate the probability distribution of the outcome to the levels of the exposure variables via the values of one or more *parameters*. For example, in Example 24.2, we used Poisson regression to compare rates of myocardial infarction according to whether men in the Caerphilly study were current smokers or never/ex-smokers. The regression model had two *parameters*: the *log of the rate* in the never/ex-smokers, and the *log of the rate ratio* comparing current smokers with never/ex-smokers.

In most of the chapter, we will show how likelihood theory can be used to reproduce results that we derived earlier in the book using properties of the normal distribution, and approximations to the normal distribution. The strength of the likelihood approach, however, lies in the way it can be generalized to any statistical model, for any number of parameters. It provides the basis for fitting logistic, Poisson and Cox regression models. For this reason it is of great import-ance in modern medical statistics.

This chapter is conceptually fairly sophisticated, and may be skipped at a first reading. An understanding of likelihood is not essential to the conduct of the majority of statistical analysis. However, this chapter does provide insights into understanding how regression models are fitted, the different ways that we can test hypotheses about the parameters of regression models, the meaning of some of the 'small print' items obtained on regression outputs, such as the iteration number, and why problems may be encountered. We recommend Clayton and Hills (1993), for a fuller explanation of the ideas presented here, and Royall (1997) for a discussion of different approaches to statistical inference based on likelihood.

28.2 LIKELIHOOD

Example 28.1

We will illustrate the idea of likelihood through an example, in which we are interested in estimating the risk of household transmission of tuberculosis (TB). We have tuberculin tested 12 household contacts of an index case of TB. Three of the twelve tested positive; the other nine tested negative. Using the notation introduced in Part C for binary outcomes, we have $d = 3$ and $h = 9$. The sample proportion, p equals $3/12$ or 0.25. As always, we are not interested in this sample result in its own right but rather in what it tells us more generally about the risk of household transmission (π). Putting this another way, given that the sample proportion was 0.25, what can we deduce from this concerning the most likely value for π? Intuitively we would answer this question with $\pi = 0.25$, and we would be correct. We will now explain the mathematical basis for this, which can be extended to deriving estimates in more complicated situations.

The approach we use is to calculate the probability, or **likelihood**, of our observed result for different values of π: the likelihood gives a comparative measure of how compatible our data are with each particular value of π. We then find the value of π that corresponds to the largest possible likelihood. This value is called the **maximum-likelihood estimate (MLE)** of the parameter π.

> $$\text{MLE} = \frac{\text{the value of the parameter that } \textit{maximizes}}{\text{the likelihood of the observed result}}$$

In this case, the likelihoods are calculated using the formula for the binomial distribution, described in Chapter 14. Figure 28.1 shows how the value of the likelihood varies with different values of π, and Table 28.1 shows the details of

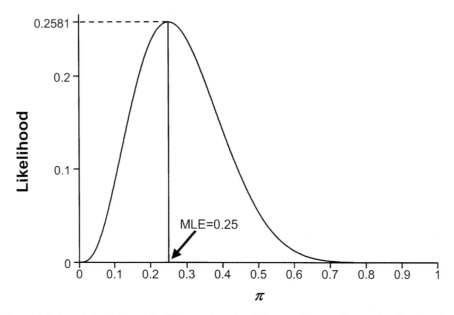

Fig. 28.1 Values of the likelihood for different values of π, if $d = 3$ and $h = 9$, showing that the maximum likelihood estimate is 0.25.

Table 28.1 Values of the likelihood of observing $d = 3$, $h = 9$ for different values of π.

Value of π	Likelihood of observed result $= \frac{12!}{3!9!} \pi^3 \times (1 - \pi)^9$
0.1	$220 \times 0.1^3 \times 0.9^9 = 0.0852$
0.2	$220 \times 0.2^3 \times 0.8^9 = 0.2362$
0.25	$220 \times 0.25^3 \times 0.75^9 = 0.2581$
0.3	$220 \times 0.3^3 \times 0.7^9 = 0.2397$
0.4	$220 \times 0.4^3 \times 0.6^9 = 0.1419$
0.6	$220 \times 0.6^3 \times 0.4^9 = 0.0125$

the calculations for a few selected values. It can be seen that the likelihood increases as π increases, reaches a maximum when $\pi = 0.25$, and then decreases. Thus, our maximum likelihood estimate is MLE $= 0.25$, agreeing with our original guess.

This result can be confirmed mathematically. The MLE can be derived by differentiating the binomial likelihood $\pi^d \times (1 - \pi)^h$ to find the value of π that maximizes it. The result is $d/(d + h)$ *or* d/n, which in this example equals $3/12$ or 0.25.

In simple situations, such as the estimation of a single mean, proportion or rate, or the comparison of two means, proportions or rates, the MLE is given by the sample value for the parameter of interest (in other words the usual estimate). This is the case here; the MLE for the within-household risk of TB transmission equals the proportion who tested tuberculin positive in the sample of 12 household contacts of the index case.

28.3 LIKELIHOOD RATIOS AND SUPPORTED RANGES

As well as concluding that 0.25 is the most likely value for the true probability π of the risk of household transmission of TB in our example, it is useful to know what other values of π are compatible with the data. We now describe how to use **likelihood ratios**, or more specifically their *logarithmic* equivalent, to give us a range of likely values for the population parameter (in this case π), which we wish to estimate.

In our example, the maximum likelihood equals 0.2581, and the corresponding maximum likelihood estimate is $\pi = 0.25$. The likelihood for any other value of π will be less than this. How much less likely is assessed using the **likelihood ratio (LR)**:

$$\text{Likelihood ratio (LR)} = \frac{\text{Likelihood for } \pi}{\text{Likelihood at the MLE}}$$

Figure 28.2 shows how the likelihood ratio varies across the range of possible values and Table 28.2 shows the details of the calculation for a few selected values

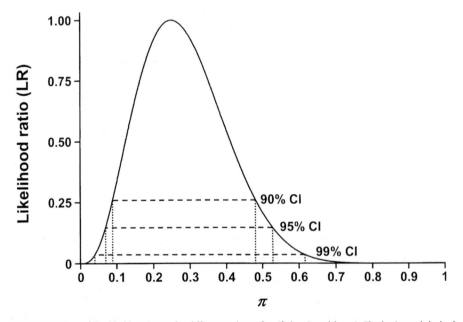

Fig. 28.2 Values of the likelihood ratio for different values of π, if $d = 3$ and $h = 9$. The horizontal dashed lines show the supported ranges corresponding to 90%, 95% and 99% confidence intervals (see Table 28.3), and the dotted vertical lines show the corresponding confidence limits.

Table 28.2 Values of the likelihood of observing $d = 3$, $h = 9$, and corresponding likelihood ratio, for different values of π.

Value of π	Likelihood	Likelihood ratio
0.1	0.0852	$0.0852/0.2581 = 0.3302$
0.2	0.2362	$0.2362/0.2581 = 0.9151$
0.25 (MLE)	0.2581	$0.2581/0.2581 = 1$
0.3	0.2397	$0.2397/0.2581 = 0.9287$
0.4	0.1419	$0.1419/0.2581 = 0.5498$
0.6	0.0125	$0.0125/0.2581 = 0.0484$

of π. By definition, the likelihood ratio equals 1 for the MLE (in this case for $\pi = 0.25$) and less than one for all other values. The shape of the curve of the likelihood ratio is *exactly* the same as that of the likelihood in Figure 28.1, since we have simply divided the likelihood by a constant amount, namely the maximum likelihood, which in this case equals 0.2581.

The likelihood ratio provides a convenient measure of the amount of support for a particular value(s) of π. The likelihood ratios for π equal to 0.2 or 0.3 are close to 1, suggesting that these values are almost as compatible with the observed data as the MLE. In contrast, the likelihood ratio for π equal to 0.6 is very small; it is therefore much less likely that the within-household transmission rate for TB is as high as 0.6. The conclusion is less immediately clear for likelihood ratios in between, such as a ratio of 0.3302 for π equal to 0.1 or 0.5498 for π equal to 0.4.

By choosing a cut-off value for the likelihood ratio, we can derive a **supported range** of parameter values. We classify values of π with likelihood ratios *above* the cut-off as supported by the data, and those with likelihood ratios *below* the cut-off as not supported by the data. This concept of a **supported range** of values is intuitively simple; the choice of the cut-off value is the critical issue. Although supported ranges arise from a different philosophical basis to confidence intervals, the two turn out to be closely linked. We will show below that, providing the sample size is sufficiently large, different choices of cut-off for the likelihood ratio correspond to different choices of confidence level, as illustrated in Figure 28.2. For example, a likelihood ratio of 0.1465 gives a supported range that approximately coincides with the 95% confidence interval for π, calculated in the usual way (see Table 28.3).

28.4 CONFIDENCE INTERVALS BASED ON THE LOG LIKELIHOOD RATIO AND ITS QUADRATIC APPROXIMATION

We work with the *logarithm* of the likelihood ratio to derive confidence intervals, rather than the likelihood ratio itself because, provided the sample size is sufficiently large, the log LR can be approximated by a quadratic equation, which is easier to handle mathematically than the likelihood ratio. Using the rules of logarithms (see the box on p. 156):

$$\log(LR) = \log(\text{likelihood for } \pi) - \log(\text{likelihood at the MLE})$$

Abbreviating this formula by using the letter L to denote log likelihood gives:

$$\log(LR) = L(\pi) - L(\text{MLE})$$

Note that, as in earlier parts of this book, we use logarithms to the base e (natural logarithms); see Section 13.2 for an explanation of logarithms and the exponential function.

The log(LR) corresponds to a *difference* in log likelihoods. Its maximum occurs at the MLE and equals zero. Figure 28.3(a) shows the log(LR) for the data in Example 28.1 on within-household transmission of TB. Figure 28.3(b) shows how the shape of the curve would change for a larger sample size (120 instead of 12), but with the same MLE of 0.25. The dashed lines in Figure 28.3 show the best quadratic approximations to these particular log likelihoods. For the small sample size in Figure 28.3(a) the quadratic approximation has a relatively poor fit, while for the larger sample size in Figure 28.3(b) there is a close fit between the log likelihood and the quadratic approximation.

The **quadratic approximation** is chosen to meet the log(LR) at the MLE and to have the *same curvature* as the log(LR) at this point. It is symmetrical about this point and its maximum value is zero. It can be shown that its equation can be written in the following way:

$$\text{Log(LR)} = -\frac{1}{2}\left(\frac{\text{MLE} - \theta}{S}\right)^2$$

where θ represents the parameter that we wish to estimate and $-1/S^2$ is the curvature at the maximum. In our example θ would be π, the within-household risk of transmission of TB. In Example 6.1, θ would be μ, the mean sprayable surface area of houses that we wished to estimate in order to be able to calculate how much insecticide would be needed to spray the whole area as part of the malaria control programme. In this case, we had a quantitative outcome which we assumed was normally distributed.

The quadratic approximation plays a key role in parameter estimation because:

1 In simple situations, such as the estimation of a single mean, proportion or rate, or the comparison of two means, proportions or rates:
   - the MLE equals the sample value for the parameter of interest (see Section 28.2);
   - the denominator S equals the usual estimate of the **standard error**.

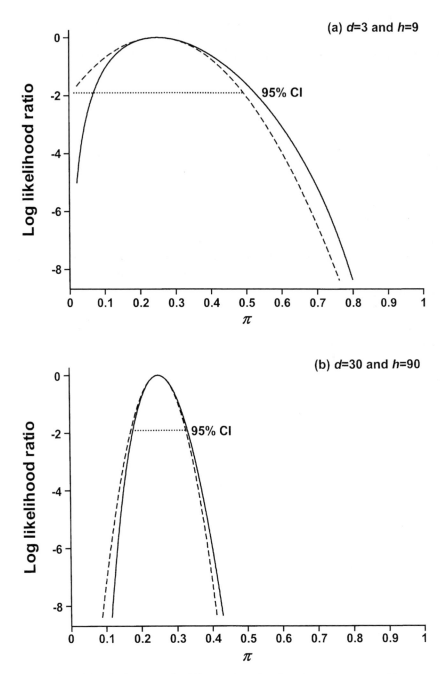

Fig. 28.3 Values of the likelihood ratio for different values of π, if (a) $d = 3$ and $h = 9$, or (b) $d = 30$ and $h = 90$. The dashed lines show the best quadratic approximations to the log likelihood ratio curves, fitted at the MLE ($\pi = 0.25$) and the dotted lines show the 95% confidence intervals based on the quadratic approximations.

2 When the underlying distribution is **normal**, the quadratic equation gives an *exact* fit to the log(LR).

3 When the sample size is sufficiently large, then the quadratic equation gives a *close* fit to the log(LR), regardless of the underlying probability distribution. This arises from the **Central Limit Theorem** (see Section 5.2), which shows that the normal distribution provides a good approximation to the *sampling distribution* of the parameter of interest, whatever its underlying distribution, provided that the sample size is sufficiently large.

4 The closest quadratic approximation to the log(LR) can be found using a process known as iteration, as explained in Section 28.6. This involves calculating the likelihood ratio, and its log, only at selected points of the curve. It avoids the need to calculate the whole of the curve.

These facts together mean that the quadratic approximation provides a method to derive MLEs and corresponding confidence intervals that avoids the need for complicated mathematics, and that works in situations with complex underlying distributions, as well as giving the same results as standard methods in simple situations.

Since fitting a quadratic approximation to the log(LR) is equivalent to using a normal approximation for the sampling distribution for the parameter θ that we wish to estimate, the **95% confidence interval** based on the quadratic approximation must be:

$$95\% \text{ CI} = \text{MLE} - 1.96 \times S \text{ to MLE} + 1.96 \times S$$

Link between confidence intervals and supported ranges

At the end of Section 28.3, we noted that a likelihood ratio of 0.1465 gives a supported range that approximately coincides with the 95% confidence interval. We will now derive this link.

Since the quadratic approximation for log(LR) is:

$$\text{Log(LR)} = -\frac{1}{2}\left(\frac{\text{MLE} - \theta}{S}\right)^2$$

And since,

$$\text{MLE} - \text{lower } 95\% \text{ CL} = \text{MLE} - (\text{MLE} - 1.96 \times S) = 1.96S$$

and

$$\text{MLE} - \text{upper } 95\% \text{ CL} = \text{MLE} - (\text{MLE} + 1.96 \times S) = -1.96S$$

the **values of the log(LR) curve at the 95 % confidence limits** (CL) are both:

$$\text{Log(LR) for 95\% CI} = -\frac{1.96^2}{2} = -1.9208$$

since the S's in the numerator and denominator cancel out, and since $(-1.96)^2 = 1.96^2$. Antilogging this gives the cut-off value of the **likelihood ratio corresponding to the 95 % confidence interval**:

$$\text{LR for 95\% CI} = e^{-1.9208} = 0.1465$$

Table 28.3 summarizes the cut-off values of the likelihood ratio and its logarithm corresponding to 90 %, 95 % and 99 % confidence intervals. Note that there is only a close agreement between standard confidence intervals and supported ranges based on these cut-offs when the quadratic approximation gives a close fit to the log(LR).

Table 28.3 Cut-off values for the likelihood ratio, and its logarithm, corresponding to 90%, 95% and 99% confidence intervals, assuming that the underlying distribution is normal or approximately normal.

	90% CI	95% CI	99% CI
% point of normal distribution	1.6449	1.96	2.5763
Cut-off value for log(LR)	−1.3529	−1.9208	−3.3187
Cut-off value for LR	0.2585	0.1465	0.0362

Information and standard error

The quantity $1/S^2$ (the multiplier of $\frac{1}{2}(\text{MLE} - \theta)^2$ in the quadratic approximation) is known as the **information** in the data. The larger the value for the information, the more sharply curved are the log(LR), its quadratic approximation, the likelihood ratio and the likelihood curves. The more information that the data contain about the parameter, the smaller is its standard error, the more precise is our estimate, and the narrower is the confidence interval.

28.5 LIKELIHOOD IN THE COMPARISON OF TWO GROUPS

Example 28.2
So far we have described the principles of likelihood in the simplest context of a single sample and a single parameter to be estimated. We will now illustrate its

of lower respiratory infections among children living in poor compared to good housing conditions was 2.01. We noted that the formula for the profile log likelihood shown in Figure 28.4 is:

$$L = d_1 \log\left(\frac{\theta T_1}{T_0}\right) - d \log\left(1 + \frac{\theta T_1}{T_0}\right) + \text{constant}$$

Calculating this for $\theta = 1$ (null) and $\theta = 2.01$ (MLE) gives:

$$L_{\text{null}} = 33 \times \log\left(\frac{1 \times 355}{518}\right) - 57 \times \log\left(1 + \frac{1 \times 355}{518}\right) + \text{constant}$$

$$= (33 \times -0.37786) - (57 \times 0.52196) + \text{constant} = -42.2211 + \text{constant}$$

$$L_{\text{MLE}} = 33 \times \log\left(\frac{2.01 \times 355}{518}\right) - 57 \times \log\left(1 + \frac{2.01 \times 355}{518}\right) + \text{constant}$$

$$= (33 \times 0.32028) - (57 \times 0.86605) + \text{constant} = -38.7956 + \text{constant}$$

The difference between these is the log(LR):

$$L_{\text{null}} - L_{\text{max}} = -42.2211 + 38.7956 = -3.4255$$

This is shown in Figure 28.4, in which the values of the log likelihood ratio at the null value ($\theta = 1$) and the MLE ($\theta = 2.01$) are depicted by the horizontal dotted lines.

The likelihood ratio statistic is:

$$\text{LRS} = -2 \times (L_{\text{null}} - L_{\text{max}}) = -2 \times -3.4255 = 6.8510$$

The corresponding P-value, derived from the χ^2 distribution with 1 d.f., is $P = 0.0089$. There is therefore good evidence against the null hypothesis, suggesting that poor housing conditions did increase the rate of respiratory infections among the Guatamalan children.

Wald tests

The Wald test is similar to the likelihood ratio test, but is based on the value of the *fitted quadratic approximation* to the log likelihood ratio at the null value of the parameter of interest, rather than the actual value of the log likelihood ratio at this point. Recall from Section 28.4 that the quadratic approximation to the log likelihood ratio is of the form:

$$\text{Log(LR)}_{\text{quad}} = -\frac{1}{2}\left(\frac{\text{MLE} - \theta}{S}\right)^2$$

The **Wald test likelihood ratio statistic** based on the quadratic approximation is therefore:

of lower respiratory infections among children living in poor compared to good housing conditions was 2.01. We noted that the formula for the profile log likelihood shown in Figure 28.4 is:

$$L = d_1 \log\left(\frac{\theta T_1}{T_0}\right) - d\log\left(1 + \frac{\theta T_1}{T_0}\right) + \text{constant}$$

Calculating this for $\theta = 1$ (null) and $\theta = 2.01$ (MLE) gives:

$$L_{\text{null}} = 33 \times \log\left(\frac{1 \times 355}{518}\right) - 57 \times \log\left(1 + \frac{1 \times 355}{518}\right) + \text{constant}$$
$$= (33 \times -0.37786) - (57 \times 0.52196) + \text{constant} = -42.2211 + \text{constant}$$
$$L_{\text{MLE}} = 33 \times \log\left(\frac{2.01 \times 355}{518}\right) - 57 \times \log\left(1 + \frac{2.01 \times 355}{518}\right) + \text{constant}$$
$$= (33 \times 0.32028) - (57 \times 0.86605) + \text{constant} = -38.7956 + \text{constant}$$

The difference between these is the log(LR):

$$L_{\text{null}} - L_{\text{max}} = -42.2211 + 38.7956 = -3.4255$$

This is shown in Figure 28.4, in which the values of the log likelihood ratio at the null value ($\theta = 1$) and the MLE ($\theta = 2.01$) are depicted by the horizontal dotted lines.

The likelihood ratio statistic is:

$$\text{LRS} = -2 \times (L_{\text{null}} - L_{\text{max}}) = -2 \times -3.4255 = 6.8510$$

The corresponding P-value, derived from the χ^2 distribution with 1 d.f., is $P = 0.0089$. There is therefore good evidence against the null hypothesis, suggesting that poor housing conditions did increase the rate of respiratory infections among the Guatamalan children.

Wald tests

The Wald test is similar to the likelihood ratio test, but is based on the value of the *fitted quadratic approximation* to the log likelihood ratio at the null value of the parameter of interest, rather than the actual value of the log likelihood ratio at this point. Recall from Section 28.4 that the quadratic approximation to the log likelihood ratio is of the form:

$$\text{Log(LR)}_{\text{quad}} = -\frac{1}{2}\left(\frac{\text{MLE} - \theta}{S}\right)^2$$

The **Wald test likelihood ratio statistic** based on the quadratic approximation is therefore:

- profile log likelihood(s) that are very non-quadratic.

Logistic, Poisson and Cox regression all use logarithmic transformations of the parameters in order to make the profile log likelihoods approximately quadratic in form. The likelihood for simple and multiple regression is based on the normal distribution, and has an exact quadratic form; the maximum likelihood estimates obtained are equivalent to those obtained using the least squares approach (see Chapters 10 and 11).

28.7 USING LIKELIHOOD FOR HYPOTHESIS TESTING

We will now describe how the likelihood approach can be used to provide a general means of hypothesis testing. As explained in Chapter 8, a hypothesis test is based on calculating a **test statistic** and its corresponding **P-value** (also known as a **significance level**), in order to assess the strength of the evidence against the **null hypothesis** (of *no* association between exposure and outcome in the population). The *smaller* the P-value, the *stronger* is the evidence against the null hypothesis.

There are three different types of tests based on the log likelihood:

1 The **likelihood ratio test**, based on the value of the log likelihood ratio at the null value of the parameter.
2 The **Wald test**, which is similar but uses the value of the *fitted quadratic approximation* to the log likelihood ratio at the null, rather than the actual value of the log likelihood ratio at this point.
3 The **score test**, based on fitting an alternative quadratic approximation to the log likelihood ratio, which has the same gradient and curvature at the *null* value of the parameter, rather than at the MLE.

Likelihood ratio tests

The likelihood ratio test is based on the value of the log likelihood ratio at the null value of the parameter, using the fact that it can be shown that *providing the log likelihood ratio curve is close to a quadratic*:

$$-2 \times \log(\text{likelihood ratio}) \text{ has a } \chi^2 \text{ distribution with 1 d.f.}$$

We therefore work with minus twice the log(likelihood ratio); this is called the **likelihood ratio statistic (LRS)**:

$$\text{LRS} = -2 \times \log(\text{LR}) = -2 \times (L_{\text{null}} - L_{\text{MLE}}) \text{ is } \chi^2 \text{ with 1 d.f.}$$

In Example 28.2, based on the data from the Guatemalan morbidity study presented in Table 23.1, we found that the MLE for the rate ratio of the incidence

7 The 95% confidence interval is calculated from the MLE and the standard error of the log(rate ratio), using an *error factor*, as explained in Chapter 23. In this example,

$$S = \sqrt{(1/d_0 + 1/d_1)} = \sqrt{(1/33 + 1/24)} = 0.2683, \text{ giving}$$

$$EF = \exp(1.96 \times 0.2683) = 1.69$$

$$\text{Thus, } 95\% \text{ CI} = 2.01/1.69 \text{ to } 2.01 \times 1.69 = 1.19 \text{ to } 3.39$$

With 95% confidence, the rate of acute lower respiratory infections among children living in poor housing is between 1.19 and 3.39 times the rate among children living in good housing.

28.6 LIKELIHOOD IN MORE COMPLICATED MODELS

In most of this chapter, we show how likelihood theory can be used to reproduce results that we derived earlier in the book using properties of the normal distribution, and approximations to the normal distribution. The strength of the likelihood approach, however, lies in the way it can be generalized to any statistical model, for any number of parameters.

Thus the likelihood approach is used to derive maximum likelihood estimates (MLEs) and standard errors of the parameters in a regression model. Since the MLE for any one parameter will depend on the values of the other parameters, it is usually not possible to write down equations for what each of the MLEs will be. Instead, they are fitted by a computer program using a process known as **iteration**:

1 This starts with a guess for the MLEs of the parameters; for example, some programs use the null values corresponding to no effects of the exposure parameters on the outcome as the starting point.

2 Next, the value of the log likelihood is calculated using these 'guesstimates'.

3 The value of each of the parameters is then perturbed in both directions, and the values of the log likelihood calculated to obtain the gradient and curvature of the log likelihood curve at this point.

4 The gradient and curvature are then used to fit the best (multi-dimensional) quadratic approximation to the log likelihood curve at this particular point.

5 The maximum of the fitted quadratic is then located.

6 The whole process is then repeated using this maximum as the best guess for the MLEs.

7 The iteration stops when subsequent steps yield the same values for the guess for the MLEs. The fit is said to have **converged**. Some programs will record the number of iteration steps it required to obtain this convergence.

8 Occasionally the program fails to achieve convergence. The main causes of this are:

- insufficient data to support the estimation of the number of parameters there are in the model;

This is called the **profile log likelihood** for θ. In our hill analogy, it is equivalent to slicing through the hill at its peak and working with the resulting cross-section.

4 Figure 28.4 shows the profile log likelihood ratio for various values of the rate ratio using this re-expression. Note that the rate ratio is plotted on a **log scale**, and that doing this makes the log likelihood ratio curve close to a quadratic.

5 The log likelihood (and corresponding likelihood) is maximized when

$$\lambda_0 = 24/518, \text{ the observed rate in the unexposed group;}$$

$$\theta = \lambda_1/\lambda_0 = 2.01, \text{ the observed rate ratio}$$

These MLEs are the same as the estimates obtained directly from the data in Example 23.1.

6 Because the rate ratio is plotted on a log scale, the equation of the quadratic approximation is:

$$\text{Log(LR)} = -\frac{1}{2}\left(\frac{\log(\text{MLE}) - \log(\theta)}{S}\right)^2, \text{ where } S = \text{s.e. of the } log \text{ rate ratio}$$

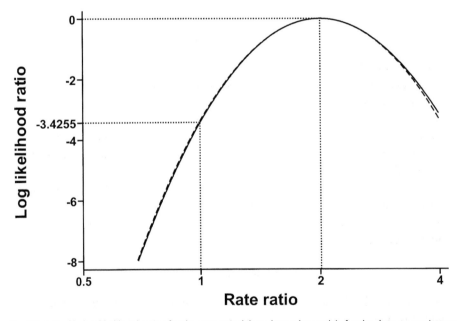

Fig. 28.4 Profile log likelihood ratios for the rate ratio (plotted on a log scale), for the data on respiratory infections in Guatemalan children. The dashed line shows the best quadratic approximation to the log likelihood ratio at the maximum, and the dotted lines show the values of the log likelihood ratio corresponding to the null value (1) and the maximum-likelihood estimate (2.01) of the rate ratio.

extension to the comparison of two exposure groups, using the data from the Guatemala morbidity study presented in Table 23.1. This table compared the incidence rate, $\lambda_1 = 33/355$, of lower respiratory infections among children aged less than 5 years living in poor housing conditions, to the rate, $\lambda_0 = 24/518$ among those living in good housing. The rate ratio was:

$$\text{rate ratio}\,(\theta) = \lambda_1/\lambda_0 = \frac{33/355}{24/518} = 2.01$$

As explained in Chapter 24 on Poisson regression, we can re-express this as:

$$\text{rate in exposed group} = \text{rate in unexposed group} \times \text{exposure rate ratio}$$

giving us the basis for a model which expresses the rate in each group in terms of two *model parameters*. These are:
- the *baseline rate*, λ_0, in the unexposed group;
- the *exposure rate ratio*, θ.

Applying the likelihood approach means that we want to find the most likely values of these two parameters given the observed data. In other words we want to find their *maximum likelihood estimates* (MLEs). It can be shown that:

1 Using the distribution of the numbers of infections in each of the two groups, we can derive a formula for the log likelihood (L) of the observed data for various combinations of the two parameters. This is:

$$L = (d_0 + d_1)\log(\lambda_0) + d_1\log(\theta) - \lambda_0 T_0 - \theta\lambda_0 T_1 + \text{constant}$$

where d_1 and d_0 are the number of observed infections and T_1 and T_0 are the child-years of follow up in the exposed (poor housing) and unexposed (good housing) groups respectively.

2 As we have two parameters we have a log likelihood surface rather than a curve. This can be thought of as like the map of a hill; the two parameters correspond to the two axes of the map, and contours on the hill correspond to values of the log likelihood ratio. We want to find the MLEs (equivalent to finding the peak of the hill) and the curvature at this point in order to fit a three-dimensional quadratic approximation to the surface (of the hill).

3 In this case it is possible to show that the value of λ_0 that maximizes the log likelihood is:

$$\lambda_0 = (d_0 + d_1)/(T_0 + \theta T_1)$$

and that substituting this formula for λ_0 into the equation for log likelihood and rearranging it gives:

$$L = d_1 \log\!\left(\frac{\theta T_1}{T_0}\right) - (d_0 + d_1)\log\!\left(1 + \frac{\theta T_1}{T_0}\right) + \text{constant}$$

the **values of the log(LR) curve at the 95 % confidence limits** (CL) are both:

$$\text{Log(LR) for 95\% CI} = -\frac{1.96^2}{2} = -1.9208$$

since the S's in the numerator and denominator cancel out, and since $(-1.96)^2 = 1.96^2$. Antilogging this gives the cut-off value of the **likelihood ratio corresponding to the 95 % confidence interval**:

$$\text{LR for 95\% CI} = e^{-1.9208} = 0.1465$$

Table 28.3 summarizes the cut-off values of the likelihood ratio and its logarithm corresponding to 90 %, 95 % and 99 % confidence intervals. Note that there is only a close agreement between standard confidence intervals and supported ranges based on these cut-offs when the quadratic approximation gives a close fit to the log(LR).

Table 28.3 Cut-off values for the likelihood ratio, and its logarithm, corresponding to 90%, 95% and 99% confidence intervals, assuming that the underlying distribution is normal or approximately normal.

	90% CI	95% CI	99% CI
% point of normal distribution	1.6449	1.96	2.5763
Cut-off value for log(LR)	−1.3529	−1.9208	−3.3187
Cut-off value for LR	0.2585	0.1465	0.0362

Information and standard error

The quantity $1/S^2$ (the multiplier of $\frac{1}{2}(\text{MLE} - \theta)^2$ in the quadratic approximation) is known as the **information** in the data. The larger the value for the information, the more sharply curved are the log(LR), its quadratic approximation, the likelihood ratio and the likelihood curves. The more information that the data contain about the parameter, the smaller is its standard error, the more precise is our estimate, and the narrower is the confidence interval.

28.5 LIKELIHOOD IN THE COMPARISON OF TWO GROUPS

Example 28.2
So far we have described the principles of likelihood in the simplest context of a single sample and a single parameter to be estimated. We will now illustrate its

$$\text{LRS}_{\text{Wald}} = -2 \times \log(\text{LR})_{\text{quad}} = \left(\frac{\text{MLE} - \theta_{\text{null}}}{S}\right)^2 = \left(\frac{\text{MLE}}{S}\right)^2, \text{ if } \theta_{\text{null}} = 0$$

For the data in Example 28.2 (and 23.1), the quadratic approximation to the log(LR) has been fitted using the log(rate ratio). Therefore:

$$\theta = \log(\text{rate ratio})$$
$$\text{MLE} = \log(2.01) = 0.6963$$
$$S = 0.2683 \text{ (see Section 28.5 above)}$$

$$\text{LRS}_{\text{Wald}} = \left(\frac{0.6963}{0.2683}\right)^2 = 6.7352$$
$$P = 0.0094 \text{ (derived from } \chi^2 \text{ with 1 d.f.)}$$

In this example, the Wald and likelihood ratio tests yield very similar results, as the quadratic approximation gives a close fit to the log likelihood ratio curve.

More commonly, the Wald test is carried out as a z-test, using the *square root* of the likelihood ratio statistic. This has a particularly convenient form:

$$\textbf{Wald statistic, } z = \frac{\text{MLE}}{S}, \text{ if } \theta_{\text{null}} = 0$$

and follows a standard normal distribution, since a χ^2 distribution with 1 d.f. is equivalent to the square of a standard normal distribution. This is the basis for the Wald tests described for logistic regression (Chapter 19), Poisson regression (Chapter 24) and Cox regression (Chapter 27).

For the data in Example 28.2, this formulation gives:

$$z = \frac{0.6963}{0.2683} = 2.5952 \text{ (equivalent to } \sqrt{6.7352})$$

As before, $P = 0.0094$.

Score tests

Much of the reasoning in this chapter has derived from fitting a quadratic approximation to the log likelihood ratio, chosen to have the same value and curvature at the MLE. The **score test** uses an alternative quadratic approximation, chosen to have the same value, gradient and curvature as the log likelihood ratio at the *null* value of the parameter rather than at its MLE. Its form is similar to that of the log likelihood ratio and Wald tests:

$$\text{Score test} = -2 \times \log(\text{LR})_{\text{quad fitted at null}} = \frac{U^2}{V}$$

where U = gradient and V = −curvature of the fitted $\log(\text{LR})$ at θ_{null}

The Mantel–Haenszel statistics derived in Chapters 18 and 23 are of this form:

$$\chi^2_{\text{MH}} = \frac{U^2}{V}$$

and are score tests. U, the gradient of the log likelihood at the null value of the parameter, is also known as the **score**, and V (minus the curvature) is also known as the **score variance**. The standard chi-squared statistic (see Chapter 17)

$$\chi^2 = \Sigma \frac{(O - E)^2}{E}$$

can also be shown to be a special form of the score test.

Choice of method

All three methods described in this section for calculating a *P*-value are *approximate*. The exception is the special (and unusual) case when the parameter of interest is the mean, μ, for a normal distribution, for which we *know* the standard deviation, σ. In this instance, the three methods coincide, as the log likelihood ratio is *exactly* quadratic, and yield an *exact P*-value.

The three methods will give quite different answers unless the quadratic approximations provide a good fit to the log likelihood ratio curve over the region of the curve between the MLE and the null value. In general it is possible to get a reasonably close fit provided the sample size is sufficiently large, and provided an appropriate scale is used for the parameter(s) of interest. In particular, for odds, rates, odds ratios and rate ratios, it is generally preferable to use a **logarithmic transformation**, as was done in Example 28.2.

The values of the Wald and score tests are both derived from the quadratic approximation, which is influenced by the particular scale used for the parameter. Their values will therefore depend on what, if any, transformation is used. In contrast, the likelihood ratio test yields the same results whatever scale is used for the parameter of interest, since a change of scale simply changes the shape of the log(LR) curve in the horizontal direction, but does not affect the height of the curve, or the relative heights between two values of the parameter. This is a considerable advantage.

However, if the three methods yield very different results, even after using an appropriate scale for the parameter(s), then it is usual to advise the use of exact *P*-values (see Clayton & Hills, 1993, for details), although these are not without their own difficulties.

Note that when the MLE and the null values are far apart, all three methods will always yield very small *P*-values. Thus, although it may not prove possible to obtain good quadratic approximations, and although the *P*-values may therefore differ numerically, this is unlikely to substantially affect the conclusions.

28.8 LIKELIHOOD RATIO TESTS IN REGRESSION MODELS

Hypothesis testing in regression models can be carried out using either **Wald tests** or **likelihood ratio tests**. We favour **likelihood ratio tests** for all but the simplest of cases, for the following reasons:

- the lack of dependence of the likelihood ratio statistic on the scale used for the parameter(s) of interest;
- the ease with which the calculation and interpretation of likelihood ratio statistics can be carried out in more complex situations, as described below;
- in contrast, although Wald tests are directly interpretable for exposure variables which are represented by a *single* parameter in the regression model (see Examples 19.1 and 24.1), they are less useful for a categorical variable, which is represented by a series of indicator variables in the regression model (see Section 29.4).

The likelihood ratio test described above for a single exposure is a special case of a more general likelihood ratio test that applies to more complex situations involving several model parameters. An example is in regression modelling where we have estimated the effect of a categorical exposure variable using k indicator variables and wish to test the null hypothesis that the exposure has no association with the outcome. In such situations we wish to test the joint null hypothesis that k parameters equal their null values. The likelihood ratio test is based on comparing the log likelihoods obtained from fitting the following two models:

1 L_{exc}, the log likelihood of the model *excluding* the parameter(s) to be tested;
2 L_{inc}, the log likelihood of the model *including* the parameter(s) to be tested.

Then the **likelihood ratio statistic (LRS)** has a χ^2 distribution with degrees of freedom equal to the number of parameters *omitted* from the model:

$$LRS = -2 \times \log(LR) = -2 \times (L_{exc} - L_{inc}) \text{ is } \chi^2 \text{ with } k \text{ d.f.}$$

Thus L_{inc} is the value of the log likelihood when all parameters equal their MLEs, and L_{exc} the value of the log likelihood when the k chosen parameters equal their null values and the other parameters equal their MLEs for the *restricted* model, excluding these parameters.

The likelihood ratio can be used to compare any two models where one is a restricted form of the other. Its use in regression modelling will be described in detail in Chapter 29.

CHAPTER 29

Regression modelling

29.1 INTRODUCTION

In previous chapters we have described simple and multiple linear regression for the analysis of numerical outcome variables, logistic regression for the analysis of binary outcome variables, and Poisson and Cox regression for the analysis of rates and survival data from longitudinal studies, as summarized in Table 29.1. We have shown how all these types of regression modelling can be used to examine the effect of a particular exposure (or treatment) on an outcome variable, including:

- Comparing the levels of an outcome variable in two exposure (or treatment) groups.
- Comparing more than two exposure groups, through the use of indicator variables to estimate the effect of different levels of a categorical variable, compared to a baseline level (see Section 19.4).

- Estimating a linear (or dose–response) effect on an outcome of a continuous or ordered categorical exposure variable.
- Controlling for the confounding effect of a variable by including it together with the exposure variable in a regression model. We explained that this assumed that there was no interaction (effect modification) between the exposure and confounding variables. That is, we assumed that the effect of each variable on the outcome was the same regardless of the level of the other.

In this chapter, we focus on general issues in the choice of an appropriate regression model for a particular analysis. These are:

- Understanding the similarities and differences between the different types of regression models.
- Deciding between different expressions of the outcome variable, and their implication for the type of regression model.
- *Hypothesis testing* in regression models.
- Investigating *interaction* (*effect modification*) between two or more exposure variables, and understanding its implications.
- Investigating whether an exposure has a *linear* (*dose–response*) effect on the outcome variable.
- Understanding the problems caused when exposure and/or confounding variables are highly correlated. This is known as *collinearity*.
- Making the final choice of exposure/confounding variables for inclusion in the regression model.

29.2 TYPES OF REGRESSION MODEL

The different types of regression models described in this book are summarized in Table 29.1. It is useful to distinguish between:

- *Simple and multiple linear regression models*, in which the outcome variable is numerical, and whose general form for the effects of p exposure variables is:

$$y = \beta_0 + \beta_1 x_1 + \beta_2 x_2 + \ldots + \beta_p x_p$$

These are known as **general linear models**. The quantity on the right hand side of the equation is known as the **linear predictor** of the outcome y, given particular values of the exposure variables x_1 to x_p. The β's are the **regression coefficients** associated with the p exposure variables.

- *All other types of regression models*, including logistic, Poisson and Cox regression, in which we model a *transformation* of the outcome variable rather than the outcome itself. For example, in logistic regression we model the *log of the odds of the outcome*. Apart from this transformation, the general form of the model is similar to that for multiple regression:

$$\text{log odds of outcome} = \log\left(\frac{\pi}{1 - \pi}\right) = \beta_0 + \beta_1 x_1 + \beta_2 x_2 + \ldots + \beta_p x_p$$

Table 29.1 Summary of the main regression models described in Parts B to D of this book.

Type of outcome variable	Type	Chapter	Link function	Measure of exposure effect	Effects
Numerical	Linear (Simple/Multiple)	10/11	Identity	Mean difference	Additive
Binary	Logistic	19	Logit	Odds ratio	Multiplicative
Matched binary	Conditional logistic	21	Logit	Odds ratio	Multiplicative
Time to binary event	Poisson	24	Log	Rate ratio	Multiplicative
Time to binary event	Cox	27	Log	Hazard ratio	Multiplicative

These regression models are known as **generalized linear models**. The linear model for the exposure variables is said to be related to the outcome via a **link function**. For logistic regression, the link function is the logit (log odds) function, and for Poisson and Cox regressions, it is the logarithmic function.

Note that multiple regression is a special case of a generalized linear model in which the link function is the *identity* function $f(y) = y$.

- *Conditional regression models*, such as conditional logistic regression and Cox regression. These are special cases of generalized linear models in which estimation is based on the distribution of exposures within case–control strata or within risk sets. Likelihoods (see Chapter 28) for these models are known as *conditional likelihoods*.

All regression models are fitted using the maximum likelihood approach described in Chapter 28. The estimates obtained for the regression coefficients are called **maximum-likelihood estimates**. There are two important differences worth noting between multiple regression and the other types of generalized linear models:

1 Multiple regression models assume that the effect of exposures combine in an *additive* manner. In all the other generalized linear models discussed in this book it is a *log* transformation of the outcome (odds, rate or hazard) that is related to the linear predictor. This means that exposure effects are *multiplicative* (see the detailed explanation for logistic regression in Section 20.2) and that results of these models are most easily interpreted on the ratio scale.

2 Since multiple linear regression is based on the normal distribution, its log likelihood has an *exact* quadratic form (see Section 28.4). This means that Wald tests and likelihood ratio tests give identical results (see Sections 28.7 and 29.4). It also means that estimates obtained using maximum-likelihood are identical to those obtained using least-squares as described in Chapters 10 and 11.

29.3 DECIDING HOW TO EXPRESS THE OUTCOME VARIABLE

It is often the case that we have a choice of which regression model to use, depending on how the outcome variable is expressed. For example, blood pressure may be expressed as a continuous, ordered categorical or binary variable, in which case we would use linear, ordinal logistic or logistic regression respectively. Similarly, a study of factors influencing the duration of breastfeeding could be analysed using Poisson or Cox regression, or using logistic regression by defining the outcome as breastfed or not breastfed at, say, age 6 months.

In making such choices we need to balance two (sometimes opposing) considerations:

1 It is desirable to *choose the regression model that uses as much of the information in the data as possible*. In the blood pressure example, this would favour using linear regression with blood pressure as a continuous variable, since categorizing or dichotomizing it would discard some of the information collected (through using groups rather than the precise measurements). In the breastfeeding example, Cox or Poisson regression would be the preferred regression models, since the logistic regression analysis would discard important information on the precise time at which breastfeeding stopped.

2 It is often sensible to *use simpler models before proceeding to more complex ones*. For example, in examining the effect of exposures on an ordered categorical variable we might start by collapsing the variable into two categories and using logistic regression, before proceeding to use ordinal logistic regression to analyse the original outcome variable. We could then check whether the results of the two models are consistent, and assess whether the gain in precision of exposure effect estimates obtained using the original outcome variable justifies the extra complexity.

29.4 HYPOTHESIS TESTING IN REGRESSION MODELS

Hypothesis testing is used in regression models both to test the null hypothesis that there is no association between an exposure variable and the outcome, and in order to refine the model, for example by:

- Examining the assumption of no interaction (effect modification) between two or more exposure variables (see Section 29.5).
- Deciding between the different forms in which an exposure/confounder variable might be included, such as deciding between modelling the effect of a categorical exposure variable using indicator variables or including it as a *linear* (*dose–response*) effect (see Section 29.6).
- Deciding whether a variable needs to be included in the final regression model (see Section 29.8).

Hypothesis testing can be carried out using either **Wald tests** or **likelihood ratio tests**, as described in Section 28.7. The *P*-values corresponding to the different parameter estimates in computer outputs are based on Wald tests. These are directly interpretable for exposure effects that are represented by a single parameter in the regression model. Examples have been given in Example 19.1 for the logistic regression of microfilarial infection with the binary exposure area (1 = rainforest/0 = savannah) and in Example 24.1 for the Poisson regression of myocardial infarction with the binary exposure 'cursmoke' (1 = men who were current smokers at the start of the study/0 = men who were never or ex-smokers at the start of the study). When an exposure effect is assumed to be linear (see Sections 19.3 and 29.6) it is also represented by a single parameter of the regression model.

Single parameter Wald tests are, however, less useful for a categorical variable, which is represented by a series of indicator variables in the regression model. Thus in Example 24.2, the Poisson regression output (Table 24.6) for the effect of social class on the rate of myocardial infarction has six parameter estimates, the rate in the baseline group and the five rate ratios comparing the other social class groups with the baseline. Wald z statistics and P-values are given for each of these five social class groups, enabling each of them to be compared with the baseline. What is needed, however, is a combined test of the null hypothesis that social class has no influence on the rate of myocardial infarction. Some computer packages have an option for a multi-parameter Wald test to do this.

We prefer instead to use **likelihood ratio tests** for all but the very simplest of cases, both for the reasons given in Chapter 28, and for the ease with which they can be calculated in all situations. As explained in Chapter 28, the **likelihood ratio statistic (LRS)** is calculated as minus twice the difference between the log likelihoods obtained from fitting the following two models:

1 L_{exc}, the log likelihood of the model *excluding* the variable(s) to be tested;
2 L_{inc}, the log likelihood of the model *including* the variable(s) to be tested.

This follows a χ^2 distribution with degrees of freedom equal to the number of parameters omitted from the model. For a simple binary exposure the degrees of freedom will equal one, and for a categorical exposure the degrees of freedom will equal the number of groups minus one.

$$LRS = -2 \times (L_{exc} - L_{inc})$$

is χ^2 with d.f. = number of additional parameters in the model including the exposure variable(s) to be tested

Note that the value of the log likelihood is a standard part of the computer output for a regression model.

Example 29.1

We will illustrate the use of the likelihood ratio test in the context of the Caerphilly cohort study, which was introduced in Chapter 24. We will base this on the

following three different Poisson regression models for rates of myocardial infarction fitted in that chapter:
1 Table 24.4: Cursmoke comparing smokers at recruitment with never/ex-
smokers.
2 Table 24.6: Socclass comparing six social class groups.
3 Table 24.9: Model including both Cursmoke and Socclass.
The values of the log likelihoods for these three models, together with the model
including no exposure variables (the 'constant-only model') are summarized in
Table 29.2. We will refer to them as $L_{model\,1}$ to $L_{model\,4}$. The constant-only model,
which has a single parameter corresponding to the constant term, is fitted by
specifying the type of regression and the outcome, and nothing else.

   Note that the parameter estimate corresponding to the 'constant' term is
different for each of the four models. It represents the rate in the baseline group
(those non-exposed to all of the exposure variables included in the model) against
which all other comparisons are made. Its value therefore depends on which
exposure variables are included in the model.

Hypothesis test for a single parameter

Cursmoke is a binary exposure variable. Model 2 therefore has two parameters:
1 Constant: the rate of myocardial infarction in the baseline group (never/ex-
smokers), and
2 Cursmoke: the rate ratio comparing current smokers with never or ex-smokers.
The likelihood ratio statistic to test the null hypothesis that myocardial infarction
rates are not related to smoking status at recruitment (Cursmoke) is based on a
comparison of models 1 and 2. Note that as the value of L_{inc} ($L_{model\,2}$) is negative,
minus becomes a plus in the calculation.

$$LRS = -2 \times (L_{exc} - L_{inc}) = -2 \times (L_{model\,1} - L_{model\,2})$$
$$= -2 \times (-1206.985 + 1195.513) = 22.944$$

This is χ^2 with d.f. = number of additional parameters in the inclusive model
= 2 − 1 = 1.
   The corresponding P-value, derived from the χ^2 distribution on 1 degree of
freedom, equals 0.0000017. There is thus strong evidence of an association between

Table 29.2 Log likelihood values obtained from different Poisson regression models fitted to data
from the Caerphilly cohort study, as described in Chapter 24.

Model	Exposure(s) in model	No. of parameters	Log likelihood
1	None (Constant only model)	1	$L_{model\,1} = -1206.985$
2	Cursmoke (Yes/No)	2	$L_{model\,2} = -1195.513$
3	Socclass (6 groups)	6	$L_{model\,3} = -1201.002$
4	Cursmoke & Socclass	7	$L_{model\,4} = -1191.119$

current smoking and rate of myocardial infarction. The equivalent z statistic is $z = \sqrt{22.944} = 4.790$. This is similar to the corresponding Wald z statistic value of 4.680, given in the output in Table 24.5.

Hypothesis test for a categorical exposure with more than one parameter

When an exposure variable has more than two categories, its effect is modelled by introducing indicator variables corresponding to each of the non-baseline categories (as explained in Section 19.4). This is the case for Socclass, the men's social class at the start of the study. It has six categories, I = 1 (most affluent), II = 2, III non-manual = 3, III manual = 4, IV = 5, V = 6 (most deprived). Model 3 therefore has six parameters:

1 Constant: the rate of myocardial infarction in the baseline group, chosen to be III non-manual as more than half the men were in this group, and
2 Socclass: five rate ratios comparing each of the other social class groups with the baseline group.

To test the null hypothesis that social class has no effect on the rate of myocardial infarction, we compare the log likelihoods obtained in models 1 and 3. The likelihood ratio test statistic is

$$
\begin{aligned}
\text{LRS} &= -2 \times (\text{L}_{\text{exc}} - \text{L}_{\text{inc}}) = -2 \times (\text{L}_{\text{model 1}} - \text{L}_{\text{model 3}}) \\
&= -2 \times (-1206.985 + 1201.002) = 11.966
\end{aligned}
$$

d.f. = number of additional parameters in the inclusive model = 6 − 1 = 5

$$P = 0.035$$

Because the effect of social class was modelled with five parameters, the P-value corresponding to this LRS is derived from the χ^2 distribution with 5 degrees of freedom. It equals 0.035. There is thus some evidence of an association between social class and rates of myocardial infarction. An alternative way to examine the effect of social class would be to carry out a test for linear trend, as was done in Example 24.2. Investigation of linear effects is discussed in detail in Section 29.6.

As mentioned above, it is also possible to derive a P-value from a multi-parameter version of the Wald test. This multi-parameter version is a χ^2 test with the same number of degrees of freedom as the likelihood ratio test. In this example the Wald statistic is $\chi^2 = 10.25$ with d.f. = 5. The corresponding P-value is 0.069, higher than that obtained from the likelihood ratio test.

Hypothesis tests in multivariable models

Models 2 and 3 in this example are univariable models, in which we examined the **crude** or **unadjusted effects** of a single exposure variable, namely the effects of smoking and of social class. We now consider the **multivariable model** including both smoking and social class. This is number 4 in Table 29.2. As previously explained in Chapter 24, the effects in this model should be interpreted as the effect of smoking controlled for social class and the effect of social class controlled for smoking. To test the null hypothesis that there is no effect of social class after controlling for smoking, we compare:

1 the log likelihood of model 2, which includes only smoking, with

2 the log likelihood of model 4 which also includes social class, with the addition corresponding to the effect of social class controlled for smoking.

The likelihood ratio test statistic is:

$$\text{LRS} = -2 \times (L_{\text{exc}} - L_{\text{inc}}) = -2 \times (L_{\text{model 2}} - L_{\text{model 4}})$$
$$= -2 \times (-1195.513 + 1191.119) = 8.788$$
$$\text{d.f.} = \text{number of additional parameters in the inclusive model} = 7 - 2 = 5$$
$$P = 0.118$$

There is therefore no good evidence for an association between social class and rates of myocardial infarction, other than that which acts through smoking. However, we should be aware that for an ordered categorical variable such as social class a more powerful approach may be to derive a *test for trend* by including social class as a linear effect in the model, rather than as a categorical variable. Modelling linear effects is discussed in detail in Section 29.6.

29.5 INVESTIGATING INTERACTION (EFFECT MODIFICATION) IN REGRESSION MODELS

Interaction was introduced in Section 18.5, where we explained that there is an *interaction* between the effects of two exposures if the effect of one exposure varies according to the level of the other exposure. For example, the protective effect of breastfeeding against infectious diseases in early infancy is more pronounced among infants living in poor environmental conditions than among those living in areas with adequate water supply and sanitation facilities. We also explained that an alternative term for interaction is **effect modification**. In this example, we can think of this as the quality of environmental conditions *modifying* the effect of breastfeeding. Finally, we noted that the most flexible approach to examine interaction is to use regression models, but that when we are using Mantel–Haenszel methods to control for confounding an alternative is to use a χ^2 test for effect modification, commonly called a χ^2 **test of heterogeneity**. Interaction, effect modification and heterogeneity are three different ways of describing exactly the same thing.

We have also seen that regression models including the effect of two or more exposures make the assumption that there is *no interaction* between the exposures. We now describe how to test this assumption by introducing **interaction terms** into the regression model.

Example 29.2

We will explain this in the context of the onchocerciasis dataset used throughout Chapters 19 and 20, where logistic regression was used to examine the effects of area of residence (forest or savannah) and of age group on the odds of micro-filarial (*mf*) infection. We found strong associations of both area of residence and of age group with the odds of *mf* infection. We will do three things:

1 Remind ourselves of the results of the standard logistic regression model including both area and age group, which assumes that is there is *no interaction* between the two. In other words, it assumes that the effect of area is the same in each of the four age groups, and (correspondingly) that the effect of age is the same in the each of the two areas, and that any observed differences are due to sampling variation. Unless you are already familiar with how such models work, we strongly suggest that you read Section 20.2 where this is explained in detail, before continuing with this section.

2 We will then describe how to specify a regression model incorporating an interaction between the effects of area and age group, and how to interpret the regression output from such a model.

3 We will then calculate a likelihood ratio statistic using the log likelihoods of these two models to test the null hypothesis that there is no interaction between the effects of area and age group.

Model with two exposures and no interaction

Table 29.3 summarizes the results from the logistic regression model for *mf* infection including both area and age group, described in Section 20.2. Part (a) of the table shows the set of equations for the eight subgroups of the data that define the model in terms of its parameters. Note that the exposure effects represent odds ratios, and that they are *multiplicative*, since logistic regression models the *log odds*. The eight subgroups can be divided into four different types:

1 The *baseline* subgroup, consisting of those in the baseline groups of both area and age, namely those aged 5–9 years living in a savannah area. This is represented by the Baseline parameter in the model.

2 One subgroup consisting of those in the baseline group for age, but *not* for area, namely those aged 5–9 years living in a rainforest area. This subgroup is '*exposed to area but not to age*'. Its relative odds of *mf* infection compared to the baseline is modelled by the Area parameter.

3 Three subgroups corresponding to those in each of the three non-baseline age groups, but who are in the baseline group for area, namely those living in savannah areas aged 10–19 years, 20–39 years, or 40 years or more. These subgroups are '*exposed to age but not area*'. Their relative odds of *mf* infection compared to the baseline are modelled by the three age group parameters, Agegrp(1), Agegrp(2) and Agegrp(3), respectively.

4 Three subgroups corresponding to those in each of the three non-baseline age groups who are also in the non-baseline group for area, namely those living in rainforest areas aged 10–19 years, 20–39 years, or 40 years or more. These subgroups are '*exposed to both area and age*'. If we assume that there is *no interaction* between the two exposures, the relative odds of *mf* infection in these three subgroups compared to the baseline are modelled by multiplying together the Area parameter and the relevant age group parameter. This gives Area × Agegrp(1), Area × Agegrp(2) and Area × Agegrp(3), respectively.

The model for the odds of *mf* infection in the eight subgroups therefore contains just five parameters. This is made possible by the assumption of *no interaction*. The parameter estimates are shown in part (b) of Table 29.3. Part (c) shows the values obtained when these estimates are inserted into the equations in part (a) to give estimated values of the odds of *mf* infection according to area and age group. The observed odds of *mf* infection in each group are also shown.

Model incorporating an interaction between the two exposures

We now describe how to specify an alternative regression model incorporating an interaction between the effects of the two exposures. We no longer assume that the

Table 29.3 Results from the logistic regression model for *mf* infection, including both area of residence and age group, assuming *no interaction* between the effects of area and age group.

(a) Odds of *mf* infection by area and age group, expressed in terms of the parameters of the logistic regression model: Odds = Baseline × Area × Age group.

	Odds of *mf* infection	
Age group	Savannah areas (Unexposed)	Rainforest areas (Exposed)
0 (5–9 years)	Baseline	Baseline × Area
1 (10–19 years)	Baseline × Agegrp(1)	Baseline × Area × Agegrp(1)
2 (20–39 years)	Baseline × Agegrp(2)	Baseline × Area × Agegrp(2)
3 (≥ 40 years)	Baseline × Agegrp(3)	Baseline × Area × Agegrp(3)

(b) Parameter estimates obtained by fitting the model.

	Baseline	Area	Agegrp(1)	Agegrp(2)	Agegrp(3)
Odds ratio	0.147	3.083	2.599	9.765	17.64

(c) Odds of *mf* infection by area and age group, as estimated from the logistic regression model, and as observed.

	Savannah areas: odds of *mf* infection		Rainforest areas: odds of *mf* infection	
Age group	Estimated	Observed	Estimated	Observed
0 (5–9 years)	0.147	0.208	$0.147 \times 3.083 = 0.453$	0.380
1 (10–19 years)	$0.147 \times 2.599 = 0.382$	0.440	$0.147 \times 3.083 \times 2.599 = 1.178$	1.116
2 (20–39 years)	$0.147 \times 9.765 = 1.435$	1.447	$0.147 \times 3.083 \times 9.765 = 4.426$	4.400
3 (≥ 40 years)	$0.147 \times 17.64 = 2.593$	2.182	$0.147 \times 3.083 \times 17.64 = 7.993$	10.32

relative odds of *mf* infection in the subgroups '*exposed to both age and area*' can be modelled by multiplying the area and age effects together. Instead we introduce extra parameters, called **interaction parameters**, as shown in Table 29.4(a). These allow the effect of area to be different in the four age groups and, correspondingly, the effects of age to be different in the two areas. An interaction parameter is denoted by the exposure parameters for the subgroup written with a full stop between them. The three interaction parameters in this example are denoted Area.Agegrp(1), Area.Agegrp(2) and Area.Agegrp(3).

This new model is fitted using seven indicator variables as shown in Box 29.1. The parameter estimates for this model are shown in Table 29.4(b). Table 29.4(c) shows the values obtained when these are inserted into the equations in part (a). Note that:

1 Since this model has *eight* parameters, the same as the number of area × age subgroups, there is an exact agreement between the estimated odds of *mf* infection in each subgroup and the observed odds, as shown in Tables 29.3(c) and 20.3.

2 Including interaction terms leads to different estimates of the baseline, area and age group parameters than those obtained in the model assuming no interaction. It is important to realize that the interpretation of the area and age group parameters is also different.

- The Area parameter estimate (1.8275) is the odds ratio for area *in the baseline age group*. In the model assuming no interaction, the Area parameter estimate (3.083) is a weighted average of the odds ratios for area in the four age groups and is interpreted as the odds ratio for area after controlling for age group.

- Similarly, the age group parameter estimates represent the effect of age in the *baseline area group*, in other words the effect among those living in savannah areas.

3 The estimates for the interaction parameters are all greater than one. This corresponds to a synergistic effect between area and each of the age groups, with the combined effect more than simply the combination of the separate effects. A value of one for an interaction term is equivalent to no interaction effect. A value less than one would mean that the combined effect of both exposures is less than the combination of their separate effects.

4 The interaction parameters allow the area effect to be different in the four age groups. They can be used to calculate age-specific area odds ratios as follows:

- The Area parameter estimate equals 1.8275, and is the area odds ratio (comparing those living in rainforest areas with those living in savannah areas) in the *baseline* age group (5–9 years).

- Multiplying the Area parameter estimate by the interaction parameter estimate Area.Agegrp(1) gives the odds ratio for area in age group 1 (10–19 years):

$$\text{OR for area in age group } 1 = \text{Area} \times \text{Area.Agegrp(1)}$$
$$= 1.8275 \times 1.3878 = 2.5362$$

Table 29.4 Logistic regression model for *mf* infection, including both area of residence and age group, and *incorporating an interaction* between their effects.

(a) Odds of *mf* infection by area and age group, expressed in terms of the parameters of the logistic regression model, with the interaction parameters shown in bold: Odds = Baseline × Area × Agegroup × Area.Agegroup

	Odds of *mf* infection	
Age group	Savannah areas (Unexposed)	Rainforest areas (Exposed)
0 (5–9 years)	Baseline	Baseline × Area
1 (10–19 years)	Baseline × Agegrp(1)	Baseline × Area × Agegrp(1) × **Area.Agegrp(1)**
2 (20–39 years)	Baseline × Agegrp(2)	Baseline × Area × Agegrp(2) × **Area.Agegrp(2)**
3 (≥40 years)	Baseline × Agegrp(3)	Baseline × Area × Agegrp(3) × **Area.Agegrp(3)**

(b) Computer output showing the results from fitting the model (interaction parameters shown in bold).

	Odds ratio	z	P > |z|	95 % CI
Area.Agegrp(1)	1.3878	0.708	0.479	0.560 to 3.439
Area.Agegrp(2)	1.6638	1.227	0.220	0.738 to 3.751
Area.Agegrp(3)	2.5881	2.171	0.030	1.097 to 6.107
Area	1.8275	1.730	0.084	0.923 to 3.619
Agegrp(1)	2.1175	1.998	0.046	1.015 to 4.420
Agegrp(2)	6.9639	6.284	0.000	3.802 to 12.76
Agegrp(3)	10.500	7.362	0.000	5.614 to 19.64
Constant (Baseline)	0.2078	−5.72	0.000	0.121 to 0.356

(c) Odds of *mf* infection by area and age group, as estimated from the logistic regression model, with the interaction parameters shown in bold.

	Odds of *mf* infection	
Age group	Savannah areas	Rainforest areas
0 (5–9 years)	0.2078	0.2078 × 1.8275 = 0.380
1 (10–19 years)	0.2078 × 2.1175 = 0.440	0.2078 × 1.8275 × 2.1175 × **1.3878** = 1.116
2 (20–39 years)	0.2078 × 6.9639 = 1.447	0.2078 × 1.8275 × 6.9639 × **1.6638** = 4.400
3 (≥40 years)	0.2078 × 10.500 = 2.182	0.2078 × 1.8275 × 10.500 × **2.5881** = 10.32

Similarly,

$$\text{OR for area in age group } 2 = \text{Area} \times \text{Area.Agegrp(2)}$$
$$= 1.8275 \times 1.6638 = 3.0406$$

and

$$\text{OR for area in age group } 3 = \text{Area} \times \text{Area.Agegrp(3)}$$
$$= 1.8275 \times 2.5881 = 4.7300$$

These four age-group-specific area odds ratios are the same as those shown in Tables 20.3 and 20.4.

5 In exactly the same way, the interaction parameters can be used to calculate area-specific age group odds ratios. For example:

$$\text{OR for age group 1 in rainforest areas} = \text{Agegrp}(1) \times \text{Area.Agegrp}(1)$$
$$= 2.1175 \times 1.3878 = 2.9386$$

6 An alternative expression of these same relationships is to note that the interaction parameter Area.Agegrp(1) is equal to the *ratio* of the odds ratios for area in age group 1 and age group 0, presented in Tables 20.3 and 20.4. For example:

$$\text{Area.Agegrp}(1) = \frac{\text{OR for area in age group 1}}{\text{OR for area in age group 0}} = \frac{2.5362}{1.8275} = 1.3878$$

If there is no interaction then the area odds ratios are the same in each age group and the interaction parameter equals 1.

7 Alternatively, we can express the interaction parameter Area.Agegrp(1) as the ratio of the odds ratios for age group 1 (compared to age group 0), in area 1 and area 0:

$$\text{Area.Agegrp}(1) = \frac{\text{OR for age group 1 in area 1}}{\text{OR for age group 1 in area 0}} = \frac{2.9386}{2.1175} = 1.3878$$

(The odds ratios for age group 1 were calculated using the raw data presented in Table 20.3).

8 The other interaction parameter estimates all have similar interpretations: for example the estimate for Area.Agegrp(2) equals the ratio of the area odds ratios in age group 2 and age group 0, and equivalently it equals the ratio of the odds ratios for age group 2 (compared to age group 0) in area 1 and area 0.

9 For a model allowing for interaction between two binary exposure variables, the *P*-value corresponding to the interaction parameter estimate corresponds to a Wald test of the null hypothesis that there is no interaction. When, as in this example, there is more than one interaction parameter, the individual *P*-values corresponding to the interaction parameters are not useful in assessing the evidence for interaction: we describe how to derive the appropriate likelihood ratio test later in this section.

Table 29.5 summarizes the interpretation of the interaction parameters for different types of regression models.

Table 29.5 Interpretation of interaction parameters.

Type of regression model	Interpretation of interaction parameters
Linear	Difference between mean differences
Logistic	Ratio of odds ratios
Poisson	Ratio of rate ratios

BOX 29.1   USING INDICATOR VARIABLES TO INVESTIGATE INTERACTION IN REGRESSION MODELS

Values of the seven indicator variables used in a model to examine the interaction between area (binary variable) and age group (4 groups):

Age group	Area	Area	Age(1)	Age(2)	Age(3)	Area.Age(1)	Area.Age(2)	Area.Age(3)
5–9 years (0)	Savannah	0	0	0	0	0	0	0
	Forest	1	0	0	0	0	0	0
10–19 (1)	Savannah	0	1	0	0	0	0	0
	Forest	1	1	0	0	1	0	0
20–39 years (2)	Savannah	0	0	1	0	0	0	0
	Forest	1	0	1	0	0	1	0
≥40 years (3)	Savannah	0	0	0	1	0	0	0
	Forest	1	0	0	1	0	0	1

Likelihood ratio test for interaction

To test the null hypothesis that there is no interaction between area and age group, we need to compare the log likelihoods obtained in the two models excluding and including the interaction parameters. These are shown in Table 29.6. The likelihood ratio test statistic is:

$$\text{LRS} = -2 \times (L_{exc} - L_{inc}) = -2 \times (-692.407 + 689.773) = 5.268$$
$$\text{d.f.} = \text{number of additional parameters in the inclusive model} = 8 - 5 = 3$$
$$P = 0.153$$

Therefore this analysis provides little evidence of interaction between the effects of area and age on the odds of microfilarial infection

Table 29.6 Log likelihood values obtained from the logistic regression models for *mf* infection by area of residence and age group, (a) assuming *no* interaction, and (b) incorporating an interaction between the effects of area and age group.

Model	Exposure(s) in model	No. of parameters	Log likelihood
(a) exc	Area and Agegrp	5	−692.407
(b) inc	Area, Agegrp and Area.Agegrp	8	−689.773

Interactions with continuous variables

It is straightforward to incorporate an interaction between the effects of a continuous exposure variable (x) and a binary exposure variable (b, coded as 0 for unexposed and 1 for exposed individuals) in a regression model, by multiplying the values of the two exposures together to create a new variable ($x.b$) representing the interaction, as shown in Table 29.7. This new variable equals 0 for those unexposed to exposure b, and the value of exposure x for those exposed to b. The regression coefficient for $x.b$ then corresponds to the difference between the slope in individuals exposed to b and the slope in individuals not exposed to b, and the evidence for an interaction may be assessed either using the Wald P-value for $x.b$, or by omitting $x.b$ from the model and performing a likelihood ratio test.

To examine interactions between two continuous exposure variables w and x, it is usual to create a new variable $w.x$ by multiplying w by x. If the regression coefficient for $w.x$ is 0 (1 for models with exposure effects reported as ratios) then there is no evidence of interaction.

Table 29.7 Creating a variable to represent an interaction between a continuous and a binary exposure variable.

Continuous exposure (x)	Binary exposure (b)	Interaction variable ($x.b$)
x	0 (unexposed)	0
x	1 (exposed)	x

Confounding and interaction

Note that confounding and interaction may coexist. If there is clear evidence of an interaction between the exposure and the confounder, it is no longer adequate to report the effect of the exposure controlled for the confounder, since this assumes the effect of the exposure to be the same at each level of the confounder. This is not the case when interaction is present. Instead, we should report *separate* exposure effects for each *stratum* of the confounder. We can derive these by performing a separate regression to examine the association between the exposure and outcome variables, for each level of the confounding variable.

It is possible to derive stratum-specific effects in regression models by including appropriate indicator variables, or combining regression coefficients as was done in Table 29.4(c). This has the advantage of allowing estimation of such effects, controlled for the effects of other exposure variables. Confidence intervals for such combinations of regression coefficients need to take into account the covariance (a measure of the association) between the individual regression coefficients: some statistical packages provide commands to combine regression coefficients and derive corresponding confidence intervals.

An advantage of Mantel–Haenszel methods is that because the stratum-specific exposure effects tend to be presented in computer output, we are encouraged to look for evidence of interaction. In regression models we have to fit interaction terms explicitly to do this.

Regression models with more than two variables

The power of regression models is that, providing we make the simplifying assumption of no interactions, they allow us to examine the joint (simultaneous) effects of a number of exposure variables. For example, suppose we had four exposure variables, with 2, 3, 4 and 5 levels respectively. The number of subgroups defined by different combinations of these exposure groups would be $2 \times 3 \times 4 \times 5 = 120$. Mantel–Haenszel methods to adjust for confounding would need to stratify by all these 120 subgroups. Similarly, a regression model that included all the interactions between these four exposures would also have 120 parameters. However, a regression model that assumes no interaction between any of the exposures would contain only 11 parameters, one for the baseline (constant) term plus 1, 2, 3 and 4 parameters for each of the four exposure variables, since $(k - 1)$ parameters are needed for an exposure with k levels. Interactions between confounding variables are often omitted from regression models: this is discussed in more detail in Chapter 38.

Increasing power in tests for interaction

The interpretation of tests for interaction is difficult. As discussed in more detail in Sections 35.4 and 38.6, tests for interaction usually have *low power*, so that the absence of strong evidence that interaction is present does not imply that interaction is absent.

A further problem, in addition to that of low power, occurs in regression models with binary or time-to-event outcomes, when some subgroups contain no individuals who experienced the outcome event. If this is the case, then interaction parameters for that subgroup cannot be estimated, and statistical computer packages may then drop all individuals in such subgroups from the analysis. This means that the model including the interactions is not directly comparable with the one assuming no interaction.

A solution to both of these problems is to *combine exposure groups*, so that the interaction introduces only a small number of extra parameters. For example, to investigate possible interactions between area and age we might first combine age groups to create a binary age group variable, separating those aged 0 to 19 years from those aged 20 years or more. Note that it is perfectly permissible to examine interactions using indicator variables based on binary variables, while controlling for the exposure effects based on the original (ungrouped) variables.

Further advice on examining interactions is provided in Box 18.1 on page 188 and in Chapter 38.

29.6 INVESTIGATING LINEAR EFFECTS (DOSE–RESPONSE RELATIONSHIPS) IN REGRESSION MODELS

Exposure effects may be modelled as linear if the exposure is either a numerical or an ordered categorical variable. In modelling exposure effects as linear, we assume that the outcome increases or decreases systematically with the exposure effect, as depicted in Figure 29.1, panels (a) and (b). If the observed association is as depicted in panel (c) of Figure 29.1, then it is appropriate to conclude that there is no linear effect. However, it is essential to be aware of the possibility that there is **extra-linear variation** in the exposure–outcome relationship. An example is depicted in panel (d) of Figure 29.1. Here, a regression model assuming a linear effect would conclude that there was no association between the exposure and the outcome. This would be incorrect, because there is in fact a non-linear association: the outcome level first increases and then decreases with increasing exposure.

The interpretation of linear effects, and the methods available to examine them, depends on the type of outcome and regression model:

- in linear or multiple regression models, the linear effect corresponds to a constant increase in the *mean* of the outcome per unit increase in the exposure variable;
- in logistic regression or conditional logistic regression models, it corresponds to a constant increase in the *log odds* per unit increase in the exposure variable;
- in Poisson regression models, it corresponds to a constant increase in the *log rate* per unit increase in the exposure variable; and
- in Cox regression models, it corresponds to a constant increase in the *log hazard* per unit increase in the exposure variable.

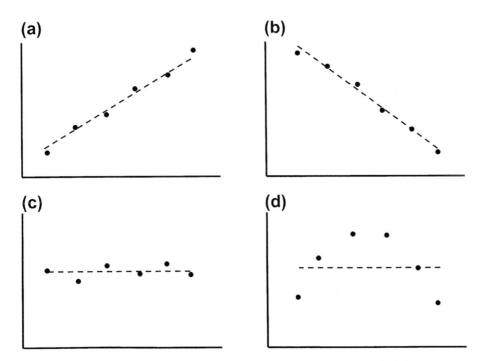

Fig. 29.1 Four possibilities for the association between outcome and exposure. Panels (a) and (b) show, respectively, positive and negative linear associations between the outcome and exposure. In panel (c) there is no association between the outcome and exposure; the estimated linear effect is zero. In panel (d) the linear effect is also zero, but there is a non-linear association between the outcome and the exposure.

When exposure effects are expressed as ratio measures, the linear effect corresponds to the amount by which the outcome is *multiplied* per unit increase in the exposure variable. For example, Table 19.11 shows that for the onchocerciasis data the log odds ratio for the linear association between microfilarial infection and age group was 0.930, corresponding to an odds ratio of 2.534 per unit increase in age group. The odds ratio comparing age group 2 with age group 0 is therefore $2.534^2 = 6.421$, and in general the odds ratio for an increase of k age groups is 2.534^k.

We saw in Chapter 10 on *linear regression* that the first step in examining the association between a numerical outcome and a numerical exposure is to draw a scatter plot. Such plots should protect us from making errors such as that depicted in panel (d) of Figure 29.1, where an assumption of a linear effect would lead to the incorrect conclusion that there is no association between the exposure and outcome.

For *logistic* and *Poisson regression*, such plots cannot be drawn without first grouping the exposure variable and then graphing the outcome (e.g. log odds, log rate) in each group. For example, the odds of a binary outcome for an individual are either $0/1 = 0$, or $1/0 = $ infinity. We cannot therefore graph the log odds for individuals, but we can calculate the log odds in groups (e.g. age groups) provided that there is at least one individual with and one without the disease outcome in each group. Therefore it is sensible to group numerical exposure variables into ordered categories in early analyses, in order to check for linearity in the measure of effect. If the exposure–outcome association appears approximately linear then the original continuous variable may be used in subsequent models. For example, Figure 19.2 shows that there is an approximately linear association between the log odds of microfilarial infection and age group in the onchocerciasis data.

In *conditional logistic regression* and *Cox regression*, in which exposure effects are calculated by comparing exposures within case–control strata or risk sets, it is not possible to draw such graphs of outcome against exposure, and it is essential to examine linearity assumptions within regression models.

Testing for a linear effect

We test the null hypothesis that there is no linear effect in the usual way using a likelihood ratio test, by comparing L_{inc}, the log likelihood from the model including the linear effect (and other exposure effects of interest), with L_{exc}, the log likelihood from the model excluding the linear effect. Standard regression output for the linear exposure effect reports the *P*-value corresponding to the Wald test of this null hypothesis.

Testing for departure from linearity

We test the *null hypothesis that the exposure effect is linear* by comparing the model assuming a linear effect with a *more general* model in which the exposure effect is not assumed to be linear. We will describe two ways of doing this:

1 for ordered categorical exposure variables, this comparison may be with a model including the exposure as a categorical variable, where indicator variables are used to estimate the difference in outcome, comparing each non-baseline category with the baseline;

2 for any ordered categorical or numerical exposure variable, we may examine the linearity assumption by introducing **quadratic** terms into the model.

Testing linearity for ordered categorical variables

The null hypothesis is that the exposure effect *is* linear. To test this, we derive a likelihood ratio statistic by comparing:

(a) L_{exc}, the log likelihood when the exposure effect is assumed to be linear (the null hypothesis);

(b) L_{inc}, the log likelihood of the model when we allow the exposure effect to be non-linear, and which therefore includes additional parameters.

Example 29.2 (continued)

We will illustrate this approach by examining the linear effect of age group in the onchocerciasis data. The two models are:

(a) A logistic regression model of the odds of *mf* infection with age group as a linear effect. This includes just two parameters, the baseline (constant) plus a linear effect for age group. Their estimates were given in Table 19.13.

(b) A logistic regression model of the odds of *mf* infection with age group as a categorical variable. This model makes no assumption about the shape of the relationship between age group and *mf* infection. It includes four parameters, the baseline and three indicator variables for comparing each of the other three age groups with the baseline group. The parameter estimates were given in Table 19.11.

Note that model (a) is a special case of the more general model (b). The log likelihood values obtained in these two models are shown in Table 29.8. The likelihood ratio test statistic is:

$$LRS = -2 \times (L_{exc} - L_{inc}) = -2 \times (-729.240 + 727.831) = 2.818$$
$$\text{d.f.} = \text{number of additional parameters in the inclusive model} = 4 - 2 = 2$$
$$P = 0.24$$

Table 29.8 Log likelihood values obtained from the logistic regression models for *mf* infection by area of residence and age group, (a) assuming a linear effect of age group, and (b) allowing for a non-linear effect of age group, by including indicator variables.

Model	Exposure(s) in model	No. of parameters	Log likelihood
(a) exc	Age group (linear, see Table 19.13)	2	−729.240
(b) inc	Agegrp (categorical, see Table 19.11)	4	−727.831

There is no evidence against the null hypothesis that the effect of age group is linear. The likelihood ratio statistic has two degrees of freedom, corresponding to the extra number of parameters needed to include age group as a categorical variable compared to including it as a linear effect.

If the likelihood ratio test does provide evidence of non-linearity, then the exposure effect should be modelled using separate indicator variables for each non-baseline exposure level, as in model (b).

Testing linearity using quadratic exposure effects

We will illustrate the second approach to testing linearity in the context of the Caerphilly study by examining the effect of fibrinogen (a numerical exposure) on the rate of myocardial infarction (MI).

Example 29.3
Fibrinogen, a factor involved in blood coagulation that has been shown to be associated with rates of cardiovascular disease in a number of studies, was measured at the baseline examination in the Caerphilly study. Its distribution is shown by the histogram in Figure 29.2(a). An initial examination of the association between fibrinogen and rates of myocardial infarction was done by:
- dividing the distribution into deciles (the lowest 10% of fibrinogen measurements, the second 10% and so on; see Section 3.3);
- calculating the median fibrinogen level in each of these deciles. These were 2.63, 3, 3.22, 3.4, 3.6, 3.8, 4, 4.25, 4.59 and 5.23;
- graphing the rate of myocardial infarction (per 1000 person-years, log scale) in each decile against median fibrinogen in each decile.

The results are shown in Figure 29.2(b). There appears to be an approximately linear association between fibrinogen and the log rate of MI.

A Poisson regression model was then fitted for the linear effect of fibrinogen (using the original, ungrouped measurement) on rates of MI. The results are

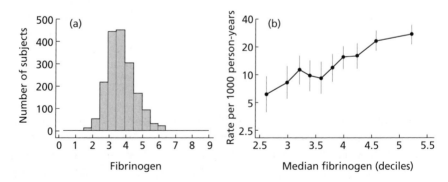

Fig. 29.2 (a) Histogram showing the distribution of fibrinogen (100g/dL) at the baseline examination of the Caerphilly study, and (b) MI rates (per 1000 person-years, log scale, with 95% confidence intervals for the rate in each group) for the median fibrinogen in each decile.

Table 29.9 Output from a Poisson regression model for the linear effect of fibrinogen on log rates of myocardial infarction in the Caerphilly study.

(a) Output on log scale

	Coefficient	s.e.	z	P > |z|	95% CI
Fibrinogen	0.467	0.054	8.645	0.000	0.361 to 0.573
Constant	−6.140	0.228	−26.973	0.000	−6.587 to −5.694

(b) Output on rate ratio scale

	Rate ratio	z	P > |z|	95% CI
Fibrinogen	1.595	8.645	0.000	1.435 to 1.773

shown in Table 29.9. The regression coefficient for fibrinogen is 0.467, corresponding to a rate ratio per unit increase of 1.595. This implies that the rate ratio for a three-unit increase in fibrinogen (from 2.5 to 5.5) is $1.595^3 = 4.057$. This is consistent with the increase seen over this range in Figure 29.2(b).

Although there is clear evidence of a linear (dose–response) association between fibrinogen and log rates of myocardial infarction, we may still wish to derive a formal test for extra-linear variation. Mathematically, the simplest departure from a linear relationship between the outcome and an exposure (x) is a **quadratic relationship**. The algebraic form of such a relationship is:

$$\text{outcome} = \beta_0 + \beta_1 x + \beta_2 x^2$$

To examine the evidence for a quadratic exposure effect, we create a new variable whose values are the squares of the exposure being examined. We then fit a regression model including *both* the exposure and the new variable (exposure squared).

Table 29.10 shows the Poisson regression output for the model including the linear effect of fibrinogen, and fibrinogen^2. There is only weak evidence (Wald P-value $= 0.091$) for a quadratic effect, so it would be reasonable to conclude that the effect of fibrinogen on log rates of MI is approximately linear. The fact that the regression coefficient for fibrinogen^2 is less than 0 (rate ratio < 1) implies that the effect of fibrinogen decreases as fibrinogen increases.

Because the linear and quadratic effects are sometimes *collinear* (see Section 29.7), it is preferable to examine the evidence for non-linearity using a likelihood ratio test comparing the models including and excluding the quadratic effect. When quadratic exposure effects are included in a model, we should not attempt to interpret the linear effect alone. In particular, the Wald P-value of 0.002 for the linear effect in Table 29.10 should *not* be interpreted as testing the null hypothesis that there is no linear effect of fibrinogen.

Table 29.10 Output from a Poisson regression model for the quadratic effect of fibrinogen on log rates of myocardial infarction in the Caerphilly study.

(a) Output on log scale

	Coefficient	s.e.	z	$P > |z|$	95% CI
Fibrinogen	1.038	0.338	3.073	0.002	0.376 to 1.700
Fibrinogen^2	−0.062	0.037	−1.688	0.091	−0.134 to 0.010
Constant	−7.383	0.757	−9.750	0.000	−8.868 to −5.899

(b) Output on rate ratio scale

	Rate ratio	z	$P > |z|$	95% CI
Fibrinogen	2.824	3.073	0.002	1.457 to 5.475
Fibrinogen^2	0.940	−1.688	0.091	0.874 to 1.010

Dose–response and unexposed groups

When examining dose–response relationships we should distinguish between the exposed group with the minimum exposure, and the unexposed group. For example, it may be that smokers in general have a higher risk of some disease than non-smokers. In addition, there may be an increasing risk of disease with increasing tobacco consumption. However, including the non-smokers with the smokers may bias our estimate of the dose–response relationship (linear effect) among smokers. This is illustrated in Figure 29.3. There are two possible ways to restrict estimation of the linear effect to exposed individuals:

1 Exclude the unexposed group, then estimate the linear effect among the exposed.
2 Include an indicator variable for exposed/unexposed together with linear effect of the exposure variable. The regression coefficient for the exposure will then estimate the linear effect among the exposed, while the regression coefficient for the indicator variable will estimate the difference between the outcome in the unexposed group and that projected by the linear effect in the exposed (dotted line in Figure 29.3).

Remarks on linear effects

1 It makes sense to model an exposure effect as linear if it is plausible that the outcome will increase (or decrease) systematically with the level of exposure. Such an exposure effect is known as a **dose–response** relationship, or **trend**.
2 A test for trend (see Section 17.5) is an approximation (based on a score test) to a likelihood ratio test of the null hypothesis that the regression coefficient for a linear effect is zero.
3 The existence of a dose–response relationship may provide more convincing evidence of a causal effect of exposure than a simple comparison of exposed with unexposed subjects.

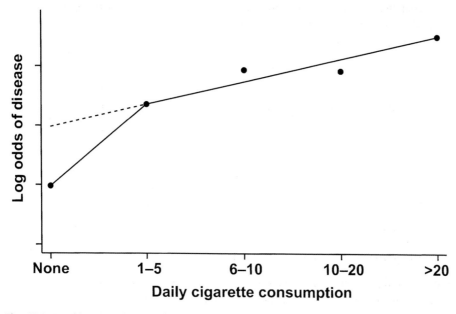

Fig. 29.3 Possible association between cigarette consumption and the log odds of a disease outcome. There is a larger difference between exposed (smokers) and unexposed (non-smokers) than would be expected given the magnitude of the dose–response relationship among the smokers.

4 Estimating a linear effect will often be the *most powerful* way to detect an association with an ordered exposure variable. This is because we only estimate one parameter, rather than a parameter for each non-baseline level. However, it is essential that this simplifying assumption, that an exposure effect may be modelled as a linear effect, be checked.

5 Modelling an exposure effect as linear will only be valid if the exposure is ordered categorical or numerical. Ideally, the category values should reflect the degree of exposure. For example, if the exposure was level of blood pressure and the four categories of exposure were obtained by grouping the blood pressures, then the category values could be the midpoints or mean of blood pressure in each of the four groups. In the absence of any genuine measurement (for instance when we model the effects of social class) it is usual to assign scores 0,1,2,3,4... to the various exposure levels.

29.7 COLLINEARITY

When two exposure variables are highly correlated we say that they are **collinear**. Collinearity can cause problems in fitting and interpreting regression models, because inclusion of two highly correlated exposure variables in a regression model can give the impression that neither is associated with the outcome, even when each exposure is strongly associated (individually) with the outcome.

We will illustrate this by examining the regression of *height* (the outcome variable) and *age* (the exposure variable) from the study of 636 children living in Lima, Peru (see Chapter 11), in the presence of an artificially constructed variable *newage*. *Newage* has been computer-generated to be *collinear* with age, by adding a random 'error' to each age, with the standard deviation of this random error made equal to 1 year. This has led to a correlation of 0.57 between *age* and *newage*, which is high but not very high.

The correlation between *height* and *age* was 0.59, and the regression coefficient was 5.15 cm/year (s.e. = 0.28). A regression of *height* on *newage* alone gives a regression coefficient of 1.61. This is much smaller than the regression coefficient for *age* (5.15) because the addition of a random error component tends to reduce the regression coefficient (see Chapter 36 for a more detailed discussion of this issue).

When both *age* and *newage* are included in the model, the regression coefficient for *age* is slightly increased (5.31) compared to the value for the model with *age* alone (5.15), while the regression coefficient for *newage* is slightly less than zero. These results are shown in the first row of Table 29.11. Thus, the joint regression has correctly identified strong evidence of an association between *height* and *age*, taking *newage* into account, and no evidence of an association between *height* and *newage*, taking *age* into account. In this artificially created example, the regression has correctly identified the joint information of *age* and *newage* being contained in *age*, since in essence *newage* is a less accurate measure of age. This level of collinearity in this particular example has not caused a problem.

We will now demonstrate how problems can occur with increasing collinearity between *age* and *newage* by decreasing the standard deviation of the random error that is added to variable *age* to create variable *newage*. The second row of Table 29.11 shows that when this standard deviation is decreased to 0.1 the correlation between *age* and *newage* is very high (0.9904). The coefficient from the regression of *height* on *newage* alone is 5.06: close to the regression coefficient for *age* alone. When both *age* and *newage* are included in the model, there is a substantial increase in the regression coefficient for *age*, while the regression coefficient for

Table 29.11 Demonstration of the effect of collinearity, using data from the study of lung disease in children in Lima, Peru. Variable *newage* is variable *age* plus a random error whose standard deviation is given in the first column in the table.

s.d. of random error	Correlation between *age* and *newage*	Regression of height on *newage*	Regression of height on *age* and *newage*		
		Coefficient (s.e.) for *newage*	Coefficient (s.e.) for *age*	Coefficient (s.e.) for *newage*	Sum of coefficients
1	0.57	1.61 (0.20)	5.31 (0.33)	− 0.17 (0.20)	5.16
0.1	0.9904	5.06 (0.28)	6.81 (2.00)	− 1.66 (1.99)	5.15
0.01	0.9999	5.16 (0.28)	21.76 (19.94)	−16.62 (19.94)	5.14

newage is clearly negative. The important thing to notice is that there is an even more dramatic increase in the standard errors of both regression coefficients.

When the standard deviation of the random error is reduced to 0.01, the correlation between *age* and *newage* is extremely high (0.9999, third row of Table 29.11). The regression coefficient for *newage* alone is almost identical to that for *age*, as would be expected because the error now contained in *newage* as a measure of age is very small. Inclusion of both variables in the model has a dramatic effect: the regression coefficient for *age* is greatly increased to 21.76, while the regression coefficient for *newage* is reduced to −16.62. The standard error of each regression coefficient is large (19.94). This joint model could lead to the erroneous conclusion that neither *age* nor *newage* is associated with the outcome variable, *height*.

The final column of the table shows that although the regression coefficients for *age* and *newage* change dramatically as the collinearity between them increases, the sum of the two coefficients remains approximately constant, and is the same as the regression coefficient for *age* alone. This suggests a solution to the problem. It is not possible simultaneously to estimate the effects of both *age* and *newage*, because each has the same association with height. However we can estimate the association of the outcome with the sum (or, equivalently, the average) of the two variables. Alternatively, we can simply choose one of the variables for inclusion in our model and exclude the other one.

In conclusion, this example demonstrates that including two strongly collinear exposure variables in a regression model has the potential to lead to the erroneous conclusion that neither is associated with the outcome variable. This occurs when collinearity is high enough to lead to dramatic increases in the standard errors of the regression coefficients. Comparing the standard errors from the single exposure models with the joint exposure model can identify whether this problem is occurring. When it does occur, it is not possible to estimate the effect of each exposure controlling for the other in a regression model.

29.8 DECIDING WHICH EXPOSURE VARIABLES TO INCLUDE IN A REGRESSION MODEL

A key challenge in analysing studies that have data on a large number of exposure variables is how to decide which of these variables to include and which to exclude from a particular regression model, since it is usually unwise or impossible to include all of them in the same model. A rough guide is that there should be at least ten times as many observations (individuals) as exposure variables in a regression model: for example, a model which includes ten variables should be based on data from at least 100 individuals. Note that each separate indicator variable counts as a separate variable.

Two important considerations will influence how the choice of exposure variables is made:

1 Are you using multiple linear regression, or a different generalized linear model?

2 Is the main aim of the model to estimate the effect of a particular exposure as accurately as possible, to predict the outcome based on the values of a number of exposures, or to develop an explanatory model of those exposures that have an influence on the outcome?

Implication of type of regression model

For **multiple linear regression**, you should aim to include *all* exposure variables that are clearly associated with the outcome when estimating the effect of a particular exposure, *whether or not they are confounders* (with the exception that variables on the causal pathway between the exposure of interest and the outcome should *not* be included; see Section 18.2). Doing this will reduce the residual sum of squares (see Chapter 10) and so will increase the precision of the estimated effect of the main exposure, and the power of the associated hypothesis test. However, this is not the case with other **generalized linear models**. For example, inclusion of additional variables in logistic regression models will tend to *increase* the standard error of the exposure effect estimate.

Estimating the effect of a particular exposure

When estimating the effect of a particular exposure, we have seen that it is important to include potential confounding variables in the regression model, and that failure to do so will lead to a biased estimate of the effect. In considering which potential confounders should be included, it is essential that careful consideration be given to hierarchical relationships between exposures and confounders, as well as to statistical associations in the data. This is explained in detail in Chapter 38 on strategies for data analysis.

Deriving a regression model to predict the outcome

Different considerations apply when the main purpose of the analysis is to derive a regression model that can be used to predict future values of the outcome variable. For example, this approach has been used in developing countries to attempt to identify whether a pregnant woman may be at risk of obstetric difficulties, based on factors such as social class, previous pregnancy outcomes, and pre-pregnancy weight and height.

The aim in developing a predictive model is to identify a set of exposure variables that give a good prediction of the outcome. The emphasis is no longer on assessing the importance of a particular exposure or on understanding the aetiology of the outcome. However, a good starting point is to include those exposure variables that are known from other studies to be strongly associated with the outcome. In addition, it may be helpful to use an automated procedure to identify which (of what are often a large number of additional variables) might be included in the model. Such procedures are usually based on the magnitude of the

P-value for each variable and are known as **stepwise selection procedures**. For example, a typical stepwise procedure might be:

1 Fit a model including all exposure variables. Now omit each variable in turn, and record the *P*-value for each likelihood ratio test. The variable with the highest *P*-value is omitted from the next step of the procedure.
2 Fit the model including all variables except that omitted in step (1). Now proceed as in step (1) to select the next variable to be omitted.
3 Continue until the *P*-value for omission of each remaining variable is less than a chosen threshold (e.g. 0.2).
4 Now consider adding, in turn, each of the variables omitted in steps (1) to (3). Add the variable with the smallest *P*-value, providing this is less than 0.2.
5 Continue until no more variables with a *P*-value of < 0.2 can be added. The resulting model is the final model to be used for prediction.

Of course, different versions of such stepwise procedures can be chosen. Such procedures may appear attractive, because they seem to provide an objective way of choosing the best possible model. However *they have serious disadvantages*, which are summarized in Box 29.2. If it is necessary to use a stepwise selection procedure, then it is advisable to use a higher *P*-value threshold, such as 0.2 rather than 0.05 (the traditional threshold for statistical significance).

BOX 29.2   PROBLEMS WITH STEPWISE VARIABLE SELECTION IN REGRESSION MODELS

1 The major problem with stepwise regression is that the derived model will give an over-optimistic impression. The *P*-values for the selected variables will be too small, confidence intervals will be too narrow and, in the case of multiple regression, the proportion of variance explained (R^2) will be too high. This is because they do not reflect the fact that the model was selected using a stepwise procedure. The higher the original number of exposure variables from which the final model was selected, the higher the chance of selecting variables with chance associations with the outcome and thus the worse this problem will be.
2 The regression coefficients will be too large (too far away from their null values). This means that the performance of the model in predicting future values of the outcome will be less good than we might expect.
3 Computer simulations have shown minor changes in the data may lead to important changes in the variables selected for the final model.
4 Stepwise procedures should never be used as a substitute for thinking about the problem. For example, are there variables that should be included because they are known from previous work to be associated with the outcome? Are there variables for which an association with the outcome is implausible?

The quality of predictions from models that have been derived using stepwise procedures should be evaluated using a separate dataset (the **test dataset**) to that which was used to derive the model (the **development dataset**). This is for two reasons:

- as explained in Box 29.2, the regression coefficients in the model will tend to be too large;
- the individuals for whom we wish to predict the outcome may differ, in a manner not captured by the variables measured, from those in the development dataset.

Developing an explanatory model for the outcome

Sometimes the focus of a study is to understand the aetiology of the outcome, and to identify those exposures or risk factors that are important influences on it. The purpose of the regression model here is halfway between that of the other two situations just described. Thus the focus is neither on identifying which confounders to include for a particular risk factor, nor is it on identifying any combination of exposures that works, as in the prediction scenario. Instead it is intended to attach meaning to the variables chosen for inclusion in the final model. For this reason, we strongly recommend that the selection procedure is based on an underlying conceptual framework (see Chapter 38 for more detail), and that formal stepwise methods are avoided because of the problems with them described in Box 29.2.

Relaxing model assumptions

30.1 INTRODUCTION

All the statistical methods presented so far have been based on assuming a specific probability distribution for the outcome, or for a transformation of the outcome. Thus we have assumed a normal distribution for numerical outcomes, a binomial distribution for binary outcomes and a Poisson distribution for rates. In this chapter we describe three types of methods that can be used when these assumptions are violated. These are:

- *non-parametric methods based on ranks*, which are used when we have a numerical outcome variable but wish to avoid specific assumptions about its distribution, or cannot find a transformation under which the outcome is approximately normal;
- *bootstrapping*, a very general technique that allows us to derive confidence intervals making only very limited assumptions about the probability distribution of the outcome;
- *robust standard errors*, which allow derivation of confidence intervals and standard errors based on the actual distribution of the outcome variable in the dataset rather than on an assumed underlying probability distribution.

30.2 NON-PARAMETRIC METHODS BASED ON RANKS

Non-parametric methods based on ranks are used to analyse a numerical outcome variable without assuming that it is approximately normally distributed. The key feature of these methods is that each value of the outcome variable is replaced by its rank after the variable has been sorted into ascending order of magnitude. For example, if the outcome values were 453, 1, 5 and 39 then analyses would be based on the corresponding ranks of 4, 1, 2 and 3.

As explained in Chapter 5, the central limit theorem tells us that as the sample size increases the sampling distribution of a mean will tend to be *normally* distributed even if the underlying distribution is non-normal. Rank methods are therefore particularly useful in a small data set when there is obvious non-normality that cannot be corrected by a suitable transformation, or when we do not wish

to transform the variable because transforming would make interpretation of the results harder. They are less powerful (efficient in detecting genuine differences) than parametric methods, but may be more *robust*, in the sense that they are less affected by extreme observations. Rank methods have three main disadvantages:

1 Their primary concern has traditionally been significance testing, since associated methods for deriving confidence limits have been developed only recently. This conflicts with the emphasis in modern medical statistics on estimation of the size of differences, and the interpretation of *P*-values in the context of confidence intervals (see Chapter 8). In particular, large *P*-values from rank order tests comparing two small samples have often been misinterpreted, in the absence of confidence intervals, as showing that there is no difference between two groups, when in fact the data are consistent either with no difference or with a substantial difference. Bootstrapping, described in Section 30.3, provides a general means of deriving confidence intervals and so overcomes this difficulty.

2 When sample sizes are extremely small, such as in comparing two groups with three persons in each group, rank tests can *never* produce small *P*-values, even when the values of the outcomes in the two groups are very different from each other, such as 1, 2 and 3 compared with 21, 22 and 23. In contrast, the *t-test* based on the normal distribution is able to detect such a clear difference between groups. It will, of course, never be possible to verify the assumption of normality in such small samples.

3 Non-parametric methods are less easily extended to situations where we wish to take into account the effect of more than one exposure on the outcome. For these reasons the emphasis in this book is on the use of parametric methods, providing these are valid.

The main rank-order methods are listed in Table 30.1 together with their parametric counterparts. The most common ones, the Wilcoxon signed rank test, the Wilcoxon rank sum test, Spearman's rank correlation and Kendall's tau, will be described using examples previously analysed using parametric methods. For a detailed account of non-parametric methods the reader is referred to Conover (1999), Siegel and Castellan (1988) or Sprent and Smeeton (2000). Details of methods to derive confidence intervals are given by Altman *et al.* (2000).

Wilcoxon signed rank test

This is the non-parametric counterpart of the paired *t*-test, and corresponds to a test of whether the median of the differences between paired observations is zero in the population from which the sample is drawn.

Example 30.1

We will show how to derive the Wilcoxon signed rank test using the data in Table 30.2, which shows the number of hours of sleep obtained by 10 patients when they

Table 30.1 Summary of the main rank order methods. Those described in more detail in this section are shown in italics.

Purpose of test	Method	Parametric counterpart
Examine the difference between paired observations	*Wilcoxon signed rank test*	Paired *t*-test
Simplified form of Wilcoxon signed rank test	Sign test	
Examine the difference between two groups	*Wilcoxon rank sum test*	Two-sample *t*-test
Alternatives to Wilcoxon rank sum test that give identical results	Mann–Whitney *U*-test Kendall's *S*-test	Two-sample *t*-test
Examine the difference between two or more groups. Gives identical results to Wilcoxon rank sum test when there are two groups	Kruskal–Wallis one-way analysis of variance	One-way analysis of variance
Measure of the strength of association between two variables	*Kendall's rank correlation (Kendall's tau)*	Correlation coefficient
Alternative to Kendall's rank correlation that is easier to calculate.	*Spearman's rank correlation*	Correlation coefficient

Table 30.2 Results of a placebo-controlled clinical trial to test the effectiveness of a sleeping drug (reproduced from Table 7.3), with ranks for use in the Wilcoxon signed rank test.

Patient	Hours of sleep		Difference	Rank (ignoring sign)
	Drug	Placebo		
1	6.1	5.2	0.9	2
2	6.0	7.9	−1.9	5
3	8.2	3.9	4.3	10
4	7.6	4.7	2.9	8
5	6.5	5.3	1.2	3
6	5.4	7.4	−2.0	6
7	6.9	4.2	2.7	7
8	6.7	6.1	0.6	1
9	7.4	3.8	3.6	9
10	5.8	7.3	−1.5	4

took a sleeping drug and when they took a placebo, and the differences between them. The test consists of five steps:

1 Exclude any differences that are zero. Put the remaining differences in ascending order of magnitude, *ignoring* their signs and give them **ranks** 1, 2, 3, etc., as shown in Table 30.2. If any differences are equal then average their ranks.

2 Count up the ranks of the positive differences and of the negative differences and denote these sums by T_+ and T_- respectively.

$$T_+ = 2 + 10 + 8 + 3 + 7 + 1 + 9 = 40$$
$$T_- = 5 + 6 + 4 = 15$$

3 If there were no difference in effectiveness between the sleeping drug and the placebo then the sums T_+ and T_- would be similar. If there were a difference then one sum would be much smaller and one sum would be much larger than expected. Denote the smaller sum by T.

$$T = \text{smaller of } T_+ \text{ and } T_-$$

In this example, $T = 15$.

4 The Wilcoxon signed rank test is based on assessing whether T is smaller than would be expected by chance, under the null hypothesis that the median of the paired differences is zero. The P-value is derived from the sampling distribution of T under the null hypothesis. A range for the P-value can be found by comparing the value of T with the values for $P = 0.05$, $P = 0.02$ and $P = 0.01$ given in Table A7 in the Appendix. Note that the appropriate sample size, n, is the number of differences that were ranked rather than the total number of differences, and does not therefore include the zero differences.

$$n = \text{number of non-zero differences}$$

In contrast to the usual situation, the *smaller* the value of T the *smaller* is the P-value. This is because the null hypothesis is that T is equal to the sum of the ranks divided by 2, so that the smaller the value of T the more evidence there is against the null hypothesis. In this example, the sample size is 10 and the 5%, 2% and 1% percentage points are 8, 5 and 3 respectively. The P-value is therefore greater than 0.05, since 15 is greater than 8.

It is more usual to derive the P-value using a computer: in this example $P = 0.20$ so there is no evidence against the null hypothesis, and hence no evidence that the sleeping drug was more effective than the placebo.

5 To derive an approximate 95% confidence interval for the median difference, we consider the averages of the $n(n + 1)/2$ possible pairs of differences. The resulting $10 \times 11/2 = 55$ possible averages for this example are shown in Table 30.3. The approximate 95% CI is given by:

95% CI (median difference) = T^{th} smallest average to T^{th} largest average
of the $n(n + 1)/2$ possible pairs of differences, where
T is the value corresponding to the 2-sided P-value of 0.05 in Table A7

Table 30.3 Fifty-five possible averages of the ten differences between patients' hours of sleep after taking a sleeping drug and their hours of sleep after taking a placebo.

	−2.0	−1.9	−1.5	0.6	0.9	1.2	2.7	2.9	3.6	4.3
−2.0	−2	−1.95	−1.75	−0.7	−0.55	−0.4	0.35	0.45	0.8	1.15
−1.9		−1.9	−1.7	−0.65	−0.5	−0.35	0.4	0.5	0.85	1.2
−1.5			−1.5	−0.45	−0.3	−0.15	0.6	0.7	1.05	1.4
0.6				0.6	0.75	0.9	1.65	1.75	2.1	2.45
0.9					0.9	1.05	1.8	1.9	2.25	2.6
1.2						1.2	1.95	2.05	2.4	2.75
2.7							2.7	2.8	3.15	3.5
2.9								2.9	3.25	3.6
3.6									3.6	3.95
4.3										4.3

In this example, $T = 8$, and so the 95% confidence interval is from the 8th smallest average to the 8th largest average. These are found from Table 30.3 to be −0.65 and 2.9 respectively.

95% confidence interval for median difference = −0.65 to 2.9

Further details of the assumptions underlying the Wilcoxon signed rank test and the confidence interval for the median difference are given in Conover (1999).

Wilcoxon rank sum test

This is one of the non-parametric counterparts of the t-test, and is used to assess whether an outcome variable differs between two exposure groups. Specifically, it examines whether the median difference between pairs of observations from the two groups is equal to zero. If, in addition, we assume that the distributions of the outcome in the two groups are identical except that they differ by a constant amount (that is, they 'differ only in location') then the null hypothesis of the test is that the difference between the medians of the two distributions equals zero.

Example 30.2
The use of the Wilcoxon rank sum test will be described by considering the data in Table 30.4, which shows the birth weights of children born to 15 non-smokers and 14 heavy smokers. It consists of three steps:
1 Rank the values of the outcome from both groups together in *ascending* order of magnitude, as shown in the table. If any of the values are equal, average their ranks.
2 Add up the ranks in the group with the smaller sample size. If there were no difference between the groups then the ranks would on average be similar. In

Table 30.4 Comparison of birth weights of children born to 15 non-smokers with those of children born to 14 heavy smokers (reproduced from Table 7.1), with ranks for use in the Wilcoxon rank sum test.

Non-smokers ($n = 15$)		Heavy smokers ($n = 14$)	
Birth weight (kg)	Rank	Birth weight (kg)	Rank
3.99	27	3.18	7
3.89	26	2.74	4
3.6*	17.5	2.9	6
3.73	24	3.27	9
3.31	10	3.65†	20.5
3.7	23	3.42	13
4.08	28	3.23	8
3.61	19	2.86	5
3.83	25	3.6*	17.5
3.41	12	3.65†	20.5
4.13	29	3.69	22
3.36	11	3.53	15
3.54	16	2.38	2
3.51	14	2.34	1
2.71	3		
	Sum = 284.5		Sum = 150.5

*Tied 17th and 18th and so ranks averaged
†Tied 20th and 21st and so ranks averaged

this case the group with the smaller sample size is the heavy smokers, and their ranks sum to 150.5. If the two groups are of the same size either one may be picked.

$T =$ sum of ranks in group with smaller sample size

3 Compare the value of T with the values in Table A8, which is arranged somewhat differently to the tables for the other tests. Look up the row corresponding to the sample sizes of the two groups, in this case row 14, 15. The range shown for $P = 0.01$ is 151 to 269: values inside this range (i.e. between 151 and 269) correspond to P-values greater than 0.01. Sums of 151 and below or 269 and above correspond to P-values less than 0.01. The sum of 150.5 in this example is just below the lower limit of 151, so the P-value is slightly less than 0.01.

As with the signed rank test, the P-value is usually derived using a computer. In this case $P = 0.0094$: there is good evidence against the null hypothesis that the median birth weight of children born to heavy smokers is the same as the median birth weight of children born to non-smokers.

Details of how to derive a confidence interval for the difference in medians (assuming that the two distributions differ only in location) are given by Conover

(1999) and in Altman *et al.* (2000). Such confidence intervals are known as **Hodges–Lehmann** estimates of shift. In this example, we find (using a computer) that the 95% CI is from -0.77 to -0.09. In Section 30.3 we see how bootstrap methods can also be used to provide a confidence interval for the difference between medians.

Rank correlations

We will now consider two rank order measures of the association between two numerical variables: Kendall's tau and Spearman's rank correlation. The parametric counterpart of these measures is the correlation coefficient, sometimes known as the **Pearson product moment correlation**, which was described in Chapter 10.

Example 30.3
We will explain these measures of association using the data in Table 30.5 on the relationship between plasma volume and body weight in eight healthy men. We will call these two quantitative variables Y and X. The Pearson correlation between these was shown in Section 10.3 to be 0.76.

To calculate **Spearman's rank correlation** coefficient r_s:
1 Independently rank the values of X and Y.
2 Calculate the Pearson correlation between the ranks, rather than between the original measurements. Other formulae for the Spearman correlation are often quoted; these give identical results. This gives a value of 0.81 in this example.

Kendall's tau (denoted by the Greek letter τ) is derived as follows:
1 Compare the ranks of X and Y between each pair of men. There are $n(n-1)/2$ possible pairs. The pairs of ranks for subjects i and j are said to be:
  (a) *concordant* if they differ in the same directions, that is if both the X and Y ranks of subject i are lower than the corresponding ranks of subject j, or both are higher. For example, the ranks of subjects 1 and 2 are concordant

Table 30.5 Relationship between plasma volume and body weight in eight healthy men (reproduced from Table 10.1), with ranks used in calculating the Spearman rank correlation.

Subject	Body weight (X) Value (kg)	Rank	Plasma volume (Y) Value (litre)	Rank
1	58.0	1	2.75	2
2	70.0	5	2.86	4
3	74.0	8	3.37	7
4	63.5	3	2.76	3
5	62.0	2	2.62	1
6	70.5	6	3.49	8
7	71.0	7	3.05	5
8	66.0	4	3.12	6

as subject 1 has a lower rank than subject 2 for both the variables. The pair 3 and 8 is also concordant: subject 3 has higher ranks than subject 8 on both variables.

(b) *discordant* if the comparison of the ranks of the two variables is in opposite directions. For example, the ranks of subjects 3 and 6 are discordant as subject 3 has a more highly ranked X value than subject 6 but a lower ranked Y value.

2 Count the number of concordant pairs (n_C) and the number of discordant pairs (n_D), and calculate τ as:

$$\tau = \frac{n_C - n_D}{n(n-1)/2}$$

In this example, Kendall's tau (derived using a computer) is 0.64. If all pairs are concordant then $\tau = 1$, while if all pairs are discordant then $\tau = -1$. More details, including an explanation of how to deal with ties, are given by Conover (1999).

All three measures of correlation have values between 1 and -1. Although Spearman's rank correlation is better known, its only advantage is that it is easier to calculate without a computer. Kendall's tau is the preferred rank measure, because its statistical properties are better and because it is easier to interpret. Given two pairs of observations (X_1, Y_1) and (X_2, Y_2) Kendall's tau is the difference between the probability that the bigger X is with the bigger Y, and the probability that the bigger X is with the smaller Y.

If X and Y are each normally distributed then there is a direct relationship between the Pearson correlation (r) and both Kendall's τ and Spearman's rank correlation (r_s):

$$r = \sin\left(\frac{\pi}{2}\tau\right) = 2\sin\left(\frac{\pi}{6}r_s\right)$$

This means that Pearson correlations of 0, $\pm 1/2$, ± 0.7071 and ± 1 correspond to Kendall τ values of 0, $\pm 1/3$, $\pm 1/2$ and ± 1 and to Spearman rank correlations of 0, ± 0.4826, ± 0.6902 and ± 1, respectively.

30.3 BOOTSTRAPPING

Bootstrapping is a way of deriving confidence intervals while making only very limited assumptions about the probability distribution that gave rise to the data. The name derives from the expression 'pull yourself up by your bootstraps', which means that you make progress through your own efforts; without external help. It is based on a remarkably simple idea: that if we take repeated samples from the data themselves, mimicking the way that the data were sampled from the population, we can use these samples to derive standard errors and confidence intervals.

The new samples are drawn *with replacement* from the original data. That is, we pick an observation at random from the original data, note down its value, then pick another observation at random from the same original data, regardless of which observation was picked first. This continues until we have a new dataset of the same size as the original one. The samples differ from each other because some of the original observations are picked more than once, while others are not picked at all.

Example 30.4

We will illustrate this using the data on birth weight and smoking, shown in Table 30.4. The median birth weight among the children born to the non-smokers was 3.61 kg, while the median among children born to the smokers was 3.25 kg. The difference in medians comparing smokers with non-smokers was therefore −0.36 kg. The *P*-value for the null hypothesis that the median birth weight is the same in smokers and non-smokers (derived in Section 30.2 using the Wilcoxon rank sum test) was 0.0094. The non-smokers and heavy smokers were recruited separately in this study, and so the bootstrap sampling procedure mimics this by sampling separately from the non-smokers and from the heavy smokers. Therefore each bootstrap sample will have 15 non-smokers and 14 heavy smokers.

This process is illustrated, for two bootstrap samples, in Table 30.6. In the first bootstrap sample observations 1, 3, 4 and 5 were not picked, observation 2 was picked four times, observations 6 and 7 were picked once and so on. In this sample the difference in median birth weight was −0.48 kg, while in the second sample the difference was −0.26 kg.

We repeat this procedure a large number of times, and record the difference between the medians in each sample. To derive confidence intervals, a minimum of around 1000 bootstrap samples is needed. Figure 30.1 is a histogram of the differences in medians derived from 1000 bootstrap samples from the birth weight data.

The simplest way to derive a 95% confidence interval for the difference between medians is to use the *percentile method* and take the range within which 95% of these bootstrap differences lie, i.e. from the 2.5[th] percentile to the 97.5[th] percentile of this distribution. This gives a 95% CI of −0.87 to −0.01 kg.

Unfortunately the percentile method, though simple, is not the most accurate method for deriving bootstrap confidence intervals. This has led to the development of **bias corrected** (BC) and **bias corrected and accelerated** (BCa) **intervals**, of which BCa intervals have been shown to have the best properties. For the birth weight data, use of the BC method gives a 95% CI of −0.80 to 0.025 kg, while the BCa method gives a 95% CI of −0.71 to 0.12 kg. More information about the use of bootstrap methods can be found in Efron and Tibshirani (1993) and in Davison and Hinkley (1997).

Table 30.6 Two bootstrap samples, based on data on birth weights (kg) of children born to 15 non-smokers and of children born to 14 heavy smokers.

	Original data			First bootstrap sample			Second bootstrap sample	
Obs. no.	Birth weight	Smoker	Original obs. no.	Birth weight	Smoker	Original obs. no.	Birth weight	Smoker
1	3.99	No	2	3.89	No	1	3.99	No
2	3.79	No	2	3.89	No	1	3.99	No
3	3.6	No	2	3.89	No	2	3.89	No
4	3.73	No	2	3.89	No	3	3.60	No
5	3.21	No	6	3.70	No	3	3.60	No
6	3.60	No	7	4.08	No	4	3.73	No
7	4.08	No	8	3.61	No	6	3.70	No
8	3.61	No	8	3.61	No	6	3.70	No
9	3.83	No	8	3.61	No	8	3.61	No
10	3.31	No	9	3.83	No	8	3.61	No
11	4.13	No	9	3.83	No	9	3.83	No
12	3.26	No	10	3.41	No	12	3.36	No
13	3.54	No	11	4.13	No	12	3.36	No
14	3.51	No	11	4.13	No	12	3.36	No
15	2.71	No	15	2.71	No	15	2.71	No
16	3.18	Yes	16	3.18	Yes	19	3.27	Yes
17	2.84	Yes	19	3.27	Yes	19	3.27	Yes
18	2.90	Yes	19	3.27	Yes	19	3.27	Yes
19	3.27	Yes	20	3.65	Yes	21	3.42	Yes
20	3.85	Yes	20	3.65	Yes	22	3.23	Yes
21	3.52	Yes	20	3.65	Yes	22	3.23	Yes
22	3.23	Yes	20	3.65	Yes	23	2.86	Yes
23	2.76	Yes	21	3.42	Yes	25	3.65	Yes
24	3.60	Yes	24	3.60	Yes	25	3.65	Yes
25	3.75	Yes	26	3.69	Yes	25	3.65	Yes
26	3.59	Yes	28	2.38	Yes	26	3.69	Yes
27	3.63	Yes	29	2.34	Yes	27	3.53	Yes
28	2.38	Yes	29	2.34	Yes	27	3.53	Yes
29	2.34	Yes	29	2.34	Yes	29	2.34	Yes

Median in non-smokers = 3.60			Median in non-smokers = 3.83			Median in non-smokers = 3.61		
Median in smokers = 3.25			Median in smokers = 3.35			Median in smokers = 3.35		
Difference in medians = −0.35			Difference in medians = −0.48			Difference in medians = −0.26		

We have illustrated the use of bootstrapping using a simple comparison of medians, but the method is quite general and can be used to derive confidence intervals for any parameter of a statistical model. For example, we might fit a regression model for the effect of smoking on birthweight, controlling for a number of other variables, then derive a bootstrap confidence interval by repeating this regression on 1000 different bootstrap samples and recording the value of the regression coefficient estimated in each. An example of the derivation of different types of bootstrap confidence interval for proportional hazards models is given by Carpenter and Bithell (2000). *If the model assumptions are not*

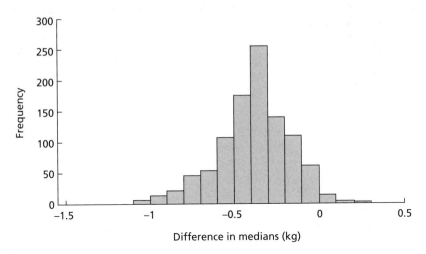

Fig. 30.1 Histogram of the differences in medians (kg) derived from 1000 bootstrap samples of the data on birth weight and smoking.

violated then the bootstrap confidence interval should be similar to the usual confidence interval reported in the regression output.

An example of the use of bootstrapping is provided by Thompson and Barber (2000), who consider the analysis of data on costs of treatment in clinical trials. Costs are often highly skewed, because a small minority of patients incur much higher costs of treatment than the rest. Because of this such data have often been analysed by log transforming the costs and performing a *t*-test. This is a valid approach, but it will lead to an estimate of the difference in mean log costs (which can be converted to a ratio of geometric mean costs, see Chapter 13). The problem is that health service planners are interested in a comparison of mean costs and not in a comparison of mean *log* costs, or in the difference in median costs that might be evaluated using non-parametric methods. Bootstrapping provides a way of deriving confidence intervals for the difference in mean costs between two groups, in circumstances when the non-normality of costs means that confidence intervals from standard methods (*t*-tests or regression) may not be valid.

30.4 ROBUST STANDARD ERRORS

It was explained in Chapter 28 that when we estimate parameters using the likelihood approach then the standard error of the parameter estimate is derived from the curvature of the likelihood at the maximum – the more information which the data provide about the parameter the more sharply curved is the likelihood and the smaller the standard error. Throughout this book we have used such *model-based* standard errors to derive confidence intervals and *P*-values.

Sometimes, we are not confident that the precise probability model underlying the likelihood is correct, and so we may not wish to rely on the likelihood to provide standard errors for our parameter estimates. Examples of this situation are when the residuals in a multiple regression model are clearly non-normal (see Chapter 12) or when the data are clustered (as discussed in Chapter 31).

An alternative approach, suggested independently by Huber (1967) and White (1980) is to estimate standard errors using the variability in the data. The formula is based on the **residuals** (the difference between the outcome and its predicted value in the regression model, see Section 12.3). Standard errors estimated in this way are known as **robust standard errors** and the corresponding variance estimate is known as the **sandwich variance estimate**, because of the mathematical form of the formula used to estimate it. If the sample size is large enough then, *providing that our basic regression model for the mean of the outcome given the level of the exposure variables is correct*, robust standard errors will be correct, even if the probability model for the outcome variable is wrong. Robust standard errors thus provide a general means of checking how reasonable are the model-based standard errors (which are calcuated assuming that the probability model is correct).

Example 30.5

In Section 11.3 we fitted a multiple regression model of lung function (FEV_1, litres) on age, height and gender among 636 children aged 7 to 10 years living in a suburb of Lima, Peru. However, in Section 12.3 we saw that there may be an association between the residuals and predicted values in this regression model: if this association is real, it would violate an assumption underlying the regression model.

Table 30.7 shows the results of re-analysing these data specifying robust standard errors, compared to the results using model-based standard errors. Note that the regression coefficients are the same whichever we use. The effect of specifying robust standard errors varies for each of the exposure variables. For age and gender (variable 'male') the standard error is only slightly increased but for height the standard error is increased by about 17%, with a corresponding reduction in the t-statistic (from 14.04 to 11.51) and an increase in the width of the confidence intervals. In this example, our conclusions are broadly similar whether we use model-based or robust standard errors.

Table 30.7 Regression coefficients, model-based standard errors and robust standard errors, each with corresponding t-statistics from the linear regression model relating FEV_1 to age, height and gender of the child in the Peru study.

FEV_1	Regression coefficient	Model-based standard error		Robust standard error	
		s.e.	t	s.e.	t
Age	0.0946	0.0152	6.23	0.0159	5.96
Height	0.0246	0.0018	14.04	0.0021	11.51
Male	0.1213	0.0176	6.90	0.0177	6.87
Constant	−2.360	0.1750	−13.49	0.208	−11.34

Analysis of clustered data

31.1 INTRODUCTION

The statistical methods discussed so far in this book are based on the assumption that the observations in a sample are **independent** of each other, that is the value of one observation is not influenced by the value of another. This assumption of independence will be violated if the data are **clustered**, that is if observations in one cluster tend to be *more similar* to each other than to individuals in the rest of the sample. Clustered data arise in three main ways:

1 **Repeated measures in longitudinal studies**. In this case the clusters are the subjects; repeated observations on the same subject will be more similar to each other than to observations on other subjects. For example:

 - in studies of asthma or other chronic diseases, episodes of disease may occur on more than one occasion in the same subject;
 - in longitudinal studies of common childhood diseases in developing countries, children may experience several episodes of diarrhoea, malaria or acute respiratory infections during the course of the study;
 - in a study of cardiovascular disease and obesity, measurements of blood pressure, body mass index and cholesterol levels may be repeated every 3 months.

2 **Multiple measures on the same subject**. For example, in dental research observations are made on more than one tooth in the same subject. In this case the clusters are again subjects.

3 **Studies in which subjects are grouped**. This occurs for example in:

 - **cluster randomized trials** (see Chapter 34), in which groups rather than individuals are randomized to receive the different interventions under trial. For example, the unit of randomization might be general practices, with all patients registered in a practice receiving the same intervention. Since patients in a general practice may be more similar to each other than to patients in other general practices, for example because some areas tend to be more deprived than others or because of exposure to a common environmental hazard, the data are clustered. In this case the cluster is the group of patients registered with a general practice;

- **family studies**, since individuals in the same family are likely to be more similar to each other than to individuals in different families, because they share similar genes and a similar environment. In this case the cluster is the family;
- surveys where **cluster sampling** is employed (see Chapter 34). For example, in order to estimate the percentage of 14-year-olds in London that work at weekends, we might select 1000 children by randomly sampling 20 schools from all the schools in London, then randomly sample 50 children from each of the selected schools. As the children within a school may be more similar to each other than to children in different schools, the data are clustered. In this case the clusters are the schools.

It is essential that the presence of clustering is allowed for in statistical analyses. The main reason for this, as we shall see, is that *standard errors may be too small* if they do not take account of clustering in the data. This will lead to confidence intervals that are too narrow, and *P*-values that are too small.

We will discuss four appropriate ways to analyse clustered data:

1 calculate **summary measures** for each cluster, and analyse these summary measures using standard methods;

2 use **robust standard errors** to correct standard errors for the clustering;

3 use **random effects** models which explicitly model the similarity between individuals in the same cluster;

4 use **generalized estimating equations (GEE)** which adjust both standard errors and parameter estimates to allow for the clustering.

We will illustrate the importance of taking clustering into account in the context of the following hypothetical example.

Example 31.1

In a study of the effect of 'compound X' in drinking water on rates of dental caries, 832 primary school children in eight different schools were monitored to ascertain the time until they first required dental treatment. Table 31.1 shows data for the first 20 children in the study (all of whom were in school 1). Since compound X is measured at the school level, it is constant for all children in the same school. The data are therefore clustered and the clusters are the eight schools.

Table 31.2 summarizes the data for each school by showing the number of children requiring dental treatment, the total child-years of follow-up, the treatment rate per 100 child-years and the level of compound X in the school's drinking water. Results from a Poisson regression analysis of these data are shown in Table 31.3. This shows strong evidence that increased levels of compound X were associated with decreased rates of dental treatment among the school children.

Table 31.1 Data on the first 20 children in a study of the relationship between rates of dental treatment and the level of compound X in drinking water.

Child's id	Years of follow up	Required dental treatment during follow up?	School number	Level of compound X in school's water supply (1000 × ppm)
1	4.62	No	1	7.1
2	3.00	No	1	7.1
3	4.44	No	1	7.1
4	3.89	No	1	7.1
5	3.08	No	1	7.1
6	2.45	Yes	1	7.1
7	2.64	Yes	1	7.1
8	4.16	No	1	7.1
9	4.25	No	1	7.1
10	2.02	Yes	1	7.1
11	3.13	No	1	7.1
12	3.49	No	1	7.1
13	4.75	No	1	7.1
14	2.39	Yes	1	7.1
15	3.66	No	1	7.1
16	3.43	No	1	7.1
17	2.63	Yes	1	7.1
18	4.21	No	1	7.1
19	2.63	Yes	1	7.1
20	2.74	No	1	7.1

Table 31.2 Total child-years of follow-up, treatment rate per 100 child-years and the level of compound X in each school's drinking water, from a study of the effect of compound X in drinking water on the 832 children attending eight primary schools.

School	Number of children requiring dental treatment	Child-years of follow-up	Rate per 100 child-years	Level of compound X (1000 × ppm)
1	46	456.3	10.08	7.1
2	19	215.1	8.83	7.6
3	17	487.8	3.49	8.2
4	46	459.9	10.00	5.4
5	15	201.2	7.46	8.4
6	20	187.7	10.66	6.8
7	58	399.1	14.53	6.2
8	20	212.5	9.41	8.9

However, treatment rates among different children in the same school may tend to be more similar than treatment rates in children in different schools for reasons unrelated to the levels of compound X in the water, for example because children in the same school are of similar social background. There would then be more observed *between-school variability* than would be expected in the absence of clustering, in which case the strength of the association between treatment rates

Table 31.3 Poisson regression of the effect of compound X in drinking water on rates of dental treatment among 832 children attending eight primary schools.

(a) Results on rate ratio scale

	Rate ratio	z	$P > \|z\|$	95% CI
Compound X	0.821	−3.47	0.001	0.734 to 0.918

(b) Results on log scale

	Coefficient	s.e.	z	$P > \|z\|$	95% CI
Compound X	−0.1976	0.0570	−3.47	0.001	−0.3094 to −0.0859
Constant	3.6041	0.3976	9.07	0.000	2.8248 to 4.3833

and levels of compound X may be exaggerated by the analysis in Table 31.3, which does not allow for such clustering.

31.2 ANALYSES USING SUMMARY MEASURES FOR EACH CLUSTER

The simplest way to analyse clustered data is to derive summary measures for each cluster. Providing that the outcomes in different clusters are independent, standard methods may then be used to compare these summary measures between clusters.

Example 31.1 (continued)

For example, we might analyse the compound X data by doing a linear regression of the log treatment rate in each school on levels of compound X in the school. Results of such a regression are shown in Table 31.4. The estimated increase in the log rate ratio per unit increase in level of compound X is −0.1866, similar to the value of −0.1976 estimated in the Poisson regression analysis in Table 31.3. However, the standard error is much larger and there is now no evidence of an association ($P = 0.177$). Note that the estimated rate ratio per unit increase in level of compound X is simply $\exp(-0.1866) = 0.830$, and that 95% confidence limits for the rate ratio may be derived in a similar way, from the 95% CI in the regression output.

The regression analysis in Table 31.4 is a valid way to take into account the clustering in the data. It suggests that the standard error for the compound X effect in the Poisson regression analysis in Table 31.3 was too small, and therefore that the assumption made in that analysis, that treatment rates among different children in the same school were statistically independent, was incorrect. Thus this analysis using summary measures has confirmed the presence of clustering within schools.

Table 31.4 Linear regression of the effect of compound X on the log of the treatment rate in each school.

	Coefficient	s.e.	t	$P > t$	95% CI
Compound X	−0.1866	0.1220	−1.53	0.177	−0.4850 to 0.1119
Constant	3.5334	0.9035	3.91	0.008	1.3227 to 5.7441

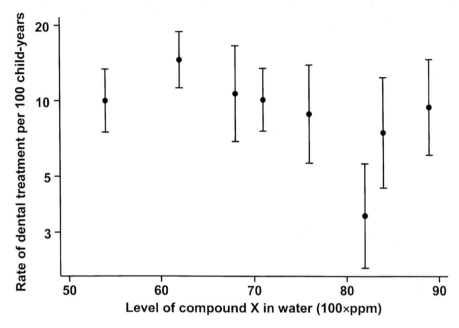

Fig. 31.1 Rate of dental treatment in each school (log scale), with corresponding 95% confidence intervals shown by the vertical lines.

Although analyses based on summary measures may be perfectly adequate in some circumstances, they can have disadvantages:

1 They do *not enable us to estimate the effect of characteristics of individuals within the cluster*. For example, rates of treatment might vary according to the age and gender of the children. Similarly, in a longitudinal study of factors associated with episodes of asthma, this approach would not allow us to examine whether subjects who had a viral infection were at increased risk of an episode of asthma during the subsequent week.

2 They take *no account of the precision with which each of the cluster measures is estimated*. In this example, the cluster measures are the rates in each school. The more events (children requiring treatment), the more precise is the estimated rate. For example, in school 5 only 15 children required treatment while in school 7, 58 children required treatment. The varying precision with which the treatment rate in each school is estimated is illustrated by the varying widths of the confidence intervals in Figure 31.1.

31.3 USE OF ROBUST STANDARD ERRORS TO ALLOW FOR CLUSTERING

As explained in the last section, the presence of clustering means that the standard errors obtained from the usual regression model will be too small. In Chapter

30 we introduced robust standard errors, which are estimated using the variability in the data (measured by the residuals) rather than the variability assumed by the statistical model. We can use a modified type of robust standard error as another approach to correct for clustering. To do this we add the residuals within each cluster together, and then use the resulting cluster-level residuals to derive standard errors that are valid in the presence of clustering.

Example 31.1 (continued)

Table 31.5 shows the results from a Poisson regression analysis based on robust standard errors that allow for within-school clustering. The rate ratio is identical to that from the standard Poisson regression analysis shown in Table 31.3, but the standard error of the log rate ratio has increased from 0.0570 to 0.1203. This analysis gives similar results to the linear regression analysis using summary measures shown in Table 31.4: there is at most weak evidence for an association between levels of compound X and treatment rates. However, *because the analysis is based on individual children we could now proceed to control for the effect of child characteristics.*

Important points to note in the use of robust standard errors to correct standard errors for clustering are:

- Robust standard errors use cluster-level residuals to take account of the similarity of individuals in the same cluster. In the presence of clustering, they will be larger than standard errors obtained from the usual regression model ignoring clustering.
- Use of robust standard errors does not affect the parameter estimate.
- Robust standard errors will be correct providing our model is correct and we have a reasonable number of clusters ($\geq$ 30).
- The log likelihood is not affected when we specify robust standard errors, and so *likelihood ratio tests do not take account of the clustering.* Wald tests must therefore be used.

Table 31.5 Poisson regression of the effect of compound X levels in drinking water on rates of dental treatment in eight primary schools, using robust standard errors to allow for the clustering.

(a) Results on rate ratio scale

	Rate ratio	z	$P > |z|$	95% CI
Compound X	0.821	−1.643	0.100	0.648 to 1.039

(b) Results on log scale

	Coefficient	s.e.	z	$P > |z|$	95% CI
Compound X	−0.1976	0.1203	−1.643	0.100	−0.4333 to 0.0381
Constant	3.6041	0.8147	4.42	0.000	2.0073 to 5.2008

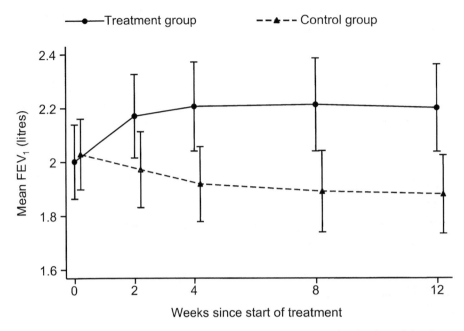

Fig. 31.2 Mean FEV$_1$ (with 95% CIs) in the treatment and control groups at baseline (0 weeks) and up to 12 weeks from the start of treatment, in a trial of 183 patients with chronic asthma.

Table 31.8 shows the results of three possible analyses of these data that take into account the fact that the means at different times are based on the same two groups of patients:

1 The first uses the average post-treatment FEV$_1$ for each patient, based on four time points for patients for whom there was complete follow-up, and on one, two or three time points for patients for whom some post-treatment measurements were missed. The linear regression of the mean post-treatment FEV$_1$ in each subject estimates that the average post-treatment FEV$_1$ is 0.2998 litres higher for those who received budesonide compared to those who received placebo. Note that this is equivalent to a *t*-test comparing the mean of the average post-treatment FEV$_1$ measurements between the treatment and control groups.

2 In the second analysis, the linear regression is based on the individual post-treatment measurements with robust standard errors used to allow for clustering of the measurements at different time points within subjects.

3 The third analysis is a random-effects linear regression of the post-treatment FEV$_1$ in each subject at each time.

The conclusions are similar in each case: treatment increased FEV$_1$ by a mean of approximately 0.3 litres. Standard errors, and hence confidence intervals and *P*-values, are also similar in the three models.

A random effects model explicitly includes both *between-cluster* and *within-cluster* variation. For a numerical outcome (as in Example 31.2) the model is:

$$y_{ij} = \beta_0 + \beta_1 x_{1ij} + \beta_2 x_{2ij} + \ldots + \beta_p x_{pij} + e_{ij} + u_j, \text{ where}$$

y_{ij} is the outcome for individual i in cluster j

x_{1ij} to x_{pij} are the values of the p exposure variables for that individual

e_{ij} is *the individual-level* random error, and is normally distributed with mean 0 and variance σ_e^2

u_j is the *cluster-level* random error, and is normally distributed with mean 0 and variance σ_u^2

This model is the same as the multiple regression model described in Section 11.4, with the addition of the cluster-level random effect u_j. The regression output for the random-effects model in Table 31.8(c) shows the estimated between-patient standard deviation ($\sigma_u = 0.6828$) and within-patient standard deviation ($\sigma_e = 0.2464$).

Table 31.8 Regression models to investigate the effect of budesonide treatment on FEV_1 in a clinical trial of 183 patients with chronic asthma. Analyses by kind permission of Dr Carl-Johan Lamm and Dr James Carpenter.

(a) Standard linear regression using the mean post-treatment FEV_1 measurements in each subject

	Coefficient	s.e.	t	$P > |t|$	95% CI
Treatment	0.2998	0.1033	2.90	0.004	0.0960 to 0.5037
Constant	1.8972	0.0729	26.04	0.000	1.7534 to 2.0409

(b) Linear regression using the post-treatment FEV_1 measurements in each subject at each time, with robust standard errors allowing for clustering within subjects

	Coefficient	Robust s.e.	t	$P > |t|$	95% CI
Treatment	0.2812	0.1044	2.69	0.008	0.0753 to 0.4872
Constant	1.9157	0.0679	28.22	0.000	1.7818 to 2.0497

(c) Random-effects linear regression

	Coefficient	s.e.	z	$P > |z|$	95% CI
Treatment	0.2978	0.1028	2.90	0.004	0.0963 to 0.4993
Constant	1.8992	0.0727	26.13	0.000	1.7567 to 2.0416
σ_u	0.6828	0.0370	18.46	0.000	0.6103 to 0.7553
σ_e	0.2464	0.0076	32.23	0.000	0.2314 to 0.2614

Intraclass correlation coefficient

The amount of clustering can be measured using the **intraclass correlation coefficient** (ICC), which is defined as the ratio of the between-cluster variance to the

total variance, which is a combination of the between- and within-cluster variances.

$$\text{Intraclass correlation coefficient, } \text{ICC} = \frac{\sigma_u^2}{\sigma_u^2 + \sigma_e^2}$$

If all the variation is explained by differences between clusters, so that there is no variation within clusters and $\sigma_e^2 = 0$, then ICC $= 1$. If σ_u^2 is estimated to be zero then there is no evidence of clustering and ICC $= 0$. In Example 31.2,

$$\text{ICC} = 0.6828^2/(0.6828^2 + 0.2464^2) = 0.885$$

so nearly 90% of the variation in FEV_1, after accounting for the effect of treatment, was between patients rather than within patients.

Although the P-value for σ_u corresponds to a Wald test of the presence of clustering, it is preferable to test for clustering using a likelihood ratio test; by comparing the log likelihood from the random-effects model (L_{inc}) with the log likelihood from a standard regression model assuming no clustering (L_{exc}).

Including cluster-level and individual-level characteristics in random effects models

The effects on the outcome variable of both cluster characteristics and of characteristics of individual observations within clusters may be included in random-effects models. For the asthma trial data, this corresponds to including characteristics of patients and of observations at different times on the same patient.

Example 31.2 (continued)
In Table 31.9 the random-effects model shown in Table 31.8(c) has been extended to include patients' FEV_1 measurements before the start of treatment (a cluster

Table 31.9 Random-effects linear regression of the effect of budesonide treatment on FEV_1 in a clinical trial of 183 patients with chronic asthma, including baseline FEV_1 and a treatment-time interaction.

	Coefficient	s.e.	z	$P > \lvert z \rvert$	95% CI
treatment	0.2695	0.0772	3.49	0.000	0.1182 to 0.4207
weeks	−0.0104	0.0035	−2.96	0.003	−0.0173 to −0.0035
treat.weeks	0.0127	0.0049	2.62	0.009	0.0032 to 0.0222
fevbase	0.7562	0.0577	13.12	0.000	0.6432 to 0.8692
constant	0.4039	0.1293	3.12	0.002	0.1504 to 0.6574
σ_u	0.4834	0.0271	17.85	0.000	0.4303 to 0.5364
σ_e	0.2445	0.0076	32.17	0.000	0.2296 to 0.2594

characteristic) and the interaction between treatment and time (a covariate that varies within clusters).

The interpretation of regression coefficients in models including interaction was explained in detail in Section 29.5. Variable *weeks* was coded as time since the 2-week measurement, so the regression coefficient for variable *treatment* estimates the treatment effect (mean difference in FEV_1) at 2 weeks (the baseline of the post-treatment groups) while the regression coefficient for variable *weeks* estimates the mean increase in FEV_1 per week in the control group (the group corresponding to the baseline value of *treatment*). The regression coefficient for the interaction parameter (variable *treat.weeks*) estimates the mean *increase* in the effect of treatment per week: thus the effect of treatment is estimated to increase by 0.0127 litres per week, between week 2 and week 12. As might be expected, there is a strong association between baseline FEV_1 and post-treatment FEV_1 (regression coefficient 0.7562 for variable *fevbase*), and controlling for baseline FEV_1 has substantially reduced the estimated between-patient standard deviation ($\sigma_u = 0.4834$, compared to 0.6828 in the model including only the effect of treatment). The intraclass correlation coefficient from this model is 0.796.

31.5 GENERALIZED ESTIMATING EQUATIONS (GEE)

Estimation of generalized linear models incorporating random effects is difficult mathematically if the outcome is non-normal, except in the case of random-effects Poisson models which exploit a mathematical 'trick' where assuming a particular distribution for the random effect leads to a well-defined 'composite' distribution for the outcome (the negative binomial distribution). For other models, in particular logistic regression models, no such trick is available and estimation of random-effects models has until recently been either unavailable or difficult and time consuming.

Generalized estimating equations (GEE) were introduced by Liang and Zeger (1986) as a means of analysing longitudinal, non-normal data without resorting to fully specified random-effects models. They combine two approaches:

1 **Quasi-likelihood estimation**, where we specify only the mean and variance of the outcome, rather than a full probability model for its distribution. In GEE, the quasi-likelihood approach is generalized to allow a choice of structures for the correlation of outcomes within clusters; this is called a 'working' correlation structure. However, it is important to understand that these correlation structures need not (and often do not) correspond to a correlation structure derived from a full, random effects, probability model for the data.

2 **Robust standard errors** are used to take account of the clustering, and the fact that the parameter estimates are not based on a full probability model.

Note that for normally distributed outcomes, parameter estimates from GEE are identical to those from standard random-effects models.

The most common choice of correlation structure, and the only one that we shall consider here, is the 'exchangeable' correlation structure in which the correl-

ation between a pair of observations in the same cluster is assumed to be the same for all pairs in each cluster.

Example 31.3

The data set we shall use to compare GEE with other approaches to the analysis of clustered data comes from a study of the impact of HIV on the infectiousness of patients with pulmonary TB (Elliott *et al., AIDS* 1993, 7:981–987). This study was based on 70 pulmonary TB patients in Zambia, 42 of whom were infected with HIV and 28 of whom were uninfected. These patients are referred to as *index cases*. The aim of the study was to determine whether HIV-infected index cases were more or less likely than HIV-negative index cases to transmit *M. tuberculosis* infection to their household contacts.

Three hundred and seven household contacts were traced, of whom 181 were contacts of HIV-infected index cases. The mean number of contacts per HIV-infected index case was 4.3 (range 1 to 13), while the mean number of contacts per HIV-uninfected case was 4.5 (range 1 to 11). All these contacts underwent a Mantoux skin test for tuberculosis infection. An induration (skin reaction) of diameter $\geq 5\,mm$ was considered to be a positive indication that the contact had tuberculosis infection. Information on a number of household level variables (e.g. HIV status of TB patient, crowding) and on a number of individual contact level variables (e.g. age of contact, degree of intimacy of contact) was recorded. If some index cases are more infectious than others, or household members share previous exposures to TB, then the outcome (result of the Mantoux test in household contacts) will be clustered within households.

Table 31.10 shows that, overall, 184/307 (59.9%) of household contacts had positive Mantoux tests, suggesting that they had tuberculosis infection. This proportion appeared lower among the contacts of HIV-infected index cases (51.9%) than among contacts of HIV-uninfected index cases (71.4%).

Table 31.11(a) shows the results from a standard logistic regression model, ignoring any clustering within households. The odds ratio comparing contacts of HIV-infected index cases with contacts of HIV-uninfected index cases was 0.432 (95% CI 0.266 to 0.701). However, as explained earlier in the chapter, ignoring within-household clustering may mean that this confidence interval is too narrow.

Table 31.10 2 × 2 table showing the association between Mantoux test status in household contacts of tuberculosis patients and the HIV status of the index case.

Mantoux test status	HIV status of index case		Total
	Positive	Negative	
Positive	94 (51.9%)	90 (71.4%)	184 (59.9%)
Negative	87 (48.1%)	36 (28.6%)	123 (40.1%)
Total	181	126	307

Table 31.11 Regression outputs (odds ratio scale) for the association between Mantoux test positivity in household contacts of tuberculosis patients, and the HIV-infection status of the index case.

(a) Standard logistic regression

	Odds ratio	z	$P > |z|$	95% CI
HIV-infected	0.432	−3.40	0.001	0.266 to 0.701

(b) Logistic regression, using robust standard errors to allow for within-household clustering

	Odds ratio	z	$P > |z|$	95% CI
HIV-infected	0.432	−2.52	0.012	0.225 to 0.829

(c) Generalized estimating equations (GEE) with robust standard errors to allow for within-household clustering

	Odds ratio	z	$P > |z|$	95% CI
HIV-infected	0.380	−2.96	0.003	0.200 to 0.721

We will now compare these results with those in parts (b) and (c) of Table 31.11 from two different methods that allow for clustering. First, part (b) shows the results specifying robust standard errors in the logistic regression model to allow for within-household clustering (see Section 31.3). This approach does not change the estimated odds ratio. However, the 95% confidence interval is now wider, and the *P*-value has increased to 0.012 from 0.001 in the standard logistic regression model.

Part (c) of Table 31.11 shows results from a GEE analysis assuming an 'exchangeable' correlation structure. As well as correcting the standard errors, confidence intervals and *P*-values to account for the clustering, the odds ratio has reduced from 0.43 to 0.38 after taking account of within-household clustering. This is because the GEE analysis gives relatively less weight to contacts in large households. Box 31.1 summarizes theoretical issues in the GEE approach to the analysis of clustered data.

31.6 SUMMARY OF APPROACHES TO THE ANALYSIS OF CLUSTERED DATA

1 If data are clustered, it is *essential* that the clustering should be allowed for in the analyses. In particular, failure to allow for clustering may mean that standard errors of parameter estimates are too small, so that confidence intervals are too narrow and *P*-values are too small.

2 It is always valid to derive summary measures for each cluster, then analyse these using standard methods. However, analyses based on such summary statistics cannot take account of exposure variables that vary between individuals in the same cluster.

BOX 31.1   THEORETICAL ISSUES IN USING GEE

- We do not need to assume that the correlation matrix in GEE is correct; hence it is known as a 'working' correlation matrix. The parameter estimates and standard errors will still be correct ('consistent') provided that the sample size is large enough.
- However, the choice of correlation matrix will affect the parameter estimates. If we assume independence, that is no clustering within groups, then the parameter estimates will be the same as for the corresponding generalized linear model. To derive parameter estimates adjusted as far as possible for the clustering, we need to specify the most realistic correlation matrix possible.
- The GEE approach treats the clustering as a nuisance of no intrinsic interest, but provides parameter estimates and standard errors corrected for the clustering. Unlike random effects models, GEE estimates are not based on a fully specified probability model for the data (except for models with an identity link function: see Section 29.2). GEE models are also known as **'population-averaged'** or **'marginal' models** because the parameter estimates refer to average effects for the population rather than to the effects for a particular individual within the population.
- The GEE approach allows flexibility in modelling correlations, but little flexibility in modelling variances. This can have serious limitations for modelling of grouped counts or proportions, such as in the compound X example above, or in a study of malaria risk if the outcome was the proportion of mosquitoes landing on a bednet that were found to be infective.
- Assumptions about the processes leading to missing data are stronger for GEE than for random-effects models. For example, consider a longitudinal study in which repeated examinations are scheduled every three months, but in which some individuals do not attend some examinations. In GEE, it is assumed that data from these examinations are *missing completely at random*, which means that the probability that an observation is missing is independent of all other observations. For random-effects models the assumption is that data are *missing at random*, which means that the probability that an observation is missing is independent of its true value at that time, but may depend on values at other times, or on the values of other variables in the dataset.

3 The likely effect of the clustering on standard errors may be assessed by specifying robust standard errors that allow for the clustering. Parameter estimates will not be affected. For such robust standard errors to be reliable we need a reasonable number of clusters (at least 30). Wald tests, rather than likelihood ratio tests, must be used.

4 Random-effects (multilevel) models allow for the presence of clustering by modifying the linear predictor by a constant amount u_j in cluster j. The random effects $\{u_j\}$ are assumed to vary randomly between clusters. Random-effects models work well for normally distributed outcomes and Poisson regression, but estimation of random-effects logistic models is difficult and computationally demanding.

5 Generalized estimating equations (GEE) modify both parameter estimates and standard errors to allow for the clustering. Again, there should be a reasonable number of clusters. The GEE approach is particularly useful in logistic regression analyses and when the focus of interest is on the estimated exposure effect and where the clustering is of no intrinsic interest.

In this chapter we have described only the simplest types of model for the analysis of clustered data. In particular the random effects models presented in Section 31.4 include a single random effect to allow for the clustering. Such models have a wealth of possible extensions: for example, we may investigate whether exposure effects, as well as cluster means, vary randomly between clusters. For more details on the analysis of clustered data and random-effects (multilevel) models, see Goldstein (1995), Donner and Klar (2000) or Bryk and Raudenbush (2001).

Systematic reviews and meta-analysis

32.1 INTRODUCTION

There has been an explosion in research evidence in past decades; over half a million articles are published annually in the biomedical literature. It is common for important issues in medical research to be addressed in several studies. Indeed, we might be reluctant to introduce a new treatment based on the result of one trial alone. This chapter focuses on how the evidence relating to a particular research question can be summarized in order to make it accessible to medical practitioners and inform the practice of **evidence-based medicine**. In particular we discuss:

- systematic reviews of the medical literature;
- the statistical methods which are used to combine effect estimates from different studies (meta-analysis);
- sources of bias in meta-analysis and how these may be detected.

Because systematic reviews and meta-analyses of medical research are mainly (though not exclusively) used in combining evidence from randomized trials, we will refer throughout to *treatment* effects, rather than to *exposure* effects.

More detail on all the statistical methods presented in this chapter can be found in *Systematic Reviews in Health Care: Meta-Analysis in Context* edited by Egger, Davey Smith and Altman (2001); see www.systematicreviews.com.

32.2 SYSTEMATIC REVIEWS

The need to summarize evidence systematically was illustrated by Antman *et al.* (1992), who compared accumulating data from randomized controlled trials of treatments for myocardial infarction (heart attack) with the recommendations of clinical experts writing review articles and textbook chapters. By the mid-1970s, based on a meta-analysis of around ten trials in more than 2500 patients, there was good evidence of a protective effect of thrombolytic therapy after myocardial infarction against subsequent mortality. However, trials continued to be performed for the next 15 years (the cumulative total patients had reached more than 48 000 by 1990). It was not until the late 1980s that the majority of textbooks and review articles recommended the routine use of thrombolytic therapy after myocardial infarction.

It is now recognized that a conventional 'narrative' literature review – a 'summary of the information available to the author from the point of view of the author' – can be very misleading as a basis from which to draw conclusions on the overall evidence on a particular subject. Reliable reviews must be *systematic* if bias in the interpretation of findings is to be avoided.

Cook *et al.* (1995) defined a **systematic review** of the literature as 'the application of scientific strategies that limit bias by the systematic assembly, critical appraisal and synthesis of all relevant studies on a specific topic'. The main feature which distinguishes systematic from narrative reviews is that they have a methods section which clearly states the question being addressed, the subgroups of interest and the *methods and criteria employed for identifying and selecting relevant studies and extracting and analysing information*. Systematic reviews are a substantial undertaking and a team with expertise in both the content area and review methodology is usually needed.

Guidelines on the conduct of systematic reviews may be found in Egger, Davey Smith and Altman (2001) and in the Cochrane Collaboration handbook. The QUOROM statement (Moher *et al.* 1999) suggests guidelines for the reporting of systematic reviews.

32.3 THE COCHRANE AND CAMPBELL COLLABORATIONS

We have seen that:
- medical practice needs to be based on the results of systematic reviews, rather than (non-systematic) 'expert reviews' of the literature;
- to perform a systematic review is a substantial undertaking

The *Cochrane Collaboration* (www.cochrane.org), which started in 1993, is an attempt to address these issues. It aims to produce systematic, periodically updated reviews of medical and public health interventions. Cochrane reviews are available in electronic form (via CD-ROM and on the internet), which means that reviews can be updated as new evidence becomes available or if mistakes have been identified. Already, more than 1000 systematic reviews are available as

part of the Cochrane Collaboration, and some 150 000 studies are indexed in the database of randomized controlled trials.

The *Campbell Collaboration* (www.campbellcollaboration.org) is a similar initiative for systematic reviews of social and educational policies and practice, some of which include an impact on health-related outcomes.

32.4 META-ANALYSIS

The statistical methods for combining the results of a number of studies are known as **meta-analysis**. It should be emphasized that not all systematic reviews will contain a meta-analysis; this will depend on whether the systematic review has located studies that are sufficiently similar to make it reasonable to consider combining their results. The increase in interest in meta-analysis is illustrated by the fact that while in 1987 there were five MEDLINE citations using the term META-ANALYSIS, this had increased to 380 by 1991, and 580 by 2001.

We will illustrate methods for meta-analysis using studies with a binary outcome and measuring treatment effects using odds ratios. Corresponding methods exist for other treatment effect estimates such as risk ratios or risk differences, and for continuous outcome measures.

Example 32.1 Effect of diuretics on pre-eclampsia in pregnancy

In an early meta-analysis, Collins *et al.* (1985) examined the results of randomized controlled trials of diuretics in pregnancy. After excluding trials in which they considered that there was a possibility of severe bias, they found nine trials in which the effect of diuretics on pre-eclampsia (a rapid increase in blood pressure or proteinuria which may have severe sequelae) was reported. Table 32.1 summarizes the results of these trials.

Table 32.1 Results of nine randomized controlled trials of diuretics in pregnancy.

	Pre-eclampsia/total		
First author	Treated patients	Control patients	Odds ratio (95% CI)
Weseley	14/131	14/136	1.043 (0.477, 2.28)
Flowers	21/385	17/134	0.397 (0.203, 0.778)
Menzies	14/57	24/48	0.326 (0.142, 0.744)
Fallis	6/38	18/40	0.229 (0.078, 0.669)
Cuadros	12/1011	35/760	0.249 (0.128, 0.483)
Landesman	138/1370	175/1336	0.743 (0.586, 0.942)
Kraus	15/506	20/524	0.770 (0.390, 1.52)
Tervila	6/108	2/103	2.971 (0.586, 15.1)
Campbell	65/153	40/102	1.145 (0.687, 1.91)

In order to make an overall assessment of the effect of diuretics on pre-eclampsia, we would like to combine the results from these nine studies into a single summary estimate of the effect, together with a confidence interval. In doing this:

- Treated individuals should only be compared with control individuals from the same study, since the characteristics of patients in the different studies may differ in important respects, for example, because of different entry criteria, or because they come from different study populations which may have different underlying risks of pre-eclampsia. Thus simply combining patients across the studies would not be an appropriate way to estimate the overall treatment effect.
- Note that even if all the studies are broadly comparable, sampling error will inevitably mean that the observed treatment effects will vary. In this example the estimated odds ratios vary from 0.229 (Fallis) to 2.971 (Tervila).
- The relative sizes of the studies should be taken into account. Note that the most extreme results (odds ratios furthest away from 1) come from the smaller studies.

In the next two sections we describe fixed-effect and random-effects approaches to meta-analysis. A **fixed-effect meta-analysis** can be conducted if it is reasonable to assume that the underlying treatment effect is the same in all the studies, and that the observed variation is due entirely to sampling variation. The fixed-effect assumption can be examined using a **test of heterogeneity** between studies, as described at the end of Section 32.5. A **random-effects meta-analysis** aims to allow for such heterogeneity, and is described in Section 32.6.

32.5 FIXED-EFFECT META-ANALYSIS

In a fixed-effect meta-analysis, we assume that the observed variation in treatment effects in the different studies is due entirely to sampling variation, and that the underlying treatment effect is the same in all the study populations. Table 32.2 shows the notation we will use for the results from study i (when we have a binary outcome, as in Example 32.1). The estimate of the odds ratio for the treatment effect in study i is

$$OR_i = \frac{d_{1i} \times h_{0i}}{d_{0i} \times h_{1i}}$$

In Example 32.1, we have nine such tables of the effects of treatment with diuretics on pre-eclampsia, one from each of the nine trials, and nine odds ratios. The

Table 32.2 Notation for the 2 × 2 table of results from study i.

	Outcome		
	Experienced event: D (Disease)	Did not experience event: H (Healthy)	Total
Group 1 (intervention)	d_{1i}	h_{1i}	n_{1i}
Group 0 (control)	d_{0i}	h_{0i}	n_{0i}
Total	d_i	h_i	n_i

summary estimate of the treatment effect is calculated as a **weighted average** (see Section 18.3) of the log odds ratios from the separate trials:

$$\log(OR_F) = \frac{\Sigma[w_i \times \log(OR_i)]}{\Sigma w_i}$$

The subscript F denotes the assumption that the effect of diuretics is the same, or *fixed*, in each study. Note that individuals are only compared with other individuals in the same study (via the study log odds ratio).

In the **inverse variance method**, the weight w_i for study i equals the inverse of the variance, v_i, of the estimated log odds ratio in that study (see Section 16.7):

$$\text{Inverse variance weights: } w_i = 1/v_i,$$

$$\text{where } v_i = 1/d_{1i} + 1/h_{1i} + 1/d_{0i} + 1/h_{0i}$$

This choice of weights minimizes the standard error of the summary log odds ratio, which is:

$$\text{s.e.}\,(\log(OR_F)) = \sqrt{\frac{1}{\Sigma w_i}}$$

This can be used to calculate confidence intervals, a z statistic and hence a P-value for the summary log odds ratio. An alternative weighting scheme is to use **Mantel–Haenszel weights** to combine the odds ratios from the individual studies. These are:

$$\text{Mantel–Haenszel weights: } w_i = d_{0i}h_{1i}/n_i$$

Example 32.1 (continued)
Results from a fixed-effect meta-analysis of the data on the effect of diuretics in pregnancy are shown in Table 32.3. This gives clear evidence that the odds of pre-eclampsia were reduced in mothers treated with diuretics. As usual, the estimated summary log odds ratio and its confidence interval have been converted to an odds ratio, for ease of interpretation.

Table 32.3 Results of a fixed-effect meta-analysis of results from nine randomized controlled trials of diuretics in pregnancy.

OR$_F$	z	P-value	95% CI
0.672	−4.455	< 0.001	0.564 to 0.800

Note on sparse data

If any of the cells in the 2×2 table for one (or more) of the contributing studies contains zero, then the formulae for the log OR$_i$ and corresponding variance, v_i, in that table break down. When this happens, it is conventional to add 0.5 to all cells in the table, and it may be preferable to use Mantel–Haenszel weights. In other circumstances the inverse-variance and Mantel–Haenszel methods will give similar results.

Forest plots

Results of meta-analyses are displayed in a standard way known as a 'forest plot', and such a plot of the diuretics data is shown in Figure 32.1. The horizontal lines correspond to the 95 % confidence intervals for each study, with the corresponding box area drawn proportional to the weight for that individual study in the meta-analysis. Hence the wider is the confidence interval the smaller is the box area. The

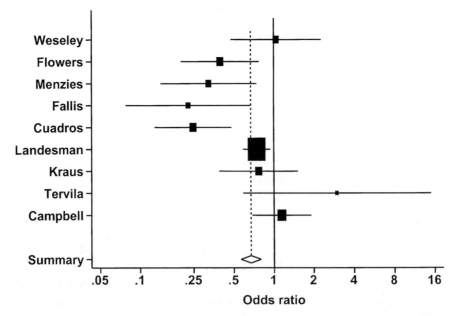

Fig. 32.1 Forest plot of the results of a fixed-effect meta-analysis of nine studies of the effect of diuretics in pregnancy.

diamond (and broken vertical line) represents the summary estimate, and the confidence interval for the summary estimate corresponds to the width of the diamond. The unbroken vertical line is at the null value (1) of the odds ratio, and is equivalent to no treatment effect. Note that the horizontal axis is plotted on a log scale, so that confidence intervals are symmetrical and an odds ratio of (e.g.) 2 is the same distance from 1 as $1/2 = 0.5$.

The exact origin of the name 'forest plot' is not clear. One possible derivation is that it allows one to avoid the pitfall of 'not being able to see the wood for the trees'.

Testing for heterogeneity between studies

The fixed-effect estimate is based on the assumption that the true effect does not differ between studies. This assumption should be checked. We can do this using a χ^2 **test of heterogeneity**, similar to that described for Mantel–Haenszel methods in Section 18.5. The greater the average distance between the log odds ratios estimated in the individual studies and the summary log odds ratio, the more evidence against the null hypothesis that the true log odds ratios are the same. The χ^2 test of heterogeneity (often denoted by Q) is based on a weighted sum of the squares of these differences:

$$\chi^2 = Q = \Sigma w_i \, [\log(OR_i) - \log(OR_F)]^2$$

$$\text{d.f.} = \text{number of studies} - 1$$

Example 32.1 (continued)
For the data on the effect of diuretics in pregnancy,

$$\chi^2 = 27.265, \ \text{d.f.} = 9{-}1 = 8, \ P = 0.001$$

There is therefore strong evidence (confirming the impression in the graph) that the effect of diuretics differs between studies.

32.6 RANDOM-EFFECTS META-ANALYSIS

If there is evidence of heterogeneity between studies, how should we proceed? Although it can be argued that it is inappropriate to calculate a summary measure (this is discussed further below), it is also possible to allow for the heterogeneity by incorporating a model for the heterogeneity between studies into the meta-analysis. This approach is called random-effects meta-analysis.

In random-effects meta-analysis, we assume that the 'true' log odds ratio in each study comes from a normal distribution:

$$\log(OR_i) \approx N(\log(OR_R), \ \tau^2)$$

whose mean equals the true 'overall' treatment effect and whose variance is usually denoted by τ^2 (τ is the Greek letter tau). We estimate this between-study variance, τ^2, from the observed data (see below) and use this to modify the weights used to calculate the **random-effects summary estimate**:

$$\log(OR_R) = \frac{\Sigma[w_i^* \times \log(OR_i)]}{\Sigma w_i^*}$$

$$w_i^* = \frac{1}{v_i + \tau^2}, \text{ where } v_i = 1/d_{1i} + 1/h_{1i} + 1/d_{0i} + 1/h_{0i}$$

The standard error of the random-effects summary estimate is calculated from the inverse of the sum of the adjusted weights:

$$\text{s.e. } (\log(OR_R)) = \sqrt{\frac{1}{\Sigma w_i^*}}$$

Estimating the between-study variance

The most commonly used formula for estimating the between-study variance, τ^2, from the observed data was put forward by DerSimonian and Laird (1986). It is based on the value of the χ^2 test of heterogeneity, represented by Q, the unadjusted weights, w_i, and the number of contributing studies, k:

$$\tau^2 = \max\left[0, \ \left(\frac{Q - (k - 1)}{W}\right)\right],$$

$$\text{where } Q = \chi^2 = \Sigma w_i \ (\log(OR_i) - \log(OR_F))^2$$

$$\text{and } W = \Sigma w_i - \left(\frac{\Sigma w_i^2}{\Sigma w_i}\right)$$

The mathematical details are included here for completeness. In practice the computer would calculate this as part of the random-effects meta-analysis routine.

Table 32.4 Comparison of fixed-effects and random-effects meta-analysis results of nine randomized controlled trials of the impact of diuretics in pregnancy on pre-eclampsia.

Method	Summary OR	95% CI	z	P-value
Fixed-effects	0.672	0.564 to 0.800	-4.455	<0.001
Random-effects	0.596	0.400 to 0.889	-2.537	0.011

Example 32.1 (continued)

For the data on the effect of diuretics in pregnancy, the estimate of the between-study variance is $\tau^2 = 0.230$, and the summary OR is $OR_R = 0.596$, somewhat smaller than the fixed-effect estimate. The confidence interval is correspondingly much wider, as can be seen in Table 32.4, which presents the results from both the fixed-effect and random-effects meta-analyses.

Comparison of fixed-effect and random-effects meta-analysis

Because of the addition of τ^2 (the estimated between-study variance) to their denominators, random-effects weights are:

1 smaller, and
2 much more similar to each other

than their fixed-effect counterparts. Table 32.5 illustrates this for the diuretics trials of Example 32.1. This results in:

3 smaller studies being given greater relative weight,
4 a wider confidence interval for the summary estimate, and
5 a larger P-value

compared to the corresponding fixed-effect meta-analysis (see Table 32.4). Thus a random-effects meta-analysis will in general be *more conservative* than its fixed-effect counterpart. This reflects the greater uncertainty inherent in the random-effects approach, because it is assumed that, in addition to sampling variation, the true effect varies between studies.

Table 32.5 Comparison of the weights used in the fixed-effect and random-effects meta-analyses of the diuretics trial data, shown in Table 32.1.

Study	Odds ratio (95% CI)	Fixed-effects weight	Random-effects weight
Weseley	1.04 (0.48 to 2.28)	6.27	2.57
Flowers	0.40 (0.20 to 0.78)	8.49	2.88
Menzies	0.33 (0.14 to 0.74)	5.62	2.45
Fallis	0.23 (0.08 to 0.67)	3.35	1.89
Cuadros	0.25 (0.13 to 0.48)	8.75	2.91
Landesman	0.74 (0.59 to 0.94)	68.34	4.09
Kraus	0.77 (0.39 to 1.52)	8.29	2.85
Tervila	2.97 (0.59 to 15.1)	1.46	1.09
Campbell	1.14 (0.69 to 1.91)	14.73	3.36

Note that the greater the estimate of τ^2, the greater the difference between the fixed-effect and random-effects weights. If τ^2 (the between-study variance) is estimated to be zero, then the fixed-effect and random-effects estimates will be identical.

Interpretation of the summary estimate from a random-effects meta-analysis

The *interpretation* of the random-effects summary estimate is in fact very different to that of the fixed-effect one. In fixed-effect meta-analysis it is *assumed* that the true effect is the same in each study and that the only reason for variation in the estimates between studies is sampling error. In other words, it is assumed that the treatment effect is universal, and the meta-analysis provides the best available estimate of it.

In random-effects meta-analysis, the estimate is of a *mean* effect about which it is assumed that the true study effects vary. There is disagreement over whether it is appropriate to use random-effects models to combine study estimates in the presence of heterogeneity, and whether the resulting summary estimate is meaningful. This will be illustrated in Example 32.2.

Example 32.2 BCG vaccination

It has been recognized for many years that the protection given by BCG vaccination against tuberculosis varies between settings. For example, the risk ratio comparing vaccinated with unvaccinated individuals in the MRC trial in the UK (conducted during the 1960s and 1970s) was 0.24 (95% CI 0.18 to 0.31), while in the very large trial in Madras, south India, there appeared to be no protection (risk ratio 1.01, 95% CI 0.89 to 1.14).

In a meta-analysis published in 1994, Colditz *et al.* used all trials in which random or systematic allocation was used to decide vaccine or placebo, and in which both groups had equivalent surveillance procedures and similar lengths of follow-up. Using a random-effects meta-analysis (having noted the highly significant heterogeneity between trials) they concluded that the risk ratio was 0.49 (95% CI 0.34 to 0.70).

While Colditz *et al.* concluded that 'the results of this meta-analysis lend added weight and confidence to arguments favouring the use of BCG vaccine', Fine (1995) reached different conclusions. Noting, like Colditz *et al.*, the strong association between latitude and estimated effect of the vaccine (BCG appeared to work better further away from the equator) he commented that 'it is invalid to combine existing data into a single overall estimate' and further that 'most of the studies of BCG have been at relatively high latitudes whereas their current use is mainly at lower latitudes'. Thus it can be argued that random-effects meta-analysis is simply a means of combining 'apples and pears': forming an average of estimates of quantities whose values we know to be different from each other.

We also saw earlier that in a random-effects meta-analysis studies are weighted more equally than in a fixed-effect meta-analysis. If a random-effects summary estimate differs from the fixed-effect estimate, this is a sign that the average estimate from the smaller studies differs from the average of the large ones. Given that small studies are more subject to publication bias than large ones (see Section 32.7), this is clearly a disadvantage of random-effects meta-analyses. While *explanations* for heterogeneity may provide useful insights into differences between studies, and may have implications for clinical practice, we should be very cautious about an approach that *adjusts* for heterogeneity without *explaining* it.

Meta-regression

While there is disagreement over whether it is appropriate to use random-effects models to combine study estimates in the presence of heterogeneity, it is clear that the investigation of **sources of heterogeneity** (such as study latitude in the example above) may yield important insights. In the case of BCG vaccination, Fine discusses how the association with latitude may be because of differential exposure to environmental mycobacteria in different populations, which may in turn yield insights into mechanisms of immunity to mycobacterial diseases.

Meta-regression can be used to examine associations between study characteristics and treatment effects. In this approach, we postulate that the treatment effect (e.g. log odds ratio) is related in a linear manner to one or more study covariates.

Then, as with random-effects meta-analysis, we incorporate an additional variance component τ^2 that accounts for unexplained heterogeneity between studies. The meta-regression procedure iterates between (i) estimating τ^2, and (ii) using this estimate in a weighted regression to estimate the covariate effects. The estimated covariate effects lead to a new estimate of τ^2, and so on. The process stops when consecutive steps in the iteration yield almost identical values for τ^2 and for the covariate effects; the model is then said to have converged.

32.7 BIAS IN META-ANALYSIS

The emphasis on the importance of sound methodology for systematic reviews arises from the observation that severe bias may result if this methodology is not applied. Summarizing the results of five biased trials will give a precise but biased result!

Causes of bias: poor trial quality

Empirical evidence that methodological quality of studies was associated with estimates of treatment effect in clinical trials was first provided in an important study by Schulz *et al.* (1995), who assessed the methodological quality of 250 controlled trials from 33 meta-analyses of treatments in the area of pregnancy and childbirth. They found that trials in which treatment allocation was inadequately concealed (see Chapter 34) had odds ratios which were exaggerated (i.e. further away from 1) by 41 % compared to trials which reported 'adequate concealment'. Trials that were not double-blind yielded 17% larger estimates of effect.

An important consequence of the recognition that the quality of a trial may affect its results was to encourage improved standards of conduct and reporting of randomized trials. In particular the CONSORT statement (see Moher, Schulz and Altman (2001), www.consort-statement.org and Chapter 34), which was published in 1996 and updated in 2001, aims to standardize the reporting of trials in medical journals.

Causes of bias: publication bias

In general, a study showing a beneficial effect of a new treatment is more likely to be considered worthy of publication than one showing no effect. There is a considerable bias that operates at every stage of the process, with negative trials considered to contribute less to scientific knowledge than positive ones:
- those who conducted the study are more likely to submit the results to a peer-reviewed journal;
- editors of journals are more likely to consider the study potentially worth publishing and send it for peer review;
- referees are more likely to deem the study suitable for publication.

This situation has been accentuated by two factors: first that studies have often been too small to detect a beneficial effect even if one exists (see Chapter 35) and second that there has been too much emphasis on 'significant' results (i.e. $P < 0.05$ for the effect of interest).

A proposed solution to the problem of publication bias is to establish registers of all trials in a particular area, from when they are funded or established. It has also been proposed that journals consider studies for publication 'blind' of the actual results (i.e. based only on the literature review and methods). It is also clear that the active discouragement of studies that do not have power to detect a clinically important effect would alleviate the problem. Publication bias is a lesser problem for larger studies, for which there tends to be general agreement that the results are of interest, whatever they are.

Funnel plots to examine bias in meta-analysis

The existence of publication bias may be examined graphically by the use of 'funnel plots'. These are simple scatter plots of the treatment effects estimated from individual studies on the horizontal axis and the standard error of the treatment effect (reflecting the study size) on the vertical axis. The name 'funnel plot' is based on the fact that the precision in the estimation of the underlying treatment effect will increase as the sample size of component studies increases. Effect estimates from small studies will therefore scatter more widely at the bottom of the graph, with the spread narrowing among larger studies. In the absence of bias the plot will resemble a symmetrical inverted funnel, as shown in panel (a) of Figure 32.2.

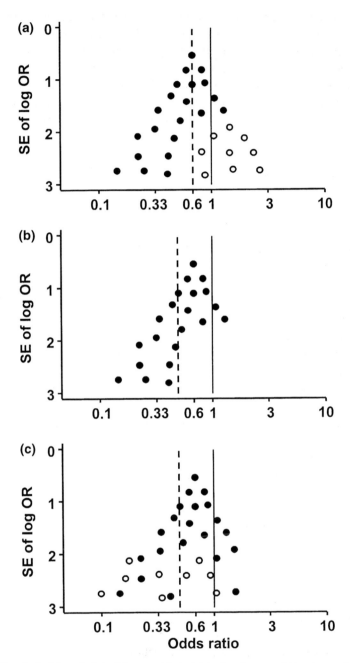

Fig. 32.2 Hypothetical funnel plots: (a) symmetrical plot in the absence of bias (open circles indicate smaller studies showing no beneficial effects); (b) asymmetrical plot in the presence of publication bias (smaller studies showing no beneficial effects are missing); (c) asymmetrical plot in the presence of bias due to low methodological quality of smaller studies (open circles indicate small studies of inadequate quality whose results are biased towards larger beneficial effects).

Relative measures of treatment effect (risk ratios or odds ratios) are plotted on a logarithmic scale. This is important to ensure that effects of the same magnitude but opposite directions, for example risk ratios of 0.5 and 2, are equidistant from 1 (corresponding to no effect). Treatment effects have generally been plotted against sample sizes. However, the statistical power of a trial is determined both by the total sample size and the number of participants developing the event of interest. For example, a study with 100 000 patients and 10 events is less likely to show a statistically significant effect of a treatment than a study with 1000 patients and 100 events. The standard error of the effect estimate, rather than total sample size, has therefore been increasingly used in funnel plots (Sterne and Egger 2001).

If there is bias, for example because smaller studies showing no statistically significant effects (open circles in the figure) remain unpublished, then such publication bias will lead to an asymmetrical appearance of the funnel plot with a gap in the right bottom side of the graph (panel (b) of Fig. 32.2). In this situation the combined effect from meta-analysis will overestimate the treatment's effect. The more pronounced the asymmetry, the more likely it is that the amount of bias will be substantial.

What factors can lead to asymmetry in funnel plots?

Publication bias has long been associated with funnel plot asymmetry, but it is important to realise that publication bias is not the only cause of funnel plot asymmetry. We have already seen that trials of lower quality may yield exaggerated estimates of treatment effects. Smaller studies are, on average, conducted and analysed with less methodological rigour than larger studies, so that asymmetry may also result from the over-estimation of treatment effects in smaller studies of lower methodological quality (panel (c) of Fig. 32.2).

Funnel plot asymmetry may have causes other than bias. Heterogeneity between trials can also lead to funnel plot asymmetry if the true treatment effect is larger (or smaller) in the smaller trials because these are conducted, for example, among high-risk patients. Such trials will tend to be smaller, because of the difficulty in recruiting such patients and because increased event rates mean that smaller sample sizes are required to detect a given effect. In addition, in some large trials, interventions may be implemented under routine conditions rather than in trial conditions where it is possible to invest heavily in assuring all aspects are perfect. This will result in relatively lower treatment effects. For example, an asymmetrical funnel plot was found in a meta-analysis of trials examining the effect of geriatric assessment programmes on mortality. An experienced consultant geriatrician was more likely to be actively involved in the smaller trials and this may explain the larger treatment effects observed in these trials.

Because publication bias is only one of the possible reasons for asymmetry, the funnel plot should be seen more as a means of examining '**small study effects**' (the tendency for the smaller studies in a meta-analysis to show larger treatment effects). The presence of funnel plot asymmetry should lead to consideration of possible explanations, and may bring into question the interpretation of the overall estimate of treatment effect from a meta-analysis.

Statistical tests for funnel plot asymmetry

Symmetry or asymmetry is generally defined informally, through visual examination, but different observers may interpret funnel plots differently. More formal statistical methods to examine associations between the studies' effects and their sizes have been proposed. Begg and Mazumdar (1994) proposed an adjusted rank correlation test for publication bias which involves calculation of the rank correlation between the treatment effect and its estimated standard error (or, equivalently, variance) in each study. Egger *et al.* (1997a) proposed a linear regression test in which the standardized treatment effect from each study, that is the treatment effect divided by its standard error, is regressed against the precision of the treatment effect. For binary outcomes, the regression equation is:

$$y_i = \beta_0 + \beta_1 x_i, \text{ where}$$

$$y_i = \log(OR_i)/\text{s.e.}\,[\log(OR_i)] = \log(OR_i) \times \sqrt{w_i}$$

$$x_i = 1/\text{s.e.}\,[\log(OR_i)] = \sqrt{w_i}$$

and evidence for bias is found if the intercept β_0 differs from zero.

This test is equivalent to a regression of the log odds ratio against standard error (Sterne *et al.* 2000). This can be seen by multiplying the regression equation above by s.e. $[\log(OR_i)]$, which gives:

$$\log(OR_i) = \beta_0 \times \text{s.e.}\,[\log(OR_i)] + \beta_1$$

where the regression accounts for between-subject heterogeneity by weighting according to the inverse of the variance of $\log(OR_i)$. The greater the association between $\log(OR_i)$ and s.e. $[\log(OR_i)]$, measured by the size of the regression coefficient β_0, the greater the evidence for funnel plot asymmetry. The test is therefore very closely related to a **meta-regression** of $\log(OR_i)$ on s.e. $[\log(OR_i)]$. There is thus the potential to include s.e.$[\log(OR_i]$ together with other study characteristics (for example measures of study quality) in a multiple meta-regression to examine competing explanations for differences between studies.

The power and sensitivity of these tests is not well established. It appears that the regression method is more powerful than the rank correlation method, but that power is low unless the amount of bias is substantial and the number of studies in the meta-analysis exceeds ten (Sterne *et al.* 2000).

32.8 META-ANALYSIS OF OBSERVATIONAL STUDIES

Although the emphasis in this chapter has been on the meta-analysis of data from randomized trials, there are many questions which can only be addressed in observational studies. These include:

- studies of the aetiology of disease (for example, does passive smoking cause lung cancer?);
- evaluations of the effectiveness of interventions that have already been introduced, such as BCG vaccination;
- evaluation of the effectiveness of an intervention on rare adverse outcomes, such as mortality, for which the sample size required for randomized controlled trials might be prohibitive;
- evaluation of the effectiveness of interventions that need to be applied on a widespread basis, such as a mass media campaign, and for which therefore it is not possible to have control groups;
- evaluation of the effectiveness of interventions in populations other than those in which they were first evaluated.

For this reason a substantial proportion of published meta-analyses are based on observational studies rather than on randomized trials.

However, the issues involved in meta-analysis of observational studies are very different, and more difficult, than for the meta-analysis of randomized trials. In particular, the appropriate control of confounding factors is of fundamental importance in the analysis and interpretation of observational studies while, in contrast, appropriate randomization should mean that confounding is not a problem in trials (providing that their size is large enough, see Chapters 34 and 35). Other types of bias, for example recall bias, may also be of greater concern in observational studies than in randomized trials.

A striking example of the potential for meta-analyses of observational studies to give misleading results was given by Egger *et al.* (1997b). They compared the results of six observational cohort studies of the association between intake of beta-carotene (a precursor of the antioxidant vitamin A) and cardiovascular mortality, with those from four randomized trials in which participants randomized to beta-carotene supplements were compared with participants randomized to placebo. As can be seen from Figure 32.3, the cohort studies indicated a strong protective effect of beta-carotene while the randomized trials suggest a moderate adverse effect of beta-carotene supplementation. An individual's diet is strongly associated with other characteristics associated with cardiovascular mortality (for example physical activity and social class) and these results suggest that failure to control for such factors, or other types of bias, led to the apparent protective effect of beta-carotene in the observational studies.

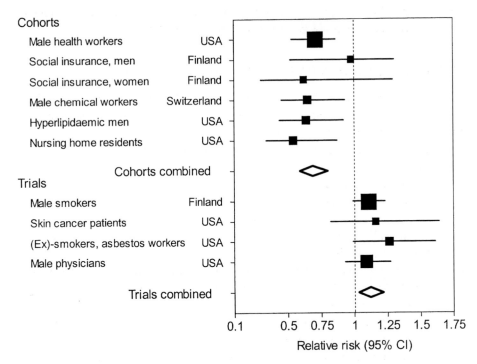

Fig. 32.3 Meta-analysis of the association between beta-carotene intake and cardiovascular mortality. Results from observational studies indicate considerable benefit whereas the findings from randomized controlled trials show an increase in the risk of death. We are grateful to Matthias Egger for permission to reproduce the figure.

This suggests that the statistical combination of studies should not, in general, be a prominent component of systematic reviews of observational studies, which should focus instead on possible sources of heterogeneity between studies and the reasons for these.

32.9 CONCLUSIONS

Systematic reviews and meta-analysis (the quantitative analysis of such reviews) are now accepted as an important part of medical research. While the analytical methods are relatively simple, there is still controversy over appropriate methods of analysis. Systematic reviews are substantial undertakings, and those conducting such reviews need to be aware of the potential biases which may affect their conclusions. However, the explosion in medical research information and the availability of reviews on-line mean that synthesis of research findings is likely to be of ever increasing importance to the practice of medicine.

CHAPTER 33

Bayesian statistics

33.1 INTRODUCTION: BAYESIAN INFERENCE

In this chapter we give a brief description of the Bayesian approach to statistical inference, and compare it to the frequentist approach which has been used in the rest of the book. The Bayesian approach is based on **Bayes' formula** for relating **conditional probabilities** (see Chapter 14):

$$\text{prob}(B \text{ given } A) = \frac{\text{prob}(A \text{ given } B) \times \text{prob}(B)}{\text{prob}(A)}$$

We have seen that a statistical model specifies how the probability distribution of an outcome variable (the data) depends on model parameters. For example, consider a trial of the effect of thrombolysis on the risk of death up to 1 year after a myocardial infarction. The data are the number of patients and number of deaths in each group, and the model parameters are the risk of death in the control group, and the risk ratio comparing the risk of death in patients given thrombolysis with the risk of death in the control group. In Chapter 28 we explained that the model parameters are fitted using the maximum likelihood approach. This is based on calculating the *conditional* probability of the observed data given model parameters.

The **Bayesian approach** to statistical inference starts with a *prior belief* about the likely values of the model parameters, and then uses the observed data to modify these. We will denote this prior belief by prob(parameters). Bayes' formula provides the mechanism to update this belief in the light of the data:

$$\text{prob}(\text{model parameters given data}) = \frac{\text{prob}(\text{data given model parameters}) \times \text{prob}(\text{parameters})}{\text{prob}(\text{data})}$$

The prior belief concerning the values of the parameters is often expressed in terms of a probability distribution, such as a normal or binomial distribution, representing a range of possible values, rather than as single values. This is called the **prior distribution**. The probability distribution of the model parameters given the data is known as the **posterior distribution**.

33.2 COMPARISON OF BAYESIAN AND FREQUENTIST STATISTICAL INFERENCE

In this book we have concentrated on the **frequentist** approach to statistical inference, in which we think of probability in terms of the proportion of times that an event would occur in a large number of similar repeated trials. In frequentist statistical inference, we think of model parameters (for instance the risk ratio for the effect of thrombolysis on the risk of death following heart attack, compared to placebo) as fixed. We use the data to make inferences about model parameters, via parameter estimates, confidence intervals and P-values.

In the Bayesian approach our inferences are based on the posterior probability distribution for the model parameters. For example, we might derive a **95 % credible interval**, based on the posterior distribution, within which there is 95 % probability that the parameter lies. Box 33.1 compares the Bayesian and frequentist approaches

---

BOX 33.1 COMPARISON OF FREQUENTIST AND BAYESIAN APPROACHES TO STATISTICAL INFERENCE

Frequentist statistics	**Bayesian statistics**
We use the data to make inferences about the true (but unknown) population value of the risk ratio.	We start with our *prior* opinion about the risk ratio, expressed as a probability distribution. We use the data to modify that opinion (we derive the *posterior* probability distribution for the risk ratio based on *both* the data and the prior distribution).
The *95 % confidence interval* gives us a range of values for the population risk ratio that is consistent with the data. 95 % of the times we derive such a range it will contain the true (but unknown) population value.	A *95 % credible interval* is one that has a 95 % chance of containing the population risk ratio.
The *P*-value is the probability of getting a risk ratio at least as far from the null value of 1 as the one found in our study.	The posterior distribution can be used to derive direct probability statements about the risk ratio, e.g. the probability that the drug *increases* the risk of death.

to statistical inference. See also the book by Royall (1997), which describes and compares different approaches to statistical inference.

If our prior opinion about the risk ratio is very vague (we consider a very wide range of values to be equally likely) then the results of a frequentist analysis are very similar to the results of a Bayesian analysis—both are based on the likelihood for the data. This is because a vague prior distribution will have little influence on the posterior probability, compared to the influence of the data:

- the 95 % confidence interval is the same as the 95 % credible interval, except that the latter has the interpretation often incorrectly ascribed to a confidence interval;
- the (1-sided) *P*-value is the same as the probability that the drug increases the risk of death (assuming that we found a protective effect of the drug).

However, the two approaches can give very different results if our prior opinion is not vague relative to the amount of information contained in the data. This issue is at the heart of a long-standing argument between proponents of the two schools of statistical inference. Bayesians may argue that it is appropriate to take external information into account by quantifying this as prior belief. Frequentists, on the other hand, may argue that our inferences should be made based only on the data. Further, prior belief can be difficult to quantify. For example, consider the hypothesis that a particular exposure is associated with the risk of a particular cancer. In quantifying our prior belief, how much weight should be given to evidence that there is a biologically plausible mechanism for the association, compared to evidence that international differences in disease rates show some association with differences in the level of the risk factor?

In some situations, Bayesian inference allows a more natural way to consider consequences of the data than does frequentist reasoning. For example:

- in a clinical trial in which an interim analysis reveals that the estimated risk of disease is identical in the treatment and control groups, Bayesian statistics could be used to ask the question 'What is the probability that there is a clinically important effect of treatment, given the data currently accrued?' This question has no meaning in frequentist statistics, since the effect of treatment is treated as a fixed but unknown quantity;
- in a trial whose aim is to examine whether a new treatment (B) is at least as clinically effective as an existing treatment (A), it is perfectly meaningful, in a Bayesian framework, to ask 'What is the probability that drug B is at least as good as drug A?' In contrast, frequentist statistics tends to focus on testing the evidence against the null hypothesis that the effect of drug B is *the same as* the effect of drug A.

33.3 MARKOV CHAIN MONTE-CARLO (MCMC) METHODS

In recent years there has been a resurgence of interest in Bayesian statistics. This has been based less on arguments about approaches to statistical inference than on a powerful means of estimating parameters in complex statistical models based on the Bayesian approach. The idea is that if we know the values of all the parameters except for one, then we can derive the *conditional distribution* of the unknown parameter, conditional on the data and the other (known) parameter values. Such a conditional distribution can be derived for each parameter, assuming that the values of all the others are known.

The **Markov Chain Monte-Carlo (MCMC)** procedure is used to generate a value for each parameter, by sampling randomly from its conditional distribution. This then acts as the 'known' value for that parameter. This process is carried out iteratively. A new parameter value is sampled from the distribution of each parameter in turn, and is used to update the 'known' values for the conditional distribution of the next parameter. The phrase 'Markov Chain' refers to the fact that the procedure is based only on the last sampled values of each parameter, while 'Monte-Carlo' refers to the random sampling of the parameter values.

After a suitable 'burn in' period (e.g. 10 000 iterations), the dependence of the procedure on the initial chioce of the parameter values is lost. The parameter values generated over the next (say) 10 000 iterations are then recorded. These correspond to the posterior distribution of the parameters, based on the data and the prior probabilities. The high speeds of modern desktop computers mean that such computationally intensive procedures can be run in reasonable amounts of time, although they are not as quick as standard (maximum-likelihood) methods.

MCMC methods can thus be used as an alternative to maximum-likelihood estimation, for models such as random-effects logistic regression where maximum-likelihood estimation is computationally difficult. This can be carried out using specialised computer software such as BUGS (available at www.mrc-bsu.cam. ac.uk/bugs), which stands for Bayesian inference Using Gibbs Sampling and allows users to specify a wide range of statistical models which are then estimated using MCMC. Note, however, that both model specification and use of the MCMC estimation procedure currently require considerably more technical knowledge than is needed to use a standard statistical software package.

STUDY DESIGN, ANALYSIS AND INTERPRETATION

Our aim in this final part of the book is to facilitate the overall planning and conduct of an analysis, and to cover general issues in the interpretation of study results. We start in Chapter 34 by explaining how to link the analysis to study design. We include guides to aid the selection of appropriate statistical methods for each of the main types of study, and draw attention to design features that influence the approach to analysis.

In the next three chapters, we address three different issues related to interpretation of statistical analyses. Chapter 35 tackles the calculation of sample size, and explains its fundamental importance in the interpretation of a study's results. Chapter 36 covers the assessment and implications of measurement error and misclassification in study outcomes and exposures. Chapter 37 outlines the different measures that are used to assess the impact of an exposure or of a treatment on the amount of disease in a population.

Finally, Chapter 38 recommends general strategies for statistical analysis.

CHAPTER 34

Linking analysis to study design: summary of methods

34.1 INTRODUCTION

The main focus of this book is on the statistical methods needed to analyse the effect of an exposure (or treatment) on an outcome. In previous parts, we have categorized these methods according to the types of outcome and exposure (or treatment) variables under consideration. These are summarized in the inside covers of the book. In this chapter, we now look more generally at how to link the analysis to the study design. In particular, we:

- summarize the range of methods available for each of the following:
     randomized controlled trials;
     other designs to evaluate the impact of an intervention;
     cross-sectional and longitudinal studies;
     case–control studies;
- highlight the key elements of each design that determine the choice of statistical method(s);
- discuss any specific issues that need to be considered in the interpretation of the results;
- draw attention to design-specific considerations that need to be built into the analysis plan, in addition to the general strategies for analysis outlined in Chapter 38.

Detailed discussions of the design of different types of study are outside the scope of this book, but are available in the following textbooks:

Clinical trials: Friedman *et al.* (1998) and Pocock (1983)
Interventions in developing countries: Smith & Morrow (1996)
Cluster randomized trials: Donner & Klar (2000) and Ukoumunne *et al.* (1999)
Case–control studies: Breslow & Day (1980) and Schlesselman & Stolley (1982)
General epidemiology: Gordis (2000), Rothman (2002), Rothman & Greenland (1998) and Szklo & Nieto (2000)

34.2 RANDOMIZED CONTROLLED TRIALS

Randomized controlled trials (RCTs) provide the best evidence on the effectiveness of treatments and health care interventions. Their key elements are:

- The comparison of a group receiving the treatment (or intervention) under evaluation, with a control group receiving either best practice, or an inactive intervention.
- Use of a **randomization** scheme to ensure that no systematic differences, in either known or unknown prognostic factors, arise during allocation between the groups. This should ensure that estimated treatment effects are not biased by confounding factors (see Chapter 18).
- **Allocation concealment**: successful implementation of a randomization scheme depends on making sure that those responsible for recruiting and allocating participants to the trial have no prior knowledge about which intervention they will receive. This is called allocation concealment.
- Where possible, a **double blind design**, in which neither participants nor study personnel know what treatment has been received until the 'code is broken' after the end of the trial. This is achieved by using a **placebo**, a preparation indistinguishable in all respects to that given to the treatment group, except for lacking the active component. If a double-blind design is not possible then outcome assessment should be done by an investigator blind to the treatment received.
- An **intention to treat analysis** in which the treatment and control groups are analysed with respect to their random allocation, regardless of what happened subsequently (see below).

It is crucial that RCTs are not only well designed but also well conducted and analysed if the possibility of systematic errors is to be excluded. It is also essential that they are reported in sufficient detail to enable readers to be able to assess the quality of their conduct and the validity of their results. Unfortunately, essential details are often lacking. Over the last decade concerted attempts to improve the quality of reporting of randomized controlled trials resulted in the 1996 **CONSORT statement** (Begg *et al.*, 1996), with a revised version in 2001 (Moher *et al.*, 2001). CONSORT stands for **CON**solidated **S**tandards **O**f **R**eporting Trials. The statement consists of a prototype flow diagram for summarizing the different phases of the trial, with the numbers involved in each (Figure 34.1), and a checklist of items that it is essential for investigators to report (Table 34.1). Details of its rationale and background together with a full description of each component can be found on the website http://www.consort-statement.org/.

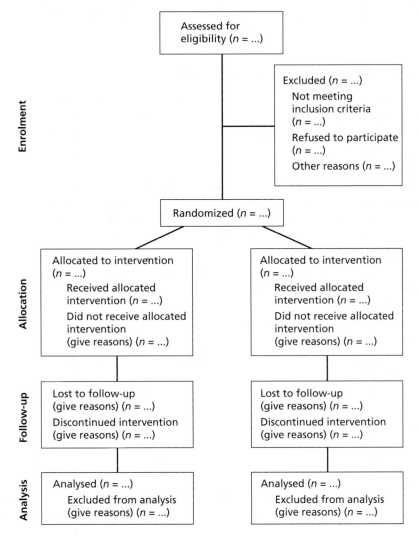

Fig. 34.1 Revised template of the CONSORT diagram showing the flow of participants through each stage of a randomized trial, reprinted with permission of the CONSORT group.

Analysis plan

In this section we will focus in particular on the features of the CONSORT statement pertinent to the **analysis plan**, key stages of which are outlined in

Table 34.1 The revised CONSORT statement for reporting randomized trials: checklist of items to include when reporting a randomized trial, reprinted with permission of the CONSORT group.

Paper section and topic	Item no.	Descriptor
TITLE AND ABSTRACT	1	How participants were allocated to interventions (e.g. 'random allocation', 'randomized', or 'randomly assigned')
INTRODUCTION		
Background	2	Scientific background and explanation of rationale
METHODS		
Participants	3	Eligibility criteria for participants and the settings and locations where the data were collected
Interventions	4	Precise details of the interventions intended for each group and how and when they were actually administered
Objectives	5	Specific objectives and hypotheses
Outcomes	6	Clearly defined primary and secondary outcome measures and, when applicable, any methods used to enhance the quality of measurements (e.g. multiple observations, training of assessors, etc.)
Sample size	7	How sample size was determined and, when applicable, explanation of any interim analyses and stopping rules
Randomization:		
Sequence generation	8	Method used to generate the random allocation sequence, including details of any restriction (e.g. blocking, stratification)
Allocation concealment	9	Method used to implement the random allocation sequence (e.g. numbered containers or central telephone), clarifying whether the sequence was concealed until interventions were assigned
Implementation	10	Who generated the allocation sequence, who enrolled participants, and who assigned participants to their groups
Blinding (masking)	11	Whether or not participants, those administering the interventions, and those assessing the outcomes were blinded to group assignment. When relevant, how the success of blinding was evaluated
Statistical methods	12	Statistical methods used to compare groups for primary outcome(s); methods for additional analyses, such as subgroup analyses and adjusted analyses
RESULTS		
Participant flow	13	Flow of participants through each stage (a diagram is strongly recommended). Specifically, for each group report the numbers of participants randomly assigned, receiving intended treatment, completing the study protocol, and analysed for the primary outcome. Describe protocol deviations from study as planned, together with reasons
Recruitment	14	Dates defining the periods of recruitment and follow-up
Baseline data	15	Baseline demographic and clinical characteristics of each group
Numbers analysed	16	Number of participants (denominator) in each group included in each analysis and whether the analysis was by 'intention-to-treat'. State the results in absolute numbers when feasible (e.g. 10/20, not 50%)
Outcomes and estimation	17	For each primary and secondary outcome, a summary of results for each group, and the estimated effect size and its precision (e.g. 95% confidence interval)

(*continued*)

Table 34.1 (*continued*)

Paper section and topic	Item no.	Descriptor
Ancillary analyses	18	Address multiplicity by reporting any other analyses performed, including subgroup analyses and adjusted analyses, indicating those pre-specified and those exploratory
Adverse events	19	All important adverse events or side effects in each intervention group
DISCUSSION		
Interpretation	20	Interpretation of the results, taking into account study hypotheses, sources of potential bias or imprecision and the dangers associated with multiplicity of analyses and outcomes
Generalizability	21	Generalizability (external validity) of the trial findings
Overall evidence	22	General interpretation of the results in the context of current evidence

Table 34.2. Although CONSORT has been designed primarily for two-group parallel designs, most of it is also relevant to a wider class of trial designs, such as equivalence, factorial, cluster and crossover trials. Modifications to the CONSORT checklist for reporting trials with these and other designs are in preparation.

Table 34.2 Outline of analysis plan for a randomized controlled trial.

1. Complete flow diagram showing number of participants involved at each phase of the trial
2. Summarize baseline characteristics of trial population
3. Compare treatment groups with respect to baseline variables – focus on subset of variables thought to be associated with main outcome(s). Avoid formal tests of the null hypothesis of no between-group differences, since the null hypothesis *must* be true if the randomization was done properly
4. Conduct *simple* analysis of main outcome(s) by *intention to treat*
   (a) Present the estimated effect of treatment together with a CI and test of the null hypothesis of no treatment effect
   (b) Consider *sensitivity analyses* examining the possible effect of losses to follow-up, if these might affect the treatment effect estimate
5. Repeat analysis including adjustment for baseline variables if appropriate
6. Carry out any subgroup analyses if there is an *a priori* justification
7. Analyse side effects and adverse outcomes
8. Analyse secondary outcomes

Participant flow

An important first stage of the analysis is to work out the flow of the number of participants through the four main phases of the trial: enrolment, allocation to intervention groups, follow-up and analysis, as shown in Figure 34.1. In particular, it is important to note the number excluded at any stage and the *reasons* for their exclusion. This information is crucial for the following reasons:

- Substantial proportions lost at any stage have important implications for the **external validity** of the study, since the resulting participants may no longer be representative of those eligible for the intervention.

- Any imbalance in losses between treatment groups has implications for the **internal validity** of the study, since they may lead to non-random differences between the treatment groups which could influence the outcome.
- Knowing the difference between the number allocated to receive an intervention, and number who actually received it (and/or adequately adhered to it), is important for the interpretation of the estimated effect, as explained below under 'intention to treat analysis'.

Analysis of baseline variables

'Baseline' information collected at enrolment is used in the analysis of a trial in the following ways:

1 To describe the characteristics of the trial participants, which is essential for assessing the generalizibility of the results.
2 To demonstrate that the randomization procedure has successfully led to comparability between trial groups.
3 To adjust treatment effects for variables strongly related to the outcome (see below).
4 To carry out subgroup analysis (see below).

In their review, 'Subgroup analysis and other (mis)uses of baseline data in clinical trials', Assmann *et al.* (2001) found that the first two objectives are often confused, and that the approach to the second is often methodologically flawed. They recommend that:

- A general and detailed description is given of the trial participants, but that the analysis of comparability between groups should be restricted to a few variables known to be strong predictors of the primary outcome(s).
- Significance tests for baseline differences are inappropriate, since any differences are either due to chance or to flawed randomization. In addition, a non-significant imbalance of a strong predictor will have more effect on the results than a significant imbalance on a factor unrelated to the outcome.

Intention to treat analysis

In an '**intention to treat**' analysis, participants are analysed according to their original group assignment, whether or not this is the intervention they actually received, and whether or not they accepted and/or adhered to the intervention. Alternatively, analysis can be based on actual intervention received, with criteria for exclusion if inadequate adherence to the intervention was achieved. This is sometimes known as a '**per protocol**' analysis. The primary analysis of a RCT should always be an intention to treat analysis, since it avoids the possibility of any bias associated with loss, mis-allocation or non-adherence of participants. For example, consider a placebo-controlled trial of a new drug with unpleasant side-effects. If the sickest patients are unable to take the new drug, they may withdraw from the assigned treatment. Such problems will not affect the placebo group, and therefore a per-protocol analysis would give a biased result by comparing the less sick patients in the drug group with all patients in the placebo group.

If there is a substantial difference between those allocated to receive an intervention and those who actually receive it (and adequately adhere to it), then we recommend that in addition analyses are carried out adjusting for actual treatment received, and that the results are compared with the intention to treat analysis. A valid method to correct for non-adherence to treatment in randomized trials was developed by Robins and Tsiatis (1991), but has not been widely used in practice, partly because it is conceptually difficult. However, software implementing the method is now available (White *et al.* 2002). It is important to report the numbers involved, and the reasons for the losses in order to assess to what extent the intention to treat analysis may lead to an underestimate of the efficacy of the intervention under ideal circumstances, and to what extent the per protocol analysis may be biased.

Adjustment for baseline variables

The analysis of the main outcome(s) should always start with simple unadjusted comparisons between treatment groups. For most randomized controlled trials, this is all that should be done. We recommend adjustment for covariates measured at baseline *only* in the following circumstances:

- Where there is clear a priori evidence about which baseline factors are likely to be strongly related to the outcome. Even where strong predictors exist, adjustment for them in the analysis is only necessary if the outcome is numerical.
- In particular, where the outcome is numerical and where a baseline measurement of it has been taken. An example would be a trial of an anti-hypertensive drug, where blood pressure is measured at baseline and following treatment. In this case the baseline measurement is likely to be strongly correlated with the outcome, and including it as a covariate in the analysis improves the precision of the treatment effect (see Section 29.8). Note that this is a better approach than taking differences from the baseline as the outcome variable, since the latter tends to overcorrect (see Snedecor & Cochran, 1989).
- Where the trial is sufficiently small that an imbalance sufficiently large to bias the treatment effect is possible. (Such a situation may occur in *cluster-randomized* trials; see below.)

Note that:

- The decision concerning covariates should *not* be made on the basis of statistically significant differences between the treatment groups at baseline, although this is often the practice (see above discussion on analysis of baseline variables).
- It is not necessary to adjust for centre in multi-centre studies, unless it is a strong predictor of outcome and the proportion of patients in the treatment group differs between centres.

Subgroup analyses

In their review, Assmann *et al.* (2001) found that the use of subgroup analyses is widespread in clinical trials, and often flawed. The choice of subgroups used is often not justified, their analysis is often inadequate and their results are given undue emphasis. They note that of all the problems that have been identified in the conduct, analysis and reporting of clinical trials, subgroup analysis remains the most over-used and over-interpreted.

- Subgroup analyses should only be conducted if there is a clear *a priori* reason to expect the treatment effect to differ between different groups of patients, such as between males and females, or between different age groups. Only a few predefined subgroups should be considered and analysis restricted to the main outcomes.
- They should include formal tests for interaction, as described in Section 29.5, and should not be based on inspection of subgroup *P*-values. A particularly common error is to assume that a small *P*-value in one subgroup, but not in another, provides evidence that the treatment effect differs between the sub-groups. If the subgroups are of different sizes then this situation may arise even if the subgroup treatment effects are identical!
- In addition, in multi-centre trials it may be useful to present the results by centre as well as overall, as a means of data quality and consistency checking between centres. The results of such analyses may be presented in a forest plot (see Chapter 32). However, this should not lead to undue emphasis being placed on any apparent differences seen, unless these are supported by strong evidence supporting their plausibility.

Crossover trials

Crossover trials are trials in which both treatments (or the active treatment and the placebo control) are given to each patient, with the order of allocation decided at random for each patient. They are suitable in situations such as trials of analgesics for pain relief or therapies for asthma, where outcomes can be measured at the end of successive time periods, and where there is unlikely to be a carry-over effect of the first treatment into the period when the second treatment is being given. To address this issue, such trials may incorporate a 'washout' period between the periods when treatments under investigation are administered.

The main advantage of crossover trials is that by accounting for between-patient variability in the outcome they may be more efficient than a corresponding trial in which treatments are randomly allocated to different individuals (**parallel group trial**). The analysis of such trials should take account of the design by using methods for paired data. For numerical outcomes, the *mean difference* between each patient's outcomes on the first and second treatment should be analysed (see Section 7.6), and the standard deviation of the mean differences should always be reported, to facilitate meta-analyses of such trials, or of trials using both crossover and parallel group designs. For binary outcomes, methods for matched pairs should be used (see Chapter 21).

Cluster randomized trials

The development, and the major use, of RCTs is in the evaluation of treatments or medical interventions (such as vaccines) applied at the individual level. In recent years, however, the use of RCTs has extended to the evaluation of health service and public health interventions. This has led to the development of **cluster randomized trials**, in which randomization is applied to clusters of people rather than individuals, either because of the nature of the intervention, or for logistical reasons. Some examples are:

- Evaluation of screening of hypertension among the elderly in the UK in which the unit of randomization was the GP practice.
- Evaluation of the impact on HIV transmission in Tanzania of syndromic management of sexually transmitted diseases, where the unit of randomization was STD clinics and their catchment populations.
- Evaluation in Glasgow of the impact on adolescent sexual behaviour of a sex education programme delivered through school, in which the schools were the unit of randomization.
- Evaluation in Ghana of the impact of weekly vitamin A supplementation on maternal mortality, where the unit of randomization is a cluster of about 120 women, the number that a fieldworker can visit in a week.

Three essential points to note are that:

1 Any clustering in the design must be taken into account in the analysis, as described in Chapter 31.

2 Because the number of clusters is often relatively small, a cluster randomized design may not exclude the possibility of imbalance in baseline characteristics between the treatment and control groups and careful consideration should be given to measurement of known prognostic factors at baseline and whether it is necessary to adjust for their effects in the analysis.

3 A cluster randomized trial needs to include more individuals than the corresponding individually randomized trial. Sample size calculations for cluster randomized trials are described in Chapter 35.

Choosing the statistical method to use

Table 34.3 provides a guide to selecting the appropriate statistical method to use. It shows how this depends on:

- the type of outcome;
- whether adjustment for baseline variables is needed;
- whether subgroup analyses are being conducted;
- and, in the case of survival outcomes, whether the proportional hazards assumption is satisfied.

Table 34.3 Analysis of clinical trials/intervention studies: summary of methods.

	Type of outcome			
	Numerical	Binary	Rate	Survival time
Data displays	Mean outcome in each group, with standard error	2×2 table, or $k \times 2$ table for a trial with k treatment groups	Number of events, person-years and rate (with confidence interval) in each group	Number of events and person-years in each group Kaplan–Meier survival curves
Measure of the effect of treatment	Difference between means t-test	Risk difference/risk ratio/odds ratio (OR): z-test/χ^2 test Number needed to treat (see Chapter 37)	Rate ratio z-test	Mantel–Cox hazard ratio Log rank test
Adjustment for baseline variables	Multiple linear regression	Mantel–Haenszel methods Logistic regression	Mantel–Haenszel methods Poisson regression	Cox regression
Analysing for different treatment effects in different subgroups	Include interaction terms in regression model			Also check for non proportional hazards (i.e. whether effect of treatment changes with time)
Special cases	Cluster randomized trial or other clustering of outcome data (see Chapter 31 for methods) Crossover trials (use methods for *matched* data)			

In addition, it highlights two special cases that need to be considered:

- whether the data are **clustered**, either in group allocation (cluster randomized trials), or in outcome measurement (repeated measures in longitudinal studies/multiple measures per subject), and
- **crossover** trials, where for each patient, treatment and control outcomes are matched.

Details of the methods can be found in the relevant sections of Parts B–E.

34.3 OTHER DESIGNS TO EVALUATE INTERVENTIONS

As discussed in Section 32.8, while the large-scale, randomized, controlled trial is the 'gold standard' for the evaluation of interventions, practical (and ethical) considerations may preclude its use. In this section, we summarize the alternative evaluation designs available, and the analysis choices involved (*see* Kirkwood *et al.*, 1997). Essentially, we have one or more of three basic comparisons at our disposal in order to evaluate the impact of interventions. These are:

1 The **pre-post comparison** involves comparing rates of the outcome of interest in several communities before the intervention is introduced (pre-intervention), with rates in the same communities after they have received the intervention (post-intervention). Such a comparison clearly requires the collection of baseline data. The plausibility of any statement attributing an impact to the intervention will be strengthened if it is demonstrated that both the prevalence of the risk factor under intervention and the rate of adverse outcome have diminished following the intervention. However, pre-post comparisons alone, without adequate concurrent controls, rarely provide compelling evidence that an intervention has successfully impacted on health, since changes in both the prevalence of risk factors and outcome are frequently observed to occur over time in the absence of any intervention. It is therefore difficult to conclude that an observed change is due to the intervention and not due to an independent secular trend. An exception to this occurs when assessing mediating factors in programmes which seek to introduce into a community a new treatment or promote a product or behaviour that did not previously exist. It will, however, still be difficult to attribute any change in health status to the programme since the improvement may still be part of a secular trend, rather than a direct consequence of the intervention.

2 The **intervention–control comparison** following the introduction of the intervention is of course at the heart of a randomized controlled trial, but this comparison may be applied in a wider context. Thus the intervention versus control comparison may be randomized or non-randomized, matched or unmatched, double-blind or open. When the comparison is double-blind and randomized, with a large number of units, as is the case with an ideally designed randomized controlled trial, the plausibility of attributing any difference in outcome observed to the intervention is high. In the absence of double-blindness or

randomization on a reasonably large scale, inference concerning the impact of the intervention becomes more problematic and it becomes essential to control for potential confounding factors.

3 **Adopters versus non-adopters comparison**: this is carried out at the individual level even if the intervention is delivered at the community level. Individuals who adopt the intervention are compared with those who do not adopt the intervention. Such a comparison is essentially a 'risk factor' study rather than an 'impact' study in that it measures the benefit to an individual of adopting the intervention rather than the public health impact of the intervention in the setting in which it was implemented. This would be the case, for example, in comparing STD incidence rates among condom users versus non-condom users following an advertising campaign. Great care needs to be taken to control potential confounding factors, since adopters and non-adopters of the intervention may differ in many important respects, including their exposure to infection. The magnitude of this problem may be assessed by a comparison of the non-adopters in the intervention area(s) with persons in control areas.

Each of these three comparisons has its merits. In the absence of a randomized controlled design, we recommend that an evaluation study include as many as possible, since they give complementary information. From Table 34.4 it can be seen that both a longitudinal design and a cross-sectional design with repeated surveys in principle allow measurement of all three of the basic types of comparison. A single cross-sectional survey can make intervention–control comparisons and adopter versus non-adopter comparisons but not pre-intervention post-intervention comparisons. The longitudinal approach can more accurately establish outcome and exposure status and the time sequence between them, but is considerably more expensive and logistically complex than the cross-sectional approach. Randomized controlled trials usually measure outcomes using a longitudinal or repeated cross-sectional design in order to maximize follow-up. However, they are not restricted to do so and, where appropriate, outcome can be measured using a single cross-sectional survey. For example, in a cluster randomized trial of the impact of a hygiene behaviour intervention, both hygiene practices and prevalence of diarrhoea could be ascertained through a single cross-sectional survey carried

Table 34.4 Matrix showing the relationship between the 'classical' study designs and the three comparisons of interest in evaluating an intervention.

Data collection	Comparisons		
	Pre-post	Intervention–control	Adopters *vs* non-adopters
Longitudinal	Yes	Yes	Yes
Cross-sectional (repeated)	Yes	Yes	Yes
Cross-sectional (single round)	No	Yes	Yes
Case-control	No	No	Yes

out, say, six months after the introduction of the intervention. A case–control evaluation can only yield an adopter versus non-adopter comparison.

The choice of analysis methods for longitudinal and cross-sectional observational studies and for case control studies are summarized in the next two sections.

34.4 LONGITUDINAL AND CROSS-SECTIONAL STUDIES

We now turn to the analysis of observational studies to investigate the association of an exposure with an outcome. In this section we cover methods relevant to cross-sectional surveys and longitudinal studies, and in the next section those relevant to case–control studies.

A **cross-sectional** study is carried out at just one point in time or over a short period of time. Since cross-sectional studies provide estimates of the features of a community at just one point in time, they are suitable for measuring prevalence but not incidence of disease (see Chapter 15 for the definition of prevalence and Chapter 22 for the definition of incidence), and associations found may be difficult to interpret. For example, a survey on onchocerciasis showed that blind persons were of lower nutritional status than non-blind. There are two possible explanations for this association. The first is that those of poor nutritional status have lower resistance and are therefore more likely to become blind from onchocerciasis. The second is that poor nutritional status is a consequence rather than a cause of the blindness, since blind persons are not as able to provide for themselves. Longitudinal data are necessary to decide which is the better explanation.

As described in Chapter 22, in a **longitudinal** study individuals are followed over time, which makes it possible to measure the incidence of disease and easier to study the natural history of disease. In some situations it is possible to obtain follow-up data on births, deaths, and episodes of disease by **continuous monitoring**, for example by monitoring registry records in populations where registration of deaths is complete. Occasionally the acquisition of data may be **retrospective**, being carried out from past records. More commonly it is **prospective** and, for this reason, longitudinal studies have often been alternatively termed **prospective studies**.

Many longitudinal studies are carried out by conducting **repeated cross-sectional surveys** at fixed intervals to enquire about, or measure, changes that have taken place between surveys, such as births, deaths, migrations, changes in weight or antibody levels, or the occurrence of new episodes of disease. The interval chosen will depend on the factors being studied. For example, to measure the incidence of diarrhoea, which is characterized by repeated short episodes, data may need to be collected weekly to ensure reliable recall. To monitor child growth, on the other hand, would require only monthly or 3-monthly measurements.

Choosing the statistical method to use

Table 34.5 provides a guide to the statistical methods available for the analysis of cross-sectional and longitudinal studies and Table 34.6 summarizes the possible

Table 34.5 Analysis of observational studies: summary of methods.

Type of exposure	Type of outcome			
	Numerical	Binary	Rate	Survival time
Binary	Difference between means t-test	Risk ratio/odds ratio (OR) χ^2 test	Rate ratio z-test	Mantel–Cox hazard ratio Log rank test
Categorical	Group means Analysis of variance Multiple linear regression	ORs against baseline Logistic regression	Rate ratios against baseline Poisson regression	Hazard ratios against baseline Cox regression
Ordered categorical (dose–response effect)	Increase in mean/group Linear regression	Increase in log odds/group Logistic regression/χ^2 test for trend	Increase in log rate/group Poisson regression	Increase in log hazard/group Cox regression
Numerical	Regression coefficient (increase in mean/unit) Linear regression	Regression coefficient (log odds ratio/unit) Logistic regression	Regression coefficient (log rate ratio/unit) Poisson regression	Regression coefficient (log hazard ratio/unit) Cox regression
Adjustment for confounders	Multiple linear regression	Mantel–Haenszel methods Logistic regression	Mantel–Haenszel methods Poisson regression	Cox regression
Special cases	Clustered data (see Chapter 31 for methods) (Repeated measures in longitudinal studies/Multiple measures per subject/ Family studies/Cluster sampling)			Non-proportional hazards

Table 34.6 Observational studies: guide to the appropriateness of types of outcome, for each study design.

	Type of outcome			
Study design	Numerical	Binary	Rate	Survival time
Longitudinal (complete follow-up)	Yes	Yes	Yes	Yes
Longitudinal (incomplete follow-up)	Yes*	Yes*	Yes	Yes
Longitudinal (repeated cross-sectional surveys)	Yes**	Yes**	Yes	Yes
Cross-sectional	Yes	Yes	No	No
Case–control	No	Yes	No	No

* Methods beyond the scope of this book
** Analyse taking into account repeated measures of outcome, using methods for clustered data (see Chapter 31).

types of outcome according to the study design. The choice of which method to use is determined by:

- the sampling scheme used to recruit participants into the study;
- whether measures are made at a single point in time, continuously over time, or at repeated points in time;
- the types of the outcome and exposure variables.

The bottom line of the guide highlights two special cases that need to be considered:

- whether the data are clustered, either because of the sampling scheme (cluster sampling or family studies), or in outcome measurement (repeated measures in longitudinal studies/multiple measures per subject); and
- in the case of survival outcomes, whether the proportional hazards assumption is satisfied.

Details of the methods can be found in the relevant sections of Parts B–E.

Types of sampling scheme and their implications

Occasionally a study includes the whole population of a confined area or institution(s), but more often only a **sample** is investigated. Whenever possible any selection should be made at random. Possible schemes include:

1 **Simple random sampling:** the required number of individuals are selected at random from the **sampling frame**, a list or a database of all individuals in the population.

2 **Systematic sampling:** for convenience, selection from the sampling frame is sometimes carried out systematically rather than randomly, by taking individuals at regular intervals down the list, the starting point being chosen at random. For example, to select a 5%, or 1 in 20, sample of the population the starting point is chosen randomly from numbers 1 to 20, and then every 20th person on the list is taken. Suppose 13 is the random number selected, then the sample would comprise individuals 13, 33, 53, 73, 93, etc.

3 **Stratified sampling:** a simple random sample is taken from a number of distinct subgroups, or **strata**, of the population in order to ensure that they are all adequately represented. If different sampling fractions are used in the different strata, simple summary statistics will not be representative of the whole population. Appropriate methods for the analysis of such studies use weights that are inversely proportional to the probability that each individual was sampled, and robust standard errors (see Chapter 30) to correct standard errors.

4 **Multi-stage or cluster sampling:** this is carried out in stages using the hierarchical structure of a population. For example, a **two-stage sample** might consist of first taking a random sample of schools and then taking a random sample of children from each selected school. The **clustering** of data must be taken into account in the analysis.

5 **Sampling on the basis of time:** for example, the 1970 British Cohort Study (BCS70) is an ongoing follow-up study of all individuals born between 5th and 11th April, 1970 and still living in Britain.

34.5 CASE–CONTROL STUDIES

In a case–control study the sampling is carried out according to *disease* rather than *exposure* status. A group of individuals identified as having the disease, the **cases**, is compared with a group of individuals not having the disease, the **controls**, with respect to their prior exposure to the factor of interest. The overriding principle is that *the controls should represent the population at risk of the disease*. More specifically, they should be individuals who, if they had experienced the disease outcome, would have been included as cases in our study. The outcome is the case–control status, and is therefore by definition a binary variable. The methods to use are therefore those outlined in Part C. These are summarized in Table 34.7. The main feature that influences the methods for analysis is whether controls were selected at random or using a matched design.

Analysis of unmatched case–control studies

For **unmatched case–control studies**, standard methods for the analysis of binary outcomes using odds ratios as the measure of association are used. Analysis of the effect of a binary exposure starts with simple 2×2 tables, and proceeds to the use of Mantel–Haenszel methods and logistic regression to control for the effect of confounding variables. These methods were described in detail in Chapters 16 to 20.

Analysis of matched case–control studies

In a **matched case–control study**, each case is matched with one or more controls, who are deliberately chosen to have the same values as the case for any potential confounding variables. There are two main reasons for matching in case–control studies:

Table 34.7 Analysis of case–control studies: summary of methods.

Sampling scheme for controls	Single exposure	Adjustment for confounding variables
Random (unmatched case–control study)	2×2 table showing exposure $\times$ case/control OR $=$ cross-product ratio Standard χ^2 test	Logistic regression or Mantel–Haenszel methods
Stratum matching (frequency matched case–control study)	Stratified analysis: 2×2 table for each stratum Mantel–Haenszel OR and χ^2 test	Logistic regression or stratified analysis, controlling for *both* the matching factor(s) and the confounding variables
Individual matching (one control per case)	2×2 table showing agreement between case–control pairs with respect to risk factor OR $=$ ratio of discordant pairs McNemar's χ^2 test	Conditional logistic regression
Individual matching (multiple controls per case)	Mantel–Haenszel OR and χ^2 test, stratifying on matched sets	Conditional logistic regression

1 Matching is often used to ensure that the cases and controls are similar with respect to one or more confounding variables. For example, in a study of pancreatic cancer occurring in subjects aged between 30 and 80 years it is likely that the cases will come from the older extreme of the age range. Controls might then be selected because they are of similar age to a case. This would ensure that the age distribution of the controls is similar to that of the cases, and may increase the efficiency of the study, for example by decreasing the width of confidence intervals compared to an unmatched study. Note that unless the matching factor is strongly associated with both the outcome *and* the exposure the increase in efficiency may not be large, and therefore may not justify the increased logistical difficulties and extra analytic complexity.

2 In some case–control studies it is difficult to define the population that gave rise to the cases. For example, a large hospital specializing in the treatment of cardiovascular disease may attract cases not just from the surrounding area but also referrals from further afield. In developing countries, there may be no register of the population in a given area, or who attend a particular health facility. An alternative way of selecting controls representative of the population that gave rise to the cases is to select them from the neighbourhood of each case. For example, controls might be selected from among subjects living in the third-closest house to that of each case.

It is essential to note that *if matching was used in the design, then the analysis must always take this into account*, as described in Chapter 21. In summary:

1 In the simple case of individually matched case–control studies with one control per case and no confounders, the methods for paired data described in Sections 21.3 and 21.4 can be used.

2 When there are several controls per case, Mantel–Haenszel methods may be used to estimate exposure odds ratios by stratifying on the case–control sets. However, they are severely limited because they do not allow for further control of the effects of confounding variables that were not also matching variables. This is because each stratum is a single case and its matched controls, so that further stratification is not possible. For example, if cases were individually matched with neighbourhood controls then it would not be possible to stratify additionally on age group. Stratification can be used to control for additional confounders only by restricting attention to those case–control sets that are homogeneous with respect to the confounders of interest.

3 The main approach is to use **conditional logistic regression** (see Section 21.5), which is a variant of logistic regression in which cases are only compared to controls in the same matched set. This allows analysis adjusting for several confounders at the same time. There is also no restriction on the numbers of cases and controls in each matched set.

4 However, if cases and controls are only **frequency matched** (e.g. if we simply ensure that the age distribution is roughly the same in the cases and controls), then the matching can be broken in the analysis, and standard logistic regression used, *providing the matching variable(s) are included in the model.* Mantel–Haenszel methods are also valid, with the analysis stratified on all matching variables.

Interpretation of the odds ratio estimated in a case–control study

For a *rare* disease, we saw in Chapters 16 and 23 that the odds ratio, risk ratio and rate ratio are numerically equal. For a *common* disease the meaning of the odds ratio estimated in a case–control study depends on the sampling scheme used to select the controls, as described by Rodrigues and Kirkwood (1990). Briefly, there are three possibilities:

1 The most usual choice is to select controls from those still disease-free at the end of the study (the denominator group in the odds measure of incidence); any controls selected during the course of the study who subsequently develop disease are treated as cases and not as controls. In this case the odds ratio estimated in the case–control study estimates the odds ratio in the population.

2 An alternative, in a case–control study conducted in a defined population, is to select controls from the disease-free population at each time at which a case occurs (**concurrent controls**). In this case the odds ratio estimated in the case–control study estimates the rate ratio in the population.

3 More rarely, the controls can be randomly selected from the initially disease-free population (if this can be defined). In this case the odds ratio estimated in the case–control study estimates the risk ratio in the population.

CHAPTER 35

Calculation of required sample size

35.1 INTRODUCTION

An essential part of planning any investigation is to decide how many people need to be studied. A formal **sample size calculation**, justifying the proposed study size and demonstrating that the study is capable of answering the questions posed, is now a component of a research proposal required by most funding agencies. Too often, medical research studies have been too small, because the sample size was decided on purely logistic grounds, or by guesswork. This is not only bad practice: it is considered by many to be unethical because of the waste of time and potential risk to patients participating in a study that cannot answer its stated research question. On the other hand, studying many more persons than necessary is also a waste of time and resources. In a clinical trial, conducting a study that is too large may also be unethical, because this could mean that more persons than necessary were given the placebo, and that the introduction of a beneficial therapy was delayed. In this chapter we will:

1 Illustrate the principles involved in sample size calculations by considering a simple example in detail.
2 Present the different formulae required for the most common sample size calculations and illustrate their application.
3 Discuss the implications of loss to follow-up, control of confounding and examination of subgroup effects.
4 Describe the principles of sample size calculation for clustered designs.
5 Define the two types of error that can occur in significance tests.
6 Illustrate the implications of study power for the interpretation of statistical significance.

35.2 PRINCIPLES OF SAMPLE SIZE CALCULATIONS

Calculating the required sample size requires that we *quantify the objectives of our study*. For example, it would not be sufficient to state simply that the objective is to demonstrate whether or not formula-fed infants are at greater risk of death than breast-fed ones. We would also need to state:

1 The *size* of the increased risk that it was desired to demonstrate since, for example, a smaller study would be needed to detect a fourfold relative risk than to detect a twofold one.

2 The *significance level (or P-value)*, that is the strength of the evidence, that we require in order to reject the null hypothesis of no difference in risk between formula- and breast-fed infants. The greater the strength of evidence required, that is the smaller the *P*-value, the larger will be the sample size needed.

3 The probability that we would like to have of achieving this level of significance. This is required since, because of sampling variation (see Section 4.5), we cannot rule out the possibility that the size of the effect observed in the study will be much smaller than the '*true*' effect. This means that we can never guarantee that a study will be able to detect an effect however large we make it, but we can increase the probability that we do so by increasing the sample size. This probability is called the **power** of the study.

For example, we might decide that a study comparing the risk of death among formula-fed and breast-fed infants would be worthwhile if there was a 90% probability of demonstrating a difference, at 1% significance, if the true risk ratio was as high as 2. We would then calculate the number of children required. Alternatively, if we knew that a maximum of 500 children were available in our study, we might calculate the power of the study given that we wanted to detect a true risk ratio of 3 at 5% significance.

The principles involved in sample size calculations will now be illustrated by considering a simple example in detail.

Example 35.1

Consider a hypothetical clinical trial to compare two analgesics, a new drug (A) and the current standard drug (B), in which migraine sufferers will be given drug A on one occasion and drug B on another, the order in which the drugs are given being chosen at random for each patient. For illustrative purposes, we will consider a simplified analysis based on the drug stated by each patient to have provided greatest pain relief. How many patients would we need in order to be able to conclude that drug A is superior?

First, we must be specific about what we mean by superiority. We will state this as an overall preference rate of 70% or more for drug A, and we will decide that we would like a 90% power of achieving a significant result at the 5% level.

Under the null hypothesis of no difference between the efficacies of the two drugs, the proportion of patients stating a preference for drug A will be 0.5 (50%). We can test the evidence that the observed preference proportion, p, differs from 0.5 using a z-test, as described in Section 15.6:

$$z = \frac{p - 0.5}{\text{s.e.}(p)} = \frac{p - 0.5}{\sqrt{(0.5 \times (1 - 0.5)/n)}} = \frac{p - 0.5}{\sqrt{(0.25/n)}}$$

This result will be significant at the 5% level ($P < 0.05$) if $z \geq 1.96$, or in other words if p is 1.96 standard errors or more away from the null hypothesis value of 0.5.

We will illustrate the principles behind sample size calculations by considering different possible sample sizes and assessing their adequacy as regards the power of our study.

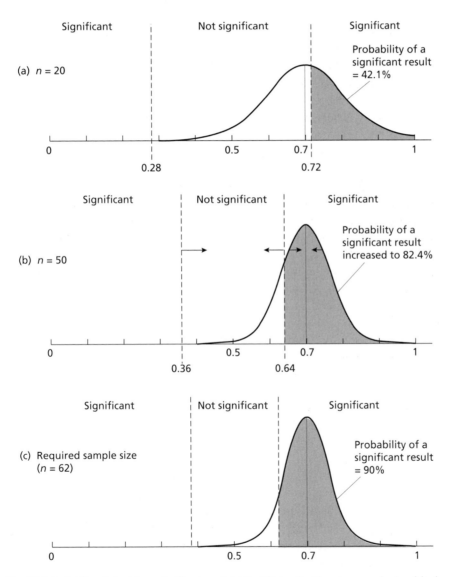

Fig. 35.1 Probability of obtaining a significant result (at the 5 % level) with various sample sizes (n) when testing the proportion of preferences for drug A rather than drug B against the null hypothesis value of 0.5, if the true value is 0.7.

(a) We will start with a sample size of $n = 20$, as depicted in Figure 35.1(a). Here:

$$\text{s.e.} = \sqrt{(0.25/20)} = 0.1118$$
$$0.5 + 1.96 \times \text{s.e.} = 0.5 + 1.96 \times 0.1118 = 0.72$$
and $\quad 0.5 - 1.96 \times \text{s.e.} = 0.5 - 1.96 \times 0.1118 = 0.28$

Thus observed proportions of 0.72 and above, or 0.28 and below, would lead to a result that is significant at the 5% level.

If the *true* proportion is 0.7, what is the likelihood of observing 0.72 or above, and thus getting a result that is significant at the 5% level? This is illustrated by the shaded area in Figure 35.1(a). The curve represents the sampling distribution, which is a normal distribution centred on 0.7 with a standard error of $\sqrt{(0.7 \times 0.3/20)} = 0.1025$. The z-value corresponding to 0.72 is:

$$\frac{0.72 - 0.7}{0.1025} = 0.20$$

The proportion of the standard normal distribution above 0.20 is found from Table A1 (in the Appendix) to equal 0.421, or 42.1%. In summary, this means that with a sample size of 20 we have only a 42.1% chance of demonstrating that drug A is better, if the true preference rate is 0.7.

(b) Consider next what happens if we increase the sample size to 50, as shown in Figure 35.1(b). The ranges of values that would now be significant have widened to 0.64 and above, or 0.36 and below. The sampling distribution has narrowed, and there is a greater overlap with the significant ranges. Consequently, the probability of a significant result has increased. It is now found to be 82.4%, but this is still less than our required 90%.

(c) Thus we certainly need to study more than 50 patients in order to have 90% power. But exactly how many do we need? We need to increase the sample size, n, to the point where the overlap between the sampling distribution and the significant ranges reaches 90%, as shown in Figure 35.1(c). We will now describe how to calculate directly the sample size needed to do this. A significant result will be achieved if we observe a value above

$$0.5 + 1.96 \times \text{s.e.} = 0.5 + 1.96 \times \sqrt{(0.5 \times 0.5/n)}$$

(or below $0.5 - 1.96 \times \text{s.e.}$). We want to select a large enough n so that 90% of the sampling distribution is above this point. The z-value of the sampling distribution corresponding to 90% is -1.28 (see Table A2), which means an observed value of

$$0.7 - 1.28 \times \text{s.e.} = 0.7 - 1.28 \times \sqrt{(0.7 \times 0.3/n)}$$

Therefore, n should be chosen large enough so that

$$0.7 - 1.28 \times \sqrt{(0.7 \times 0.3/n)} > 0.5 + 1.96 \times \sqrt{(0.5 \times 0.5/n)}$$

Rearranging this gives

$$0.7 - 0.5 > \frac{1.96 \times \sqrt{(0.5 \times 0.5)} + 1.28 \times \sqrt{(0.7 \times 0.3)}}{\sqrt{n}}$$

Squaring both sides, and further rearrangement gives

$$n > \frac{[1.96 \times \sqrt{(0.5 \times 0.5)} + 1.28 \times \sqrt{(0.7 \times 0.3)}]^2}{0.2^2}$$

$$= \frac{1.5666^2}{0.2^2} = 61.4$$

We therefore require at least 62 patients to satisfy our requirements of having a 90% power of demonstrating a difference between drugs A and B that is significant at the 5% level, if the true preference rate for drug A is as high as 0.7.

35.3 FORMULAE FOR SAMPLE SIZE CALCULATIONS

The above discussion related to sample size determination for a test that a single proportion (the proportion of participants preferring drug A to drug B) differs from a specified null value. In practice it is not necessary to go through such detailed reasoning every time. Instead the sample size can be calculated directly from a general formula, which in this case is:

$$n > \frac{[u\sqrt{\pi(1 - \pi)} + v\sqrt{\pi_{null}(1 - \pi_{null})}]^2}{(\pi - \pi_{null})^2}$$

where:

$n =$ required minimum sample size

$\pi =$ proportion of interest

$\pi_{null} =$ null hypothesis proportion

$u =$ one-sided percentage point of the normal distribution corresponding to 100% − the power, e.g. if power $= 90\%$, $(100\% - \text{power}) = 10\%$ and $u = 1.28$

$v =$ percentage of the normal distribution corresponding to the required (two-sided) significance level, e.g. if significance level $= 5\%$, $v = 1.96$.

For example, in applying this formula to the above example we have:

$$\pi = 0.7, \ \pi_{null} = 0.5, \ u = 1.28 \text{ and } v = 1.96$$

giving

$$n > \frac{[1.28 \times \sqrt{(0.7 \times 0.3)} + 1.96 \times \sqrt{(0.5 \times 0.5)}]^2}{(0.7 - 0.5)^2} = \frac{1.5666^2}{0.2^2} = 61.4$$

which is exactly the same as obtained above.

The same principles can also be applied in other cases. Detailed reasoning is not given here but the appropriate formulae for use in the most common situations are listed in Table 35.1. The list consists of two parts. Table 35.1(a) covers cases where the aim of the study is to demonstrate a specified difference. Table 35.1(b) covers situations where the aim is to estimate a quantity of interest with a specified precision.

Note that for the cases with two means, proportions, or rates, the formulae give the sample sizes required for *each* of the two groups. The total size of the study is therefore *twice* this.

Table 35.2 gives adjustment factors for **study designs with unequal size groups** (see Example 35.4). Note also that the formulae applying to rates give the required sample size in the same unit as the rates (see Example 35.3).

The use of Table 35.1 will be illustrated by several examples. It is important to realize that sample size calculations are based on our best guesses of a situation. The number arrived at is not magical. It simply gives an idea of the sort of numbers to be studied. In other words, it is useful for distinguishing between 50 and 100, but not between 51 and 52. *It is essential to carry out sample size calculations for several different scenarios, not just one.* This gives a clearer picture of the possible scope of the study and is helpful in weighing up the balance between what is desirable and what is logistically feasible.

Example 35.2

A study is to be carried out in a rural area of East Africa to ascertain whether giving food supplementation during pregnancy increases birth weight. Women attending the antenatal clinic are to be randomly assigned to either receive or not receive supplementation. Formula 4 in Table 35.1 will help us to decide how many women should be enrolled in each group. We need to supply the following information:

1 The size of the difference between mean birth weights that we would like to be able to detect. After much consideration it was decided that an increase of 0.25 kg was an appreciable effect that we would not like to miss. We therefore need to apply the formula with $\mu_1 - \mu_0 = 0.25$ kg.

2 The standard deviations of the distributions of birth weight in each group. It was decided to assume that the standard deviation of birth weight would be the same in the two groups. Past data suggested that it would be about 0.4 kg. In other words we decided to assume that $\sigma_1 = 0.4$ kg and $\sigma_0 = 0.4$ kg.

3 The power required. 95% was agreed on. We therefore need $u = 1.64$.

4 The significance level required. It was decided that if possible we would like to achieve a result significant at the 1% level. We therefore need $v = 2.58$.

Applying formula 4 with these values gives:

$$n > \frac{(1.64 + 2.58)^2 \times (0.4^2 + 0.4^2)}{0.25^2} = \frac{17.8084 \times 0.32}{0.0625} = 91.2$$

Therefore, in order to satisfy our requirements, we would need to enrol about 90 women in each group.

Example 35.3

Before embarking on a major water supply, sanitation, and hygiene intervention in southern Bangladesh, we would first like to know the average number of episodes of diarrhoea per year experienced by under-5-year-olds. We guess that this incidence is probably about 3, but would like to estimate it within ±0.2. This means that if, for example, we observed 2.6 episodes/child/year, we would like to be able to conclude that the true rate was probably between 2.4 and 2.8 episodes/child/year. Expressing this in more statistical terms, we would like our 95% confidence interval to be no wider than ±0.2. As the width of this confidence interval is approximately ±2 s.e.'s, this means that we would like to study enough children to give a standard error as small as 0.1 episodes/child/year. Applying formula 9 in Table 35.1 gives:

$$n > \frac{3}{0.1^2} = 300$$

Note that the formulae applying to rates (numbers 2, 5, 9, 12) give the required sample size in the same unit as the rates. We specified the rates as per child per year. We therefore need to study 300 child-years to yield the desired precision. This could be achieved by observing 300 children for one year each or, for example, by observing four times as many (1200) for 3 months each. It is important not to overlook, however, the possibility of other factors such as seasonal effects when deciding on the time interval for a study involving the measurement of incidence rates.

Example 35.4

A case–control study is planned to investigate whether bottle-fed infants are at increased risk of death from acute respiratory infections compared to breast-fed infants. The mothers of a group of cases (infant deaths, with an underlying respiratory cause named on the death certificate) will be interviewed about the breast-feeding status of the child prior to the illness leading to death. The results will be compared with those obtained from mothers of a group of healthy controls regarding the current breast-feeding status of their infants. It is expected that about 40% of controls ($\pi_0 = 0.4$) will be bottle-fed, and we would like to detect a difference if bottle-feeding was associated with a twofold increase of death (OR = 2).

Table 35.1 Formulae for sample size determination. (a) For studies where the aim is to demonstrate a significant difference. (b) For studies where the aim is to estimate a quantity of interest with a specified precision.

		Information needed	Formula for minimum sample size
(a) Significant result			
1 Single mean	$\mu - \mu_0$	Difference between mean, μ, and null hypothesis value, μ_0	$\dfrac{(u+v)^2\sigma^2}{(\mu-\mu_0)^2}$
	σ	Standard deviation	
	u, v	As below	
2 Single rate*	μ	Rate	$\dfrac{(u+v)^2\mu}{(\mu-\mu_0)^2}$
	μ_0	Null hypothesis value	
	u, v	As below	
3 Single proportion	π	Proportion	$\dfrac{\{u\sqrt{[\pi(1-\pi)]}+v\sqrt{[\pi_0(1-\pi_0)]}\}^2}{(\pi-\pi_0)^2}$
	π_0	Null hypothesis value	
	u, v	As below	
4 Comparison of two means (sample size of each group)	$\mu_1 - \mu_0$	Difference between the means	$\dfrac{(u+v)^2(\sigma_1^2+\sigma_0^2)}{(\mu_1-\mu_0)^2}$
	σ_1, σ_0	Standard deviations	
	u, v	As below	
5 Comparison of two rates* (sample size of each group)	μ_1, μ_0	Rates	$\dfrac{(u+v)^2(\mu_1+\mu_0)}{(\mu_1-\mu_0)^2}$
	u, v	As below	
6 Comparison of two proportions (sample size of each group)	π_1, π_0	Proportions	$\dfrac{\{u\sqrt{[\pi_1(1-\pi_1)+\pi_0(1-\pi_0)]}+v\sqrt{[2\bar\pi(1-\bar\pi)]}\}^2}{(\pi_0-\pi_1)^2}$
	u, v	As below	where $\bar\pi = \dfrac{\pi_1+\pi_0}{2}$
7 Case–control study (sample size of each group)	π_0	Proportion of controls exposed	$\dfrac{\{u\sqrt{[\pi_0(1-\pi_0)+\pi_1(1-\pi_1)]}+v\sqrt{[2\bar\pi(1-\bar\pi)]}\}^2}{(\pi_1-\pi_0)^2}$
	OR	Odds ratio	
	π_1	Proportion of cases exposed, calculated from $\pi_1 = \dfrac{\pi_0\,OR}{1+\pi_0\,(OR-1)}$	where $\bar\pi = \dfrac{\pi_0+\pi_1}{2}$
	u, v	As below	

All cases

u	One-sided percentage point of the normal distribution corresponding to 100 % – the power
	e.g. if power = 90 %, $u = 1.28$
v	Percentage point of the normal distribution corresponding to the (two-sided) significance level
	e.g. if significance level = 5%, $v = 1.96$

(b) Precision

8 Single mean	σ	Standard deviation	$\dfrac{\sigma^2}{e^2}$
	e	Required size of standard error	
9 Single rate*	μ	Rate	$\dfrac{\mu}{e^2}$
	e	Required size of standard error	
10 Single proportion	π	Proportion	$\dfrac{\pi(1 - \pi)}{e^2}$
	e	Required size of standard error	
11 Difference between two means (sample size of each group)	σ_1, σ_0	Standard deviations	$\dfrac{\sigma_1^2 + \sigma_0^2}{e^2}$
	e	Required size of standard error	
12 Difference between two rates* (sample size of each group)	μ_1, μ_0	Rates	$\dfrac{\mu_1 + \mu_0}{e^2}$
	e	Required size of standard error	
13 Difference between two proportions (sample size of each group)	π_1, π_0	Proportions	$\dfrac{\pi_1(1 - \pi_1) + \pi_0(1 - \pi_0)}{e^2}$
	e	Required size of standard error	

*In these cases the sample size refers to the same units as used for the denominator of the rate(s). For example, if the rate is expressed per person-year, the formula gives the number of person-years of observation required (*see* Example 35.3).

How many cases and controls need to be studied to give a 90% power ($u = 1.28$) of achieving 5% significance ($v = 1.96$)? The calculation consists of several steps as detailed in formula 7 of Table 35.1.

1 Calculate π_1, the proportion of cases bottle-fed:

$$\pi_1 = \frac{\pi_0 \mathrm{OR}}{1 + \pi_0 (\mathrm{OR} - 1)} = \frac{0.4 \times 2}{1 + 0.4 \times (2 - 1)} = \frac{0.8}{1.4} = 0.57$$

2 Calculate $\bar{\pi}$, the average of π_0 and π_1:

$$\bar{\pi} = \frac{0.4 + 0.57}{2} = 0.485$$

3 Calculate the minimum sample size:

$$n > \frac{[1.28\sqrt{(0.4 \times 0.6 + 0.57 \times 0.43)} + 1.96\sqrt{(2 \times 0.485 \times 0.515)}]^2}{(0.57 - 0.4)^2}$$

$$= \frac{[1.28\sqrt{0.4851} + 1.96\sqrt{0.4996}]^2}{0.17^2} = \frac{2.2769}{0.17^2} = 179.4$$

We would therefore need to recruit about 180 cases and 180 controls, giving a total sample size of 360.

What difference would it make if, rather than recruiting equal numbers of cases and controls, we decided to recruit three times as many controls as cases? Table 35.2 gives appropriate adjustment factors for the number of cases according to differing number of controls per case. For $c = 3$ the adjustment factor is 2/3. This means we would need $180 \times 2/3$, that is 120 cases, and three times as many,

Table 35.2 Adjustment factor for use in study designs to compare unequal sized groups, such as in a case–control study selecting multiple controls per case. This factor (f) applies to the smaller group and equals $(c + 1)/(2c)$, where the size of the larger group is to be c times that of the smaller group. The sample size of the smaller group is therefore fn, where n would be the number required for equal-sized groups, and that of the larger group is cfn (see Example 35.4).

Ratio of larger to smaller group (c)	Adjustment to sample size of smaller group (f)
1	1
2	3/4
3	2/3
4	5/8
5	3/5
6	7/12
7	4/7
8	9/16
9	5/9
10	11/20

namely 360, controls. Thus although the requirement for the number of cases has considerably decreased, the total sample size has increased from 360 to 540.

35.4 ADJUSTMENTS FOR LOSS TO FOLLOW-UP, CONFOUNDING AND INTERACTION

The calculated sample size should be increased to allow for possible non-response or loss to follow-up. Further adjustments should be made if the final analysis will be adjusted for the effect of confounding variables or if the examination of subgroup effects is planned.

1 It is nearly always the case that a proportion of the people originally recruited to the study will not provide data for inclusion in the final analysis: for example because they withdraw from the study or are lost to follow-up, or because information on key variables is missing. The required sample size should be adjusted to take account of these possibilities. If we estimate that $x\%$ of patients will not contribute to the final analysis then the sample size should be multiplied by $100/(100-x)$. For example if $x=20\%$, the multiplying factor equals $100/(100-20)=1.25$.

$$\text{Adjustment factor for } x\% \text{ loss} = 100/(100-x)$$

2 Smith and Day (1984) considered the effect of controlling for confounding variables, in the context of the design of case–control studies. They concluded that, for a single confounding variable, an increase in the sample size of more than 10% is unlikely to be needed. Breslow and Day (1987) suggested that for several confounding variables that are jointly independent, as a rough guide one could add the extra sample size requirements for each variable separately.

3 In some circumstances we wish to design a study to detect differences between associations in different subgroups, in other words to detect *interaction* between the treatment or exposure effect and the characteristic that defines the subgroup. The required sample size will be *at least* four times as large as when the aim is to detect the overall association, and may be considerably larger. For more details see Smith and Day (1984) or Breslow and Day (1987).

35.5 ADJUSTMENT FOR CLUSTERED DESIGNS

The analysis of studies that employ a clustered design was described in Chapter 31. These include cluster randomized trials, in which randomization is applied to clusters of people rather than individuals (see also Section 34.2), family studies and studies which employ a cluster sampling scheme (see also Section 34.4). Because individuals within a cluster may be more similar to each other than to individuals in other clusters, a cluster randomized trial needs to include more individuals than the corresponding individually randomized trial. The same is true of studies that employ a cluster rather than individual sampling scheme.

The amount by which the sample size needs to be multiplied is known as the **design effect** (Deff), and depends on **the intraclass correlation coefficient** (ICC). The ICC was defined in Section 31.4 as the ratio of the between-cluster variance to the total variance.

$$\text{Design effect (Deff)} = 1 + (n' - 1) \times \text{ICC}$$

$$\text{ICC} = \text{intraclass correlation coefficient}$$

$$n' = \text{average cluster size}$$

It can be seen that two factors influence the size of the design effect:

1 the greater the ICC, the greater will be the design effect; and
2 the greater the number of individuals per cluster, the greater will be the design effect.

The number of clusters required is given by:

$$\text{No. of clusters} = \frac{n}{n'}[1 + (n' - 1) \times \text{ICC}]$$

$$n = \text{uncorrected total sample size}$$

$$n' = \text{average cluster size}$$

Estimation of the ICC, at the time that a study is designed, is often difficult because published papers have not tended to report ICCs. Although attempts have been made to publish typical ICCs, for different situations (for example see Gulliford *et al.*, 1999), it will usually be sensible to calculate the number of clusters required under a range of assumptions about the ICC, as well as using a range of values for the cluster size. In particular, it may be useful to present the results graphically, with lines showing the number of clusters required against number of individuals per cluster, for various values of ICC.

For more details about sample size calculations for cluster randomized trials, see Donner and Klar (2000) or Ukoumunne *et al.* (1999). Alternatively, Hayes and Bennett (1999) suggested a method based on the **coefficient of variation** (standard deviation/mean) of cluster rates, proportions or means. They give guidance on how to estimate this value with or without the use of prior data on between-cluster variation, and provide formulae for both unmatched and pair-matched trials.

35.6 TYPES OF ERROR IN SIGNIFICANCE TESTS

A significance test can never prove that a null hypothesis is either true or false. It can only give an indication of the strength of the evidence against it. In using significance tests to make decisions about whether to reject a null hypothesis, we can make two types of error: we can reject a null hypothesis when it is in fact true, or fail to reject it when it is false. These are called **type I** and **type II errors** respectively (Table 35.3).

As explained in Chapter 8, the *P*-value (significance level) equals the probability of occurrence of a result as extreme as, or more extreme than, that observed if the null hypothesis were true. For example, there is a 5% probability that sampling variation alone will lead to a $P < 0.05$ (a result significant at the 5% level), and so if we judge such a result as sufficient evidence to reject the null hypothesis, there is a 5% probability that we are making an error in doing so, if the null hypothesis is true (see Figure 35.2a).

The second type of error is that the null hypothesis is not rejected when it is false. This occurs because of overlap between the real sampling distribution of the sample difference about the population difference, $d (\neq 0)$ and the acceptance region for the null hypothesis based on the hypothesized sampling distribution about the incorrect difference, 0. This is illustrated in Figure 35.2(b). The shaded area shows the proportion ($b\%$) of the real sampling distribution that would fall within the acceptance region for the null hypothesis, i.e. that would appear consistent with the null hypothesis at the 5% level. The probability that we *do not* make a type II error ($100 - b\%$) equals the **power** of the test.

If a lower significance level were used, making the probability of a type I error smaller, the size of the shaded area would be increased, so that there would be a larger probability of a type II error. The converse is also true. For a given significance level, the probability of a type II error can be reduced by increasing the power, by increasing either the sample size or the precision of the measurements (see Chapter 36). Each of the curves in Figure 35.2 would be taller and narrower, and overlap less; the size of the shaded area would therefore be reduced.

Table 35.3 Types of error in hypothesis tests.

	Reality	
Conclusion of significance test	Null hypothesis is true	Null hypothesis is false
Reject null hypothesis	*Type I error* (probability = significance level)	Correct conclusion (probability = power)
Do not reject null hypothesis	Correct conclusion (probability = 1 − significance level)	*Type II error* (probability = 1 − power)

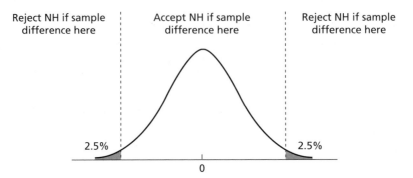

| Reject NH if sample difference here | Accept NH if sample difference here | Reject NH if sample difference here |

2.5%   2.5%

0

(a) Type I error. Null hypothesis (NH) is *true*. Population difference = 0. The curve shows the sampling distribution of the sample difference. The shaded areas (total 5%) give the probability that the null hypothesis is wrongly rejected.

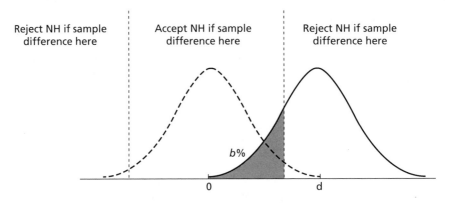

| Reject NH if sample difference here | Accept NH if sample difference here | Reject NH if sample difference here |

b%

0   d

(b) Type II error. Null hypothesis is *false*. Population difference = d≠0. The continuous curve shows the real sampling distribution of the sample difference, while the dashed curve shows the sampling distribution under the null hypothesis. The shaded area is the probability (*b*%) that the null hypothesis fails to be rejected.

Fig. 35.2 Probabilities of occurrence of the two types of error of hypothesis testing, illustrated for a test at the 5% level.

35.7 IMPLICATIONS OF STUDY POWER FOR THE INTERPRETATION OF SIGNIFICANCE TESTS

Unfortunately, significance tests are often misused, with investigators using a 5% threshold for statistical significance and concluding that any non-significant result means that the null hypothesis is true. Another common misinterpretation is that *the P-value is the probability that the null hypothesis is true.*

Table 35.4(a) demonstrates why such thinking is incorrect. It is based on considering what would happen if 1000 different null hypotheses were tested and significance at the 5% level ($P < 0.05$) used as a threshold for rejection, under the following plausible assumptions:

Table 35.4 Implications of study power for the interpretation of significance tests.

(a) Conclusions of significance tests of 1000 hypotheses, of which 10% are false, using $P = 0.05$ as threshold significance level, and conducted with 50% power (adapted from Oakes, 1986).

Conclusion of significance test	Reality		Total
	Null hypothesis true	Null hypothesis false	
Reject null hypothesis ($P < 0.05$)	45 (*Type I errors*)	50	95
Do not reject null hypothesis ($P \geq 0.05$)	855	50 (*Type II errors*)	905
Total	900	100	1000

(b) Proportion of false-positive significant results, according to the P-value used for significance, the power of the study and the proportion of studies in which the null hypothesis is truly false (adapted from Sterne and Davey Smith 2001). The result corresponding to Table 35.4(a) is in bold.

Proportion of studies in which the null hypothesis is false	Power of study	Percentage of significant results that are false-positives		
		$P = 0.05$	$P = 0.01$	$P = 0.001$
	20%	5.9	1.2	0.1
80%	50%	2.4	0.5	0.0
	80%	1.5	0.3	0.0
	20%	20.0	4.8	0.5
50%	50%	9.1	2.0	0.2
	80%	5.9	1.2	0.1
	20%	69.2	31.0	4.3
10%	50%	**47.4**	15.3	1.8
	80%	36.0	10.1	1.1
	20%	96.1	83.2	33.1
1%	50%	90.8	66.4	16.5
	80%	86.1	55.3	11.0

1 10% of the null hypotheses tested are in fact false (i.e. the effect being investigated is real), and 90% are true (i.e. the hypothesis tested is incorrect). This is conceivable given the large numbers of factors searched for in the epidemiological literature. For example by 1985 nearly 300 risk factors for coronary heart disease had been identified; it is unlikely that more than a fraction of these factors actually increase the risk of the disease.

2 The power of the test is 50%. This is consistent with published surveys of the size of clinical trials (see, for example, Moher *et al.*, 1994); a large proportion having been conducted with an inadequate sample size to address the research question.

Assumption (1) determines the column totals in the table; the null hypothesis is true in 900 of the tests and false in 100 of them. The type I error rate will be 5%, the significance level being used. This means that we will incorrectly reject 45 of the 900 true null hypotheses. Assumption (2) means that that the type II error rate equals 50% (100% – power). We will therefore fail to reject 50 of the 100 null hypotheses that are false. It can be seen from the table that of the 95 tests that result in a statistically significant result, only 50 are correct; 45 (47.4%) are type I errors (false positive results).

Table 35.4(b) extends Table 35.4(a) by showing the percentage of false positive results for different P-value thresholds under different assumptions about both the power of studies and the proportion of true null hypotheses. For any choice of significance level, the proportion of 'significant' results that are false-positives is greatly reduced as power increases. The table suggests that unless the proportion of meaningful hypotheses is very small, it is reasonable to regard P-values less than 0.001 as providing strong evidence against the null hypothesis.

CHAPTER 36

Measurement error: assessment and implications

36.1 INTRODUCTION

In this chapter we consider how to examine for errors made in measuring outcome or exposure variables, and the implications of such errors for the results of statistical analyses. Such errors may occur in a variety of ways, including:

1 **Instrumental errors**, arising from an inaccurate diagnostic test, an imprecise instrument or questionnaire limitations.

2 **Underlying variability**, leading to differences between replicate measurements taken at different points in time.

3 **Respondent errors**, arising through misunderstanding, faulty recall, giving the perceived 'correct' answer, or through lack of interest. In some instances the respondent may deliberately give the wrong answer because, for example, of embarrassment in questions connected with sexually transmitted diseases or because of suspicion that answers could be passed to income tax authorities.

4 **Observer errors**, including imprecision, misuse/misunderstanding of procedures, and mistakes.

5 **Data processing errors**, such as coding, copying, data entry, programming and calculating mistakes.

Our focus is on the detection, measurement and implications of random error, in the sense that we will assume that any errors in measuring a variable are independent of the value of other variables in the dataset. Detailed discussion of **differential bias** arising from the design or conduct of the study, such as **selection bias**, is outside the scope of this book. Readers are referred to textbooks on epidemiology and study design: recommended books are listed at the beginning of Chapter 34. We cover:

1 How to evaluate a diagnostic test or compare a measurement technique against a **gold standard**, that gives a (more) precise measurement of the true value. Often, the gold-standard method is expensive, and we wish to examine the performance of a cheaper or quicker alternative.

2 How to choose the 'best' cut-off value when using a numerical variable to give a binary classification.

3 How to assess the *reproducibility* of a measurement, including:
   • agreement between different observers using the same measurement technique,
   • the agreement between replicate measurements taken at different points in time.

4 The implications of inaccuracies in measurement for the interpretation of results.

36.2 THE EVALUATION OF DIAGNOSTIC TESTS

The analysis of binary outcome variables was considered in Part C, while methods for examining the effect of binary exposure variables are presented throughout this book. In this section we consider how to assess the ability of a procedure to correctly classify individuals between the two categories of a binary variable. For example, individuals may be classified as diseased or non-diseased, exposed or non-exposed, positive or negative, or at high risk or not.

Sensitivity and specificity

The ability of a **diagnostic test** (or procedure) to correctly classify individuals into two categories (positive and negative) is assessed by two parameters, **sensitivity** and **specificity**:

Sensitivity = proportion of true positives correctly identified as such
= 1 − false negative rate

Specificity = proportion of true negatives correctly identified as such
= 1 − false positive rate

To estimate sensitivity and specificity, each individual needs to be classified definitively (using a 'gold-standard' assessment) as true positive or true negative and, in addition, to be classified according to the test being assessed.

Example 36.1

Table 36.1 shows the results of a pilot study to assess parents' ability to recall the correct BCG immunization status of their children, as compared to health authority records. Of the 60 children who had in fact received BCG immunization, almost all, 55, were correctly identified as such by their parents, giving a sensitivity of 55/60 or 91.7%. In contrast, 15 of the 40 children with no record of BCG

Table 36.1 Comparison of parents' recall of the BCG immunization status of their children with that recorded in the health authority records.

BCG immunization according to health authority records ('gold standard' test)	BCG immunization according to parents (procedure being assessed)			
	Yes	No	Total	
Yes	55	5	60	*Sensitivity* = 55/60 = 91.7%
No	15	25	40	*Specificity* = 25/40 = 62.5%
Total	70	30	100	
	PPV = 55/70 = 78.6%	NPV = 25/30 = 83.3%		

immunization were claimed by their parents to have been immunized, giving a specificity of 25/40 or 62.5%.

Sensitivity and specificity are characteristics of the test. Their values do *not* depend on the prevalence of the disease in the population. They are particularly important in assessing **screening tests**. Note that there is an inverse relationship between the two measures, tightening (or relaxing) criteria to improve one will have the effect of decreasing the magnitude of the other. Where to draw the line between them will depend on the nature of the study. For example, in designing a study to test a new leprosy vaccine, it would be important initially to exclude any lepromatous patients. One would therefore want a test with a high success rate of detecting positives, or in other words a highly sensitive test. One would be less concerned about specificity, since it would not matter if a true negative was incorrectly identified as positive and so excluded. In contrast, for the detection of cases during the post-vaccine (or placebo) follow-up period, one would want a test with high specificity, since it would then be more important to be confident that any positives detected were real, and less important if some were missed.

Predictive values

A clinician who wishes to interpret the results of a diagnostic test will want to know the probability that a patient is truly positive if the test is positive and similarly the probability that the patient is truly negative if the test is negative. These are called the **positive** and **negative predictive values** of the test:

Positive predictive value (PPV) = proportion of test positives that are truly positive

Negative predictive value (NPV) = proportion of test negatives that are truly negative

In Example 36.1, BCG immunization was confirmed from health authority records for 55 of the 70 children reported by their parents as having received immunization, giving a PPV of 55/70 or 78.6%. The NPV was 25/30 or 83.3%.

The values of the positive and negative predictive values *depend on the prevalence of the disease in the population*, as well as on the sensitivity and specificity of the procedure used. The lower the prevalence of true positives, the lower will be the proportion of true positives among test positives and the lower, therefore, will be the positive predictive value. Similarly, increasing prevalence will lead to decreasing negative predictive value.

Choosing cut-offs

Where binary classifications are derived from a numerical variable, using a cut-off value, the performance of different cut-off values can be assessed using a **Receiver Operating Characteristic** curve, often known as a **ROC curve**. This is a plot of sensitivity against 1 − specificity, for different choices of cut-off. The name of the curve derives from its original use in studies of radar signal detection.

Example 36.2

Data from a study of lung function among 636 children aged 7 to 10 years living in a deprived suburb of Lima, Peru were introduced in Chapter 11. For each child the FEV_1 (the volume of air the child could breathe out in 1 second) was measured before and after she or he exercised on an electric treadmill for 4 minutes, and the percentage reduction in FEV_1 after exercise was calculated. This ranged from −17.9% (i.e. an increase post-exercise) to a 71.4% reduction.

A total of 60 (9.4%) of the parents (or carers) reported that their child had experienced chest tightness suggestive of asthma in the previous 12 months. There was strong evidence of an association between % reduction in FEV_1 and reported chest tightness in the child (odds ratio per unit increase in % reduction 1.052, 95% CI 1.031 to 1.075). To examine the utility of % reduction in FEV_1 as a means of diagnosing asthma, a ROC curve was plotted, as displayed in Figure 36.1, showing sensitivity (vertical axis) against 1 − specificity (horizontal axis) for different choices of cut-off values for FEV_1. In this example, we can see that if we required 75% sensitivity from our cut-off then specificity would be around 50%, while a lower cut-off value that gave around 60% sensitivity would yield a specificity of about 75%.

The overall ability of the continuous measure (in this case FEV_1) to discriminate between individuals with and without disease may be measured by the **area under the ROC curve**. If perfect discrimination were possible (the existence of a cut-off with 100% sensitivity and 100% specificity), the ROC curve would go across the top of the grid area, and yield an area of 1. This is because decreasing the specificity by lowering the cut-off would maintain sensitivity at 100%, since a lower cut-off can only capture an equal or higher percentage of cases. In contrast, if the continuous measure is not able to discriminate at all, then 100% sensitivity

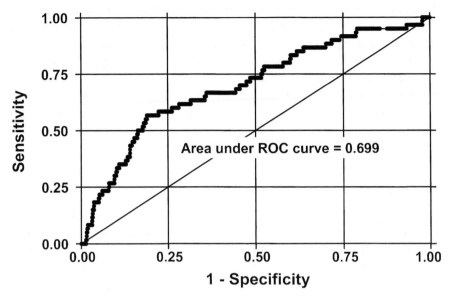

Fig. 36.1 ROC curve showing the sensitivity and specificity corresponding to different choices of cut-off for % reduction in FEV$_1$ as a test for chest tightness suggestive of asthma in children in Peru.

can only be achieved with 0% specificity and vice versa. The ROC curve will be the straight line in Figure 36.1 showing sensitivity = 1− specificity, and the area under the curve will be 0.5. In this example the area under the ROC curve is 0.699. The area under the ROC curve may also be used to quantify how well a predictor based on a number of variables (for example based on the linear predictor from a logistic regression model) discriminates between individuals with and without disease.

36.3 ASSESSING REPRODUCIBILITY OF MEASUREMENTS

In this section we describe methods to assess the extent of **reproducibility** of a measurement (also known as **reliability**), including:
- agreement between different observers using the same measurement technique;
- agreement between replicate measurements taken at different points in time.

This is particularly important for any variable that is subjectively assessed, such as in Example 36.3, or for which there may be underlying natural variation, such as the composition of a person's daily nutritional intake (see Example 36.5), which will show some day-to-day variations, as well as possible marked seasonal differences.

Kappa statistic for categorical variables

For categorical variables, the extent of reproducibility is usually assessed using a **kappa** statistic. This is based on comparing the *observed* proportion of agreement

(A_{obs}) between two readings made by two different observers, or on two different occasions, with the proportion of agreements (A_{exp}) that would be *expected* simply by chance. It is denoted by the Greek letter kappa, κ, and is defined as:

$$\kappa = \frac{A_{obs} - A_{exp}}{1 - A_{exp}}$$

If there is complete agreement then $A_{obs} = 1$ and so $\kappa = 1$. If there is no more agreement than would be expected by chance alone then $\kappa = 0$, and if there is *less* agreement than would be expected by chance alone then κ will be negative. Based on criteria originally proposed by Landis and Koch:

- kappa values greater than about 0.75 are often taken as representing excellent agreement;
- those between 0.4 and 0.75 as fair to good agreement; and
- those less than 0.4 as moderate or poor agreement.

    Standard errors for kappa have been derived, and are presented in computer output by many statistical packages. These may be used to derive a *P*-value corresponding to the null hypothesis of no association between the ratings on the two occasions, or by the two raters. In general, *such P-values are not of interest*, because the null hypothesis of no association is not a reasonable one.

    We will illustrate the calculation of kappa statistics using data from a study of the way in which people tend to explain problems with their health. We will do this first using a binary classification, and then a fuller 4-category classification.

Example 36.3: Binary classification

Table 36.2 summarizes data from a study in which 179 men and women filled in a Symptom Interpretation Questionnaire on two occasions three years apart. On the basis of this questionnaire they were classified according to whether or not they tended to provide a *normalizing* explanation of symptoms. This means discounting symptoms, externalizing them and explaining them away as part of normal experience. It can be seen that while 76 participants were consistently classified as normalizers, and 47 as non-normalizers, the classification changed for a total of 56 participants. More participants were classified as normalizers on the second than the first occasion.

    The *observed* proportion of agreement between the assessment on the two occasions, denoted by A_{obs} is therefore given by:

$$A_{obs} = (76 + 47)/179 = 123/179 = 0.687 \ (68.7\%)$$

Part (b) of Table 36.2 shows the number of agreements and disagreements that would be expected between the two classifications on the basis of chance alone. These expected numbers are calculated in a similar way to that described for the

Table 36.2 Classification of 179 men and women as 'symptom normalizers' or not, on two measurement occasions three years apart. Data kindly provided by Dr David Kessler.

(a) Observed numbers

First classification	Second classification		Total
	Normalizer	Non-normalizer	
Normalizer	76	17	93
Non-normalizer	39	47	86
Total	115	64	179

(b) Expected numbers

First classification	Second classification		Total
	Normalizer	Non-normalizer	
Normalizer	59.7	33.3	93
Non-normalizer	55.3	30.7	86
Total	115	64	179

chi-squared test in Chapter 17. The overall proportion classified as normalizers on the second occasion was 115/179. If this classification was unrelated to that on the first, then one would expect this same proportion of second occasion normalizers in each first occasion group, that is $115/119 \times 93 = 59.7$ classified as normalizers on both occasions, and $115/119 \times 86 = 55.3$ of those classified as non-normalizers on the first occasion classified as normalizers on the second. Similarly $64/179 \times 93 = 33.3$ of those classified as normalizers on the first occasion would be classified as non-normalizers on the second, while $64/179 \times 86 = 30.7$ would be classified as non-normalizers on both occasions. The *expected* proportion of chance agreement is therefore:

$$A_{exp} = (59.7 + 30.7)/179 = 0.505 \ (50.5\%)$$

Giving a kappa statistic of:

$$\kappa = (0.687 - 0.505)/(1 - 0.505) = 0.37$$

This would usually be interpreted as representing at most moderate agreement between the two classifications made over the three-year follow-up period.

Example 36.4: Categorical classification
Table 36.3(a) shows a more complete version of the data presented in Table 36.2, with each participant now assessed as belonging to one of four groups according to the way in which they tended to explain symptoms. Those classed as non-normalizers (see earlier explanation) have been divided into *somatizers*, those who

Table 36.3 Classification of the dominant style for explaining symptoms of 179 men and women as normalizers, somatizers, psychologizers or no dominant style, on two measurement occasions three years apart. Data kindly provided by Dr David Kessler.

(a) Observed numbers

Dominant style at first classification	Dominant style at second classification				Total
	Normalizer	Somatizer	Psychologizer	None	
Normalizer	76	0	7	10	93
Somatizer	2	0	3	1	6
Psychologizer	17	1	15	8	41
None	20	3	5	11	39
Total	115	4	30	30	179

(b) Expected numbers of agreements

Dominant style at first classification	Dominant style at second classification				Total
	Normalizer	Somatizer	Psychologizer	None	
Normalizer	59.7				93
Somatizer		0.1			6
Psychologizer			6.9		41
None				0.2	39
Total	115	4	30	30	179

tend to explain their symptoms as indicating a potentially more serious physical illness, *psychologizers*, those who tend to give psychological explanations for their symptoms, and those with no dominant style. The *observed* proportion of agreement between the two occasions using the four category classification is:

$$A_{\text{obs}} = (76 + 0 + 15 + 11)/179 = 123/179 = 0.570 \ (57.0\%)$$

The expected numbers for the various combinations of first and second occasion classification can be calculated in exactly the same way as argued in the two-category example. For the kappa statistic, we need these only for the numbers of agreements; these are shown in Table 36.3(b).

$$A_{\text{exp}} = (59.7 + 0.1 + 6.9 + 0.2)/179 = 72.9/179 = 0.407 \ (40.7\%)$$

giving

$$\kappa = \frac{A_{\text{obs}} - A_{\text{exp}}}{1 - A_{\text{exp}}} = (0.570 - 0.407)/(1 - 0.407) = 0.27$$

representing poor to moderate agreement.

As the *number* of categories increases, the value of kappa will tend to decrease, because there are more opportunities for misclassification. Further, for ordinal measures we may wish to count classification into adjacent categories as *partial* agreement. For instance, classification into adjacent categories might count as 50% agreement, such as normalizers classified as somatizers and vice versa in Table 36.3. This is done using a **weighted kappa** statistic, in which the observed and expected proportions of agreement are modified to include partial agreements, by assigning a weight between 0 (complete disagreement) and 1 (complete agreement) to each category. Kappa statistics can also be derived when there are more than two raters: for more details see Fleiss (1981) or Dunn (1989).

Numerical variables: reliability and the intraclass correlation coefficient

We now describe how to quantify the amount of measurement error in a numerical variable. As with the kappa statistic, this may be done using replicate measurements of the variable: for example measurement of blood pressure made on the same patient by two observers at the same time, or using the same automated measuring device on two occasions one week apart.

The **reliability** of a measurement is formally defined as the ratio of the variance of the 'true' (underlying) values between individuals to the variance of the observed values, which is a combination of the variation between individuals (σ_u^2) and measurement error (σ_e^2). It can be measured using the **intraclass correlation coefficient** (ICC), defined in Section 31.4 in the context of random-effects models:

$$\text{Intraclass correlation coefficient (ICC)} = \frac{\sigma_u^2}{\sigma_u^2 + \sigma_e^2}$$

$$\sigma_u^2 = \text{variance between true measurements}$$

$$\sigma_e^2 = \text{measurement error variance}$$

Here the 'clusters' are the individuals on whom measurements are made, and the observations within clusters are the repeated measurements on the individuals. ICC can range from 0 to 1, with the maximum of 1 corresponding to complete reliability, which is when there is no measurement error, $\sigma_e^2 = 0$. The smaller the amount of measurement error, the smaller will be the increase in the variability of the observed measurements compared to the true measurements and the closer will be the reliability (and ICC) to 1. If all individuals have the same 'true' value, then $\sigma_u^2 = 0$ and ICC $= 0$; all observed variation is due to measurement error.

The intraclass correlation coefficient may be estimated using a one-way analysis of variance (see Chapter 11), or by using a simple random-effects model (see Chapter 31). When there are paired measurements, the ICC can also be derived by calculating the Pearson (product moment) correlation with each pair entered twice, once in reverse order.

Example 36.5

As part of a case–control study investigating the association between asthma and intake of dietary antioxidants (measured using food frequency questionnaires), replicate measurements of selenium intake were made 3 months after the original measurements, for 94 adults aged between 15 and 50 years. Figure 36.2 is a scatter plot of the pairs of measurements; note that because estimated selenium intake was positively skewed the measurements are plotted on a log scale (see Chapter 13). While there is clearly an association between the measurements on the first and second occasions, there is also substantial between-occasion variability.

The mean and standard deviation of log selenium intake (measured in log (base e) μg/week) in the 94 subjects with repeat measurements were 3.826 (s.d. = 0.401) on the first occasion and 3.768 (s.d. = 0.372) on the second occasion. There was some evidence that measured intake declined between the two measurements (mean reduction 0.058, 95 % CI −0.008 to 0.125, $P = 0.083$). The estimated components of variance were:

Within-subject (measurement error) variance, $\sigma_e^2 = 0.0535$

Between-subject variance, $\sigma_u^2 = 0.0955$

Total variance $= \sigma_u^2 + \sigma_e^2 = 0.1491$

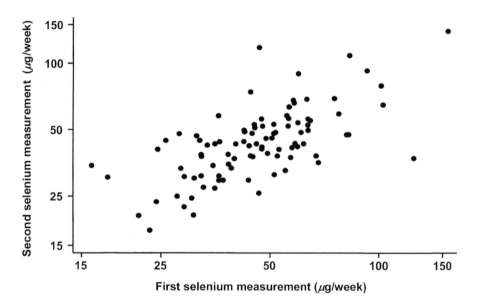

Fig. 36.2 Scatter plot of weekly selenium intake (μg/week) on a log scale among 94 participants in a study of asthma and intake of antioxidant vitamins, measured using a food frequency questionnaire on two occasions three months apart. Data displays and analyses from the FLAG study (Shaheen SO, Sterne JAC, Thompson RL, Songhurst CE, Margetts BM, Burney PGJ (2001) *American Journal of Respiratory and Critical Care Medicine* **164**: 1823–1828).

Therefore,

$$\text{ICC} = \frac{\sigma_u^2}{\sigma_u^2 + \sigma_e^2} = 0.0955/0.1491 = 0.6410$$

Thus in this example, 64.1% of the total variability was between-subject variability, indicating fairly good reliability of assessing selenium intake using a single application of a food frequency questionnaire.

Links between weighted kappa and the intraclass correlation coefficient

For ordered categorical variables, there is a close link between the weighted kappa statistic (defined above) and the intraclass correlation coefficient. If the variable has k categories, and the weight, w_{ij}, for a subject in category i at the first measurement and j at the second measurement is chosen to be:

$$w_{ij} = 1 - \frac{(i-j)^2}{(k-1)^2}$$

then the value of the weighted kappa will be very close to the ICC. For example, for an ordered categorical variable with four categories the weights would be

$$w_{11} = w_{22} = w_{33} = w_{44} = 1 - \frac{0}{3^2} = 1$$

$$w_{12} = w_{21} = w_{23} = w_{32} = w_{34} = w_{43} = 1 - \frac{1^2}{3^2} = 0.889$$

$$w_{13} = w_{31} = w_{24} = w_{42} = 1 - \frac{2^2}{3^2} = 0.556$$

$$w_{14} = w_{41} = 1 - \frac{3^2}{3^2} = 0$$

36.4 NUMERICAL VARIABLES: METHOD COMPARISON STUDIES

We will now consider analyses appropriate to **method comparison studies**, in which two different methods of measuring the same underlying (true) value are compared. For example, lung function might be measured using a spirometer, which is expensive but relatively accurate, or with a peak flow meter, which is cheap (and can therefore be used by asthma patients at home) but relatively inaccurate. The appropriate analysis of such studies was described, in an influential paper, by Bland and Altman (1986).

Example 36.6

We will illustrate appropriate methods for the analysis of method comparison studies using data on 1236 women who participated in the British Women's

Regional Heart Study. The women were asked to report their weight as part of a general questionnaire, and their weight was subsequently measured using accurate scales. Figure 36.3 is a scatter plot of self-reported versus measured weight.

The two measures are clearly strongly associated: the Pearson correlation between them is 0.982. It is important to note, however, that the correlation measures the strength of association between the measures and *not* the agreement between them. For example, if the measurements made with the new method were exactly twice as large as those made with the standard method then the correlation would be 1, even though the new method was badly in error. Further, the correlation depends on the range of the true quantity in the sample. The correlation will be greater if this range is wide than if it is narrow.

The diagonal line in Figure 36.3 is the **line of equality**: the two measures are in perfect agreement only if all measurements lie along this line. It can be seen that more of the points lie below the line than above it, suggesting that self-reported weight tends to be lower than measured weight.

Bland and Altman suggested that the extent of agreement could be examined by plotting the *differences* between the pairs of measurements on the vertical axis, against the *mean* of each pair on the horizontal axis. Such a plot (often known as a **Bland–Altman plot**) is shown in Figure 36.4. If (as here) one method is known to be accurate, then the mean difference will tell us whether there is a systematic **bias** (a tendency to be higher or lower than the true value) in the other measurement. In

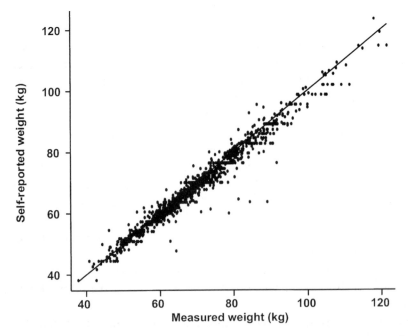

Fig. 36.3 Scatter plot of self-reported versus measured weight (kg) in 1236 women who participated in the British Regional Women's Heart Study. The solid line is the *line of equality*. Data displays and analyses by kind permission of Dr Debbie Lawlor and Professor Shah Ebrahim.

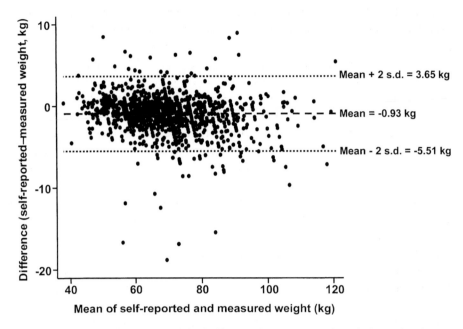

Fig. 36.4 Scatter plot (Bland–Altman plot) of self-reported minus measured weight (vertical axis) against mean of self-reported and measured weight (horizontal axis) in 1236 women who participated in the British Regional Women's Heart Study. The dashed horizontal line corresponds to the mean difference (−0.93 kg) while the dotted horizontal lines correspond to the 95% limits of agreement.

this example, mean self-reported weight was 68.88 kg, while the mean measured weight was 69.85 kg. The mean difference between self-reported and measured weight was −0.93 kg (95 % CI −1.07 to −0.80 kg). There was thus a clear tendency for the women to under-report their weight, by an average of 0.93 kg. This is shown by the dashed horizontal line in Figure 36.4.

The dotted horizontal lines in Figure 36.4 correspond to the **95 % limits of agreement**, given by the mean difference plus or minus twice the *standard deviation* of the differences. If the differences are normally distributed then approximately 95 % of differences will lie within this range. In this example the 95 % limits of agreement are from −5.51 kg to 3.65 kg. Inspection of Figure 36.4 also shows that the differences were negatively skewed; there were more large negative differences than large positive ones. Further, there was a tendency for greater (negative) differences with greater mean weight.

Note that *the difference should not be plotted against either of the individual measurements*, because of the problem of '**regression to the mean**' described in Section 36.5.

Having calculated the mean difference and the 95 % limits of agreement, it is for the investigator to decide whether the methods are sufficiently in agreement for one (perhaps the cheaper method) to be used in place of the other. In this example, the systematic underreporting of weight in questionnaires, and the reduced accuracy, would have to be considered against the increased cost of inviting women to a visit at which their weight could be measured accurately.

36.5 IMPLICATIONS FOR INTERPRETATION

The problems that may result from errors that occur when measuring outcome or exposure variables are summarized in Table 36.4. Each type of problem will be addressed in the sub-sections below. Note that the focus here is on random errors, in the sense that we are assuming that any errors in measuring a variable are independent of the values of other variables in the dataset.

Table 36.4 Summary of implications of random misclassification and measurement error.

	Type of error	
Type of variable	Misclassification (binary/categorical variable)	Measurement error (numerical variable)
Outcome	Regression dilution bias	Regression to the mean
Exposure	Regression dilution bias Potential problems if adjusting for confounders	

Regression dilution bias

Regression dilution bias means that the estimated regression coefficient of the exposure-effect estimate has been biased towards the null value of no exposure effect, so that the magnitude of the association between the exposure and outcome will tend to be underestimated:

1 For a numerical *exposure* variable, the degree of bias depends on the intraclass correlation coefficient (ICC). For linear regression the relationship is:

$$\text{Estimated coefficient} = \text{correct coefficient} \times \text{ICC}$$

For other regression models, such as logistic regression and Cox regression, the same relationship holds approximately, providing that the correct coefficient is not too large, and that the measurement error variance is not too large compared to the variance between true measurements. Frost and Thompson (2000) compare a number of methods to correct for regression dilution bias.

2 The estimated effect of a categorical (or binary) *exposure* variable can be corrected using replicate measurements on some or all individuals. However, methods to do this are more complex than those for numerical exposure variables, because *the errors will be correlated with the true values*. For example, if the true value of a binary variable is 0 then the size of the error is either 0 or 1, while if the true value is 1 then the size is 0 or −1. For this reason, applying

methods appropriate for numerical exposure variables will *overcorrect* the regression dilution in the effect of a binary exposure variable. Appropriate methods for this situation are reviewed by White *et al.* (2001).

3 For a binary *outcome* variable, if the sensitivity and specificity with which it was measured are known then estimated odds ratios from logistic regression may be corrected, as described by Magder and Hughes (1997).

4 Measurement error in a numerical *outcome* variable does *not* lead to regression dilution bias, although the greater the measurement error the lower the precision with which exposure-outcome associations are estimated.

As mentioned above, correcting for regression dilution bias requires that we make *replicate measurements* on some or all subjects. If each subject-evaluation costs the same amount, then we must trade off the benefits of increasing the number of *subjects* in our study with the benefits of increasing the number of *measurements per subject*. Phillips and Davey Smith (1993) showed that it will sometimes be better to recruit a smaller number of subjects with each evaluated on more than one occasion, because this leads to more precise estimates of subjects' exposure levels and hence to reduced bias in exposure effect estimates. They suggested that attempts to anticipate and control bias due to exposure measurement error should be given at least as high a priority as that given to sample size assessment in the design of epidemiological studies.

Before applying any method to correct regression coefficients for measurement error, it is important to be aware of the potential problems associated with measurement error in a number of exposure variables included in multivariable models, as described in the next sub-section.

The effects of measurement error and misclassification in multivariable models

When there are measurement errors in a *number* of exposure variables, and we wish to control for the possible confounding effects of each on the other, the effects are less straightforward to predict than is the case when we are considering the association between an outcome and a *single* exposure variable. For example, consider the situation in which:

1 the correct (underlying) value of exposure A is associated with the disease outcome, but is measured with substantial error;

2 the correct (underlying) value of exposure B is not associated with the disease outcome after controlling for exposure A; and

3 the amount of measurement error in exposure B is much less than the measurement error in exposure A.

In this situation, including A and B in a multivariable model may give the misleading impression that B is associated with the outcome, and that A is not associated with the outcome after controlling for B: the opposite of the true situation if there were no measurement error.

Such possible problems are frequently ignored. Note that the bias caused by differing amounts of measurement error in the two exposure variables may act in either direction, depending on:

1 the direction of the association between the two variables;
2 the relative amounts of error in measuring them; and
3 whether the measurement errors are correlated.

Regression to the mean

Regression to the mean refers to a phenomenon first observed by Galton when he noticed that the heights of sons tended to be closer to the overall mean than the heights of their fathers. Thus, tall fathers tended to have sons shorter than themselves, while the opposite was true for short fathers.

The same phenomenon occurs whenever two repeat measurements are made, and where they are subject to measurement error. Larger values of the first measurement will, on average, have positive measurement errors while smaller values of the first measurement will, on average, have negative measurement errors. This means that the repeat measurement will tend to be smaller if the first measurement was larger, and larger if the first measurement was smaller. It follows that the size of the first measurement will be negatively associated with the difference between the two measurements.

The implications of this will be explained in more detail by considering the repeated measurement of blood pressure and the assessment of anti-hypertensive drugs in reducing blood pressure. For a more detailed discussion of regression to the mean, and methods to correct for it, see Hayes (1988).

Example 36.7

Figure 36.5 shows the relationship between two diastolic blood pressure readings taken 6 months apart on 50 volunteers, while Figure 36.6 is a scatter plot of the difference between the two readings (vertical axis) against the initial reading (horizontal axis). This gives the impression that there is a downward gradient, so that those with a high initial level have a reduced blood pressure 6 months later, while the opposite is true for those with an initial low level. However, for the reasons explained above, this downward gradient may be the result of measurement error. If there is *no* association between the *true* reduction and the *true* initial value, the regression coefficient β_{obs} for the *observed* association between the difference and the initial value is given by:

$$\beta_{obs} = ICC - 1$$

in absence of 'true' association

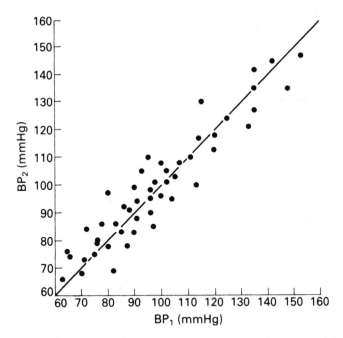

Fig. 36.5 The relationship between two diastolic blood pressure readings taken six months apart on 50 volunteers, showing little change on average. The straight line is the relationship that would be seen if the readings on the two occasions were the same.

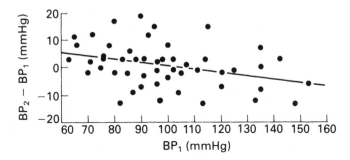

Fig. 36.6 Change in diastolic blood pressure plotted against initial value. An artificial negative correlation ($r = -0.35$, d.f. $= 48$, $P = 0.013$) is observed. The straight line is the regression line corresponding to this association.

Thus the greater the measurement error variance, the smaller is the ICC and so the greater is the slope of this apparent negative association.

Thus measurement error has important implications when the focus of interest is *change* in outcome measurement, for example in a clinical trial to evaluate the ability of an anti-hypertensive drug to reduce blood pressure:

1 If, as is often the case, the trial is confined to people with high initial diastolic blood pressure, say 120 mmHg or above, then it can be seen from Figure 36.6 that their repeated blood pressure measurements would show an average

reduction, even in the absence of any treatment. It is therefore essential to have a control group, and to compare any apparent reduction in the treatment group with that in the control group.

2 Analyses investigating whether the size of any change in blood pressure is related to the initial value must correct for *regression to the mean*. Blomqvist (1977) suggested that the true regression coefficient can be estimated from the observed regression coefficient using:

$$\beta_{true} = \frac{\beta_{obs} + (1 - \text{ICC})}{\text{ICC}}$$

To apply this method in practice requires an external estimate of the within-person (measurement error) variance.

3 Oldham (1962) suggested plotting the difference, $BP_2 - BP_1$, against the *average* of the initial and final blood pressure readings, $\frac{1}{2}(BP_1 + BP_2)$, rather than against the initial reading as shown in Figure 36.7, to correct for regression to the mean. (Note the similarity with Bland–Altman plots, described in Section 36.4.) The correlation is attenuated to -0.19, suggesting that much or all of the apparent association between blood pressure reduction and initial blood pressure was caused by regression to the mean. However, there are at least two circumstances when this can give misleading results. The Oldham plot will show a positive association when the true change is unrelated to the initial level, if:

- the true change differs between individuals; or
- individuals have been selected on the basis of high initial values.

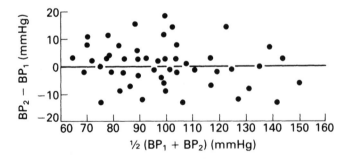

Fig. 36.7 Change in diastolic blood pressure plotted against the average of the initial and final readings, The correlation is attenuated to -0.19, suggesting little or no relationship between $BP_2 - BP_1$ and blood pressure.

CHAPTER 37

Measures of association and impact

37.1 INTRODUCTION

In this chapter we focus on the different measures that are used to assess the **impact** of an exposure or of a treatment on the amount of disease in a **population**. We start by summarizing the three different ratio measures of the association between an exposure (or treatment) and outcome, used throughout the book, and show how these relate to measures of impact.

37.2 MEASURES OF ASSOCIATION

Table 37.1 summarizes the three ratio measures that we use to assess the strength of the association between an exposure (or treatment) and an outcome. These are the risk ratio, the rate ratio and the odds ratio.

Risk ratios

A risk ratio > 1 implies that the risk of disease is higher in the exposed group than in the unexposed group, while a risk ratio < 1 occurs when the risk is lower in the exposed group, suggesting that exposure may be protective. A risk ratio of 1 occurs when the risks are the same in the two groups and is equivalent to no association between the exposure and the disease. The further the risk ratio is from 1, the stronger the association. See Chapter 16 for methods to derive confidence intervals for the RR.

Table 37.1 Summary of ratio measures of the association between exposure and disease, and the different study designs in which they can be estimated.

Definitions of different ratio measures	Study design(s) in which they can be estimated			
	Longitudinal (complete follow-up)	Longitudinal (incomplete follow-up)	Cross-sectional	Case–control
Risk ratio = $\dfrac{\text{risk in exposed group}}{\text{risk in unexposed group}}$	Yes	No	Yes	No
Rate ratio = $\dfrac{\text{rate in exposed group}}{\text{rate in unexposed group}}$	Yes	Yes	No	No
Odds ratio = $\dfrac{\text{odds in exposed group}}{\text{odds in unexposed group}}$	Yes	No	Yes	Yes

Odds ratios

Interpretation of odds ratios is the same as that for risk ratios (see above), but the odds ratio is always further away from 1 than the corresponding risk ratio. Thus:

- if $RR > 1$ then $OR > RR$;
- if $RR < 1$ then $OR < RR$.

For a rare outcome (one in which the probability of the event not occurring is close to 1) the odds ratio is approximately equal to the risk ratio (since the odds is approximately equal to the risk).

Rate ratios

While the calculation of the risk is based on the population at risk at the start of the study, the rate is based on the total person-years at risk during the study and reflects the changing population at risk. This was illustrated for a cohort study in Figure 22.2. When the outcome is not rare, the risk ratio will change over time, so that the rate ratio (providing that it is constant over time) may be a more appropriate measure of the association between exposure and disease. In particular, if all subjects experience the disease outcome by the end of the study, then the risk ratio will be 1 even if the time to event was much greater in the exposed than the unexposed group (or vice versa).

Comparison of the rate ratio, risk ratio and odds ratio

It was shown in Chapters 16 and 23 that for a rare outcome

$$\text{Risk} \approx \text{Odds} \approx \text{Rate} \times \text{Time}$$

so that
$$\text{Risk ratio} \approx \text{Odds ratio} \approx \text{Rate ratio}$$

For a **common disease**, however, the *three measures are different*, and will lead to three different measures of association between exposure and disease. The preferred choice in longitudinal studies is to use rate ratios (or hazard ratios when data on times to event occurrences are available and disease rates change over time: see Chapter 26). The rate ratio is the only choice when follow-up is incomplete, or individuals are followed for differing lengths of time. The use of risk ratios is more appropriate, however, when assessing the protective effect of an exposure or intervention, such as a vaccine, which it is believed offers full protection to some individuals but none to others, rather than partial protection to all (Smith *et al.*, 1984).

The risk ratio and odds ratio can both be estimated from longitudinal studies with complete follow-up and from cross-sectional studies. Although the risk ratio would generally be regarded as more easily interpretable than the odds ratio, the odds ratio is often used because the statistical properties of procedures based on the odds ratio are generally better. In case–control studies the odds ratio is always used as the measure of effect.

37.3 MEASURES OF THE IMPACT OF AN EXPOSURE

We now show how ratio measures (of the strength of the association between exposure and disease) relate to measures of the impact of exposure. The formulae we present apply identically whether risks or rates are used.

Attributable risk

The risk ratio assesses how much more likely, for example, a smoker is to develop lung cancer than a non-smoker, but it gives no indication of the magnitude of the excess risk in absolute terms. This is measured by the **attributable risk**:

> Attributable risk (AR) = risk among exposed − risk among unexposed
> = the **risk difference** (see Section 16.3)

Example 37.1

Table 37.2 shows hypothetical data from a cohort study to investigate the association between smoking and lung cancer. Thirty-thousand smokers and 60 000 non-smokers were followed for a year, during which time 39 of the smokers and six of the non-smokers developed lung cancer. Thus the risk ratio was:

Table 37.2 Hypothetical data from a one year cohort study to investigate the association between smoking and lung cancer. The calculations of relative and attributable risk are illustrated.

	Lung cancer	No lung cancer	Total	One year risk
Smokers	39	29 961	30 000	1.30/1000
Non-smokers	6	59 994	60 000	0.10/1000
Total	45	89 955	90 000	
$RR = \frac{1.30}{0.10} = 13.0$		$AR = 1.30 - 0.10 = 1.20/1000$	$Prop\ AR = \frac{1.20}{1.30} = 0.923$ or 92.3 %	

$$RR = \frac{39/30000}{6/60000} = \frac{1.30}{0.10} = 13.0$$

so that there was a very strong association between smoking and lung cancer. The attributable risk of lung cancer due to smoking, given by the difference between the risks among smokers and non-smokers, was:

$$AR = 1.30 - 0.10 = 1.20 \text{ cases per } 1000 \text{ per year}$$

Attributable risk is sometimes expressed as a proportion (or percentage) of the total incidence rate among the exposed, and is then called the **proportional attributable risk**, the attributable proportion (exposed), the attributable fraction (exposed) or the **aetiologic fraction (exposed)**.

$$\text{Proportional AR} = \frac{\text{risk among exposed} - \text{risk among unexposed}}{\text{risk among exposed}}$$
$$= \frac{(RR - 1)}{RR}$$

In the example, the proportional attributable risk was $1.20/1.30 = 0.923$, suggesting that smoking accounted for 92.3 % of all the cases of lung cancer among the smokers.

Comparing attributable and relative measures

Example 37.2

Table 37.3 shows the relative and attributable rates of death from selected causes associated with heavy cigarette smoking. The association has been most clearly demonstrated for lung cancer and chronic bronchitis, with rate ratios of 32.4 and 21.2 respectively. If, however, the association with cardiovascular disease,

Table 37.3 Relative and attributable rates of death from selected causes, 1951–1961, associated with heavy cigarette smoking by British male physicians. Data from Doll & Hill (1964) *British Medical Journal* 1, 1399–1410, as presented by MacMahon & Pugh (1970) *Epidemiology – Principles and Methods*. Little, Brown & Co., Boston (with permission).

Cause of death	Age-standardized death rate (per 1000 person-years)		RR	AR
	Non-smokers	Heavy smokers		
Lung cancer	0.07	2.27	32.4	2.20
Other cancers	1.91	2.59	1.4	0.68
Chronic bronchitis	0.05	1.06	21.2	1.01
Cardiovascular disease	7.32	9.93	1.4	2.61
All causes	12.06	19.67	1.6	7.61

although not so strong, is also accepted as being causal, elimination of smoking would save even more deaths due to cardiovascular disease than due to lung cancer: 2.61 compared to 2.20 for every 1000 smoker-years at risk. Note that the death rates were age standardized to take account of the differing age distributions of smokers and non-smokers, and of the increase in death rates with age (see Chapter 25).

In summary, the risk (or rate) ratio measures the strength of an association between an exposure and a disease outcome. The attributable risk (or rate), on the other hand, gives a better idea of the excess risk of disease experienced by an individual as the result of being exposed.

Population attributable risk

It is important to realize that the overall impact of an exposure on disease in the population also depends on how prevalent the exposure is. In population terms a rare exposure with a high associated risk ratio may be less serious in the total number (or proportion) of deaths that it will cause than a very common exposure with a lower associated risk ratio. The impact at the population level is assessed by the excess overall risk (or rate) in the population as compared with the risk (or rate) among the unexposed. The resulting measure is the **population attributable risk**:

Population AR = overall risk − risk among unexposed

This may also be expressed as a proportion (or percentage) of the overall risk. The resulting measure is the **population proportional attributable risk**, alternatively named the **aetiologic fraction (population)** or the attributable fraction (population).

$$\text{Population proportional AR} = \frac{\text{overall risk} - \text{risk among unexposed}}{\text{overall risk}}$$
$$= \frac{\text{prevalence}_{\text{exposure}}(\text{RR} - 1)}{1 + \text{prevalence}_{\text{exposure}}(\text{RR} - 1)}$$

Figure 37.1 shows how the value of the population proportional attributable risk increases independently with the prevalence of the exposure and with the size of the risk ratio. If all the population are exposed (prevalence $= 100\%$), then the value of the population proportional attributable risk is the same as the proportional AR (exposed) defined above.

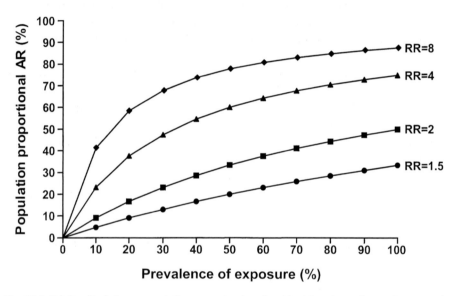

Fig. 37.1 Relationship between population proportional attributable risk and prevalence of exposure for various values of the risk ratio.

Potential impact of reducing prevalence of exposure

The population attributable and proportional attributable risks give a measure of the burden of disease in the population associated with a particular exposure. They also give a measure of the impact that would be achieved by a totally successful intervention which managed to eliminate the exposure. This is a theoretical maximum impact that is unlikely to be realized in practice. For example, it is unlikely that any approach to control smoking would result in all smokers giving up. If the intervention *reduces* the prevalence of exposure by $r\%$, then the actual impact will be as follows:

$$\text{Percentage impact} = r\% \times \text{Population proportional AR}$$

Example 37.3

Figure 37.2 illustrates the difference between potential impact and population proportional attributable risk in a hypothetical population of 1000 children, followed for one year without loss to follow-up. There are 400 children exposed to a risk factor that is associated with a three-fold risk of death, and 600 children who are not exposed. The 600 children in the unexposed group experience a mortality rate of 50/1000/year which means that $600 \times 50/1000 = 30$ of them will die during the year. If the 400 children in the exposed group were at the same risk as the unexposed children, then $400 \times 50/1000 = 20$ of them would die. However, they are at 3 times this risk. Their mortality rate is therefore 150/child/year, which translates into $400 \times 150/1000 = 60$ deaths during the year, an excess of 40 deaths associated with exposure. Thus if it were possible to eliminate exposure to the risk factor, the total number of deaths per year would be reduced by 40, giving a total of 50 rather than 90 deaths a year. The population proportional attributable risk, which is the percentage of deaths attributable to exposure, equals 40/90, or 44%.

Suppose now that an intervention took place which successfully reduced the prevalence of exposure by one half, that is from 40% to 20%. The right hand panel in Figure 37.2 shows that there would then be 70 deaths a year. As the size of the exposed group would be halved, the number of excess deaths

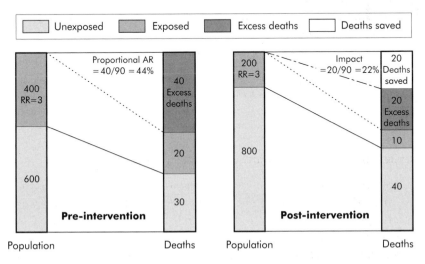

Fig. 37.2 Example showing potential impact of an intervention, assuming (i) 40% of population exposed pre-intervention, (ii) RR associated with exposure equals 3, (iii) mortality rate among unexposed equals 50/1000/year, and (iv) the intervention reduces the prevalence of exposure by 50%.

would also be halved, and would now be 20 rather than 40. Such an intervention would therefore prevent 20 of the pre-intervention total of 90 deaths. That is, its impact would be 20/90, or 22%.

37.4 MEASURES OF THE IMPACT OF A TREATMENT OR INTERVENTION

Efficacy

The **efficacy** of a treatment or intervention is measured by the proportion of cases that it prevents. Efficacy is directly calculated from the risk ratio (or rate ratio) comparing disease outcome in the treated versus control group. For a successful treatment (or intervention) this ratio will be less than 1.

$$\text{Efficacy} = 1 - \text{RR}$$

Example 37.4

Table 37.4 shows the *hypothetical* results from a randomized controlled trial of a new influenza vaccine. A total of 80 cases of influenza occurred in the placebo group. If this group had instead received vaccination one would have expected only 8.3% (the rate experienced by the vaccinated group) of them to have developed influenza, that is $220 \times 0.083 = 18.3$ cases. The saving would therefore have been $80 - 18.3 = 61.7$ cases, giving an efficacy of $61.7/80 = 77.2\%$.

The efficacy can be calculated directly from the risk ratio, which gives the risk in the vaccinated group as a proportion of the risk in the control group. If the vaccination had no effect, the risks would be the same and the risk ratio would equal 1. In this case, the risk is considerably lower in the vaccine group. The risk ratio equals 0.228, considerably less than 1. In other words the risk of influenza in the vaccine group is only 0.228 or 22.8% of that in the placebo group. The vaccine has therefore prevented 77.2% of influenza cases.

Table 37.4 Results from an influenza vaccine trial, previously presented in Table 16.2.

	Influenza		
	Yes	No	Total
Vaccine	20 (8.3%)	220 (91.7%)	240
Placebo	80 (36.4%)	140 (63.6%)	220
Total	100 (21.7%)	360 (78.3%)	460

$$\text{RR} = \frac{20/240}{80/220} = \frac{0.083}{0.364} = 0.228; \quad \text{Efficacy} = 1 - 0.228 = 0.772, \text{ or } 77.2\%$$

The **confidence interval for efficacy** is calculated from the confidence interval for risk ratio, as follows. Recall from Section 16.5 that:

$$95\% \text{ CI (RR)} = RR/EF \text{ to } RR \times EF,$$
$$\text{where } EF = \exp[1.96 \times \text{s.e.}(\log RR)]$$
$$\text{and s.e.}(\log RR) = \sqrt{[(1/d_1 - 1/n_1) + (1/d_0 - 1/n_0)]}$$

Since efficacy equals one minus RR, its 95% confidence interval is obtained by subtracting each of the RR confidence limits from one.

$$95\% \text{ CI (Efficacy)} = 1 - RR \times EF \text{ to } 1 - RR/EF$$

Note that the lower efficacy limit is obtained from the upper RR limit, and the upper efficacy limit from the lower RR limit. In this example:

$$\text{s.e.}(\log RR) = \sqrt{[(1/20 - 1/240) + (1/80 - 1/220)]} = 0.2319$$
$$EF = \exp(1.96 \times 0.2319) = \exp(0.4546) = 1.5755$$
$$95\% \text{ CI (RR)} = RR/EF \text{ to } RR \times EF = 0.228/1.5755 \text{ to } 0.228 \times 1.5755$$
$$= 0.145 \text{ to } 0.359$$

$$95\% \text{ CI (Efficacy)} = 1 - RR \times EF \text{ to } 1 - RR/EF = 1 - 0.359 \text{ to } 1 - 0.145$$
$$= 0.641 \text{ to } 0.855$$

Thus the 95% confidence interval for the efficacy of this influenza vaccine is from 64.1% to 85.5%.

Number needed to treat

An additional way of measuring the impact of treatment, which has become popular in recent years, is the **number needed to treat** (NNT). This is the number of patients who we must treat in order to prevent one adverse event. It is defined as:

$$\text{Number needed to treat (NNT)} = \frac{1}{|\text{risk difference}|}$$

The vertical bars in the formula mean the *absolute* value of the risk difference, that is the size of the risk difference ignoring its sign. NNT is best used to illustrate the likely impact of treatment given a range of possible risks of the outcome event in the treated population.

Example 37.5

Consider the effect of a new treatment that reduces the risk of death following myocardial infarction by 25% (risk ratio $=0.75$). The impact of using such a treatment will depend on the frequency of death following myocardial infarction. This is illustrated in Table 37.5, which shows that if the risk of death is 0.5 then 125 lives will be saved by treating 1000 patients with the new treatment, while if this risk of death is 0.02 then only five lives will be saved. The reduction in the number of deaths is simply the risk difference multiplied by the number of patients (risk difference = risk of event in treated patients minus risk of event in control patients). Therefore the risk difference measures the impact of treatment in *reducing* the risk of an adverse event in the same way that the attributable risk measures the impact of exposure in *increasing* the risk of an adverse event.

The values of the NNT are also shown in the table. When the risk of death in the absence of treatment is 0.5, the NNT equals $1/0.125 = 8$. Thus we will prevent one death for every eight patients treated. If, on the other hand, the risk of death in the absence of treatment is only 0.02, the NNT equals $1/0.005 = 200$, meaning that we will prevent one death for every 200 patients treated.

Table 37.5 Number of deaths in 1000 patients suffering a myocardial infarction according to whether a new treatment is used, assuming different risks of death in the absence of the new treatment and a treatment risk ratio of 0.75.

Risk of death			Number of deaths			
Current treatment (a)	New treatment (b) = 0.75 × (a)	Risk difference (c) = (b) − (a)	Current treatment (d) = 1000 × (a)	New treatment (e) = 1000 × (b)	Reduction in number of deaths (f) = (d) − (e)	NNT (g) = 1/|(c)|
0.5	0.375	−0.125	500	375	125	8
0.1	0.075	−0.025	100	75	25	40
0.02	0.015	−0.005	20	15	5	200

Number needed to harm

It is important to distinguish between beneficial effects of a treatment (risk ratio <1, risk difference <0) and harmful effects (risk ratio >1, risk difference >0). If the treatment is harmful then the NNT is referred to as the **number needed to harm** (NNH). This can be useful to assess the adverse impact of a treatment which has known side effects. For example, if our treatment for myocardial infarction was known to increase the risk of stroke, we might compare the number of patients treated to cause one stroke (NNH) with the number of patients treated to prevent one death (NNT).

Note that if the treatment has no effect (risk ratio $= 1$, risk difference $= 0$) then the NNT is $1/0 = \infty$ (infinity). This has a sensible interpretation: if the treatment is ineffective then we will not prevent any outcome events however many patients we treat. However problems can arise when deriving confidence intervals for the NNT, if one limit of the CI is close to the point of no treatment effect.

37.5 ESTIMATES OF ASSOCIATION AND IMPACT FROM MULTIVARIABLE ANALYSES

In most circumstances, multivariable analyses are based on ratio measures of the effect of exposure or treatment. This is because, both on theoretical grounds and on the basis of experience, the assumption of no interaction between the exposure and confounding variables is more likely to hold (at least approximately) for ratio measures. In the context of randomized trials, there is good empirical evidence that meta-analyses based on risk differences tend to be more heterogeneous than meta-analyses based on risk ratios or odds ratios (see Engels *et al.*, 2000; or Egger *et al.*, 2001, pages 313–335).

It is therefore usually sensible to derive a *ratio* estimate of the strength of association in a multivariable analysis of an observational study or meta-analysis of randomized trials, whatever measure of impact is required. Estimates of NNT or NNH are then derived by considering a range of levels of risk in the unexposed group, and/or prevalence of exposure.

CHAPTER 38

Strategies for analysis

38.1 INTRODUCTION

It is essential to plan and conduct statistical analyses in a way that maximizes the quality and interpretability of the findings. In a typical study, data are collected on a large number of variables and it can be difficult to decide which methods to use and in what order. In this final chapter we present general guidelines on strategies for data analysis.

38.2 ANALYSIS PLAN

The formulation of a written plan for analysis is recommended. The extent to which it is possible to plan analyses in detail will depend on the type of study being analysed:

- For a randomized controlled trial (RCT), which by its nature addresses a set of clearly defined questions, the analysis plan is usually specified in detail. It will include the precise definition of primary and secondary outcomes, the statistical method to be used, guidelines on whether to adjust for baseline variables and, possibly, a small number of planned subgroup analyses. See Section 34.2 for a description of the analysis of RCTs.
- For an observational study, which is exploratory in nature, it is often not possible to completely specify a plan for the analysis. However it is helpful to write down, in advance, the main hypothesis or hypotheses to be addressed. This will include the definitions of the outcome and exposure variables that will be needed to answer these question(s), the variables thought a priori to be possible confounders of the exposure–outcome association(s) and a small number of possible effect modifiers.

Well-written analysis plans both serve as a guide for the person conducting the analysis and, equally importantly, aid the interpretation and reporting of results. For example, if we find evidence of a subgroup effect (interaction) we should report whether this was specified *a priori* or whether it is an unexpected finding.

38.3 DATA CHECKING

Careful checking and editing of the data set are essential before statistical analysis commences. The first step is to examine the distribution of each of the variables to check for possible errors. For categorical variables, this means checking that all observations relate to allowed categories, and that the frequencies in each category make sense. For numerical variables, **range checks** should be performed to search for values falling outside the expected range. Histograms can also be used to look for '**outliers**' that look extreme relative to the rest of the data.

The next step is to conduct **consistency checks**, to search for cases where two or more variables are inconsistent. For example, if sex and parity are recorded, a cross-classification of the two can be used to check that no males were recorded with a parity of one or more. Scatter plots can be useful for checking the consistency of numerical variables, for example of weight against age, or weight against height. Further outliers can be detected in this way.

Possible errors should be checked against the original records. In some cases it may be possible to correct the data. In other cases, it may be necessary to insert a missing value code if it is certain that the data were in error (for example an impossible birth weight). In borderline cases, where an observation is an outlier but not considered impossible, it is generally better to leave the data unchanged. Strictly speaking, the analysis should then be checked to ensure that the conclusions are not affected unduly by the extreme values (either using sensitivity analyses in which the extreme values are excluded, or by examining influence statistics; see Section 12.3). Note that when numerical values are grouped into categories before analysis, a small number of outliers are unlikely to have a marked influence on the results.

For studies in which individuals are classified as with and without disease, checks should generally be made separately in the two groups, as the distributions may be quite different.

38.4 INITIAL ANALYSES

Descriptive analysis

Once the data have been cleaned as thoroughly as possible, the distributions of each of the variables should be re-examined (see Chapter 3), both (i) as a final check that required corrections have been made, and (ii) to gain an understanding of the characteristics of the study population. Individuals with and without disease should again be examined separately.

Specifying variables for analysis

In addressing a particular question we will need to specify both the *outcome variable* and the *exposure variable* or variables (see Section 2.4). In observational studies, the control of confounding (see Chapter 18) is a key issue in the analysis, and so we should identify:

1 variables believed in advance to confound the exposure–outcome association (*a priori* confounders); and
2 other variables to be investigated as possible confounders, since a plausible argument can be made concerning their relationship with the exposure and outcome variables, but for which there is little or no existing evidence.

We should also specify any variables considered to be possible *effect-modifiers*: in that they modify the size or even the direction of the exposure–outcome association. As described in Sections 18.4 and 29.5, effect modification is examined using tests for interaction.

In practice, variables may play more than one role in an analysis. For example, a variable may confound the effect of one of the main exposures of interest, but its effect may also be of interest in its own right. A variable may be a confounder for one exposure variable and an effect-modifier for another. Many studies have an exploratory element, in that data are collected on some variables which may turn out to be important exposures, but if they do not they may still need to be considered as potential confounders or effect-modifiers.

Data reduction

Before commencing formal statistical analyses, it may be necessary to derive new variables by *grouping* the values of some of the original variables, as explained in Section 2.3. Note that *the original variables should always be retained in the dataset*; they should never be overwritten.

Grouping of *categorical* exposure variables is necessary when there are large numbers of categories (for example, if occupation is recorded in detail). If there is an *unexposed* category, then this should generally be treated as a separate group (e.g. non-smokers). The *exposed* categories should be divided into several groups; four or five is usually sufficient to give a reasonable picture of the risk relationship.

Grouping of *numerical* exposure variables may be necessary in order to:

1 use methods based on stratification (see Chapters 18 and 23), as recommended for the initial examination of confounding (see below);
2 use graphical methods to examine how the level of a non-numerical outcome changes with exposure level (see Section 29.6); and
3 to examine whether there is a linear association between a numerical *exposure* variable and a non-numerical outcome (see Section 29.6).

Note that grouping entails *loss of information*: after checking linearity assumptions or performing initial analyses using the grouped variable it may be appropriate to use the original variable, or a transformation of the original variable (see Chapter 13), in the final analysis.

One strategy for numerical exposures is to divide the range of the variable using, say, quintiles, to give five groups with equal numbers of subjects in each group. This helps to ensure that estimates of effect for each category are reasonably precise, but can sometimes obscure an important effect if a few subjects with very high levels are grouped with others with more moderate levels. Alternatively, cut-off points may be chosen on the basis of data from previous studies, the aim being to define categories within which there is thought to be relatively little variation in risk. Using standard cut-off points has the advantage of making comparisons between studies easier. For example, Table 38.1 shows the different possibilities for including body mass index (BMI), defined as weight/(height^2), in an analysis to examine its association with a disease outcome.

For variables included in the analysis as *confounders*, three or four categories may be sufficient to remove most of the confounding. However, more categories will be needed if the confounding is strong, as would often be the case with age, for example. It is often necessary to examine the strength of the association between the potential confounder and the outcome variable before deciding on the number of categories to be used in analysis. The weaker the association, the more one may combine groups. However it would be unwise to combine groups with very different risks or rates of disease.

A further consideration is that for analyses of binary or time-to-event outcomes, groups in which there are no, or very few, outcome events must be combined with others before inclusion in analysis.

Table 38.1 Possible ways of deriving variables based on measured body mass index (BMI).

Choice
(i) Original variable
(ii) A transformation of the original variable (for example log BMI)
(iii) Quintiles of BMI, coded 1–5
(iv) Quintiles of BMI, coded as the median BMI in each quintile
(v) Standard cut-offs for BMI focusing on high levels of BMI as risky (<25 = normal; 25–30 = overweight; ≥ 30 = obese)
(vi) Standard cut-offs including an underweight group (<20 = underweight; 20–25 = normal; 25–30 = overweight; ≥ 30 = obese)

Univariable analyses

It is usually helpful to begin with a univariable analysis, in which we examine the association of the outcome with each exposure of interest, ignoring all other variables. This is often called the **crude association** between the exposure and the outcome. Although later analyses, controlling for the effects of other variables, will supersede this one, it is still a useful stage of the analysis because:

1 Examination of simple tables or graphs, as well as the estimated association, can give useful information about the data set. For example, it can show that there were very few observations, or very few outcome events, in particular exposure categories.

2 These analyses will give an initial idea of those variables that are strongly related to the disease outcome.

3 The degree to which the crude estimate of effect is altered when we control for the confounding effects of other variables is a useful indication of the amount of confounding present (or at least, the amount that has been measured and successfully removed).

For exposures with more than two levels, one of the levels has to be chosen as the baseline (see Section 19.2). Often this will be the *unexposed group* or, if everyone is exposed to some extent, the group with the lowest level of exposure. If there are very few persons in this group, however, this will produce exposure effect estimates with large standard errors. It is then preferable to choose a larger group to be the baseline group.

38.5 ALLOWING FOR CONFOUNDING

This section should be read in conjunction with Section 29.8, which describes general issues in the choice of exposure variables for inclusion in a regression model.

In any observational study, the control of confounding effects will be a major focus of the analysis. We have two tools available for this task: classical (Mantel–Haenszel) methods based on stratification, and regression modelling. We have emphasized the similarities between the two approaches (see Chapters 20 and 24), so they should not be seen as in conflict. Regression methods *controlling* for the effect of a categorical variable involve exactly the same assumptions, and hence give essentially the same results, as Mantel–Haenszel methods *stratifying* on the categorical variable.

A major reason for using classical methods in the initial phase of the analysis is that the output encourages us to examine the exposure–outcome association in each stratum, together with the evidence for interaction (effect modification). In contrast, it is easy to use regression models without checking the assumption that there is no interaction between the effects of the different variables in the model.

However, regression models are generally the best approach when we wish to control for the effects of a number of confounding variables, because stratifying on the cross-classification of all the confounders is likely to produce a large number of strata. As explained in Section 29.5, by assuming in regression models that there is no interaction between the effects of confounding variables, we can greatly reduce the number of strata (the number of parameters used to model the effect of the confounders). In addition, dose–response effects can be examined more flexibly in regression models (see Section 29.6).

The need for external knowledge in assessment of confounding

As explained in Chapter 18, a confounding variable, C, is one that is associated with both the exposure variable (E) and the outcome variable (D), and is not on the part of the causal chain leading from E to D. It is important to realize that *external knowledge is more important than statistical strategies* in choosing appropriate confounders to be controlled for in examining a particular exposure–outcome association. *This is because statistical associations in the data cannot, on their own, determine whether it is appropriate to control for the effects of a particular variable.*

Example 38.1

In their article on the appropriate control of confounding in studies of the epidemiology of birth defects, Hernán *et al.* (2002) considered the following example. Should we control for C, a binary variable which records the event that the pregnancy ended in stillbirth or therapeutic abortion, when examining the association between folic acid supplementation in early pregnancy (the exposure variable, E) and the risk of neural tube defects (the outcome, D) using data from a case–control study? They pointed out that controlling for C would *not* be the correct analysis, although:

1 controlling for the effect of C leads to a substantial change in the estimated association between E and D; and
2 C is strongly associated with both E and D, and is not on the causal pathway between them.

The reason is that C is affected by both E and D, rather than having any influence on either of them. Therefore C, in this instance, cannot confound the E–D association. Yet it is not uncommon to find epidemiological analyses controlling for C in situations such as this. Note that restricting the analysis to live births (i.e. considering only one of the strata defined by C) will also produce a biased estimate of the E–D association in this situation.

This example shows that careful consideration of the likely *direction of associations* between E, D and C is required in order to decide whether it is appropriate to control for C in estimating the E–D association. Figure 38.1 gives examples of circumstances in which C will and will not confound the E–D association.

Example 38.2

Because of the frequent introduction of new antiretroviral drugs for treatment of HIV-infected persons, and the large number of different possible combinations of these, many relevant questions about the effect of different drugs or drug combinations have not been addressed in randomized trials with 'hard' outcomes such as development of AIDS or death. There is therefore great interest in using longitudinal studies of HIV-infected individuals to address these questions.

Consider a comparison of drug regimens A and B. Because antiretroviral therapy may involve taking a large number of pills per day, and may have serious

(a) Situations in which C is a confounder for the E-D association.
(◄─►) non-causal association; (──►) causal association.

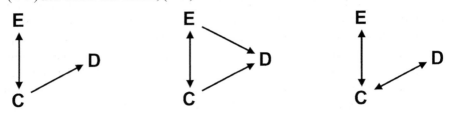

(b) Situations in which C is not a confounder for the E-D association.

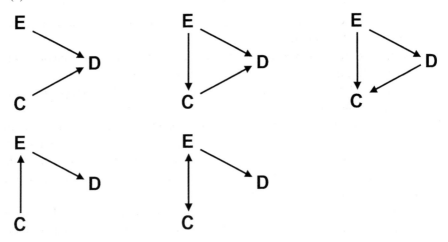

Fig. 38.1 Circumstances in which C will and will not confound an exposure–disease (E–D) association. (Adapted from *Case Control Studies MEB2* by James J. Schlesselman, copyright 1982 by Oxford University Press, Inc., with permission.)

side-effects, adherence to the prescribed regime is likely to be associated both with the probability of progressing to AIDS (D) and with the drug regimen (E). However, in this example *the drug regimen used is likely to influence adherence to therapy*. It would not, therefore, be appropriate to control for adherence in estimating the E–D association, as it will be on the pathway between them.

Example 38.3
The 'fetal origins' hypothesis suggests that there are associations between prenatal growth, reflected in measures such as birthweight, and adult heart disease. Huxley *et al.* (2002) reviewed 55 studies that had reported associations between birthweight (exposure) and later systolic blood pressure (outcome). Almost all of the reported regression coefficients were adjusted for adult weight. However, these need to be interpreted with caution since adult weight is on the causal pathway between birthweight and blood pressure. Removing the adjustment for adult weight, in 12 studies, halved the size of the estimated association.

Choosing confounders

Taking into account the need to combine external knowledge with statistical associations, we recommend the following strategy for choosing confounders:

1 Formulating a conceptual, hierarchical framework for the relationships between the different variables and the disease outcome is strongly recommended, as described by Victora *et al.* (1997) in the context of determinants of childhood diarrhoea mortality. This is particularly useful both as a way of summarizing existing knowledge and for clarifying the direction of any associations.

2 As a general rule, variables that are known *a priori* to be important confounders, based on previous work should be controlled for in the analysis.

3 In addition, other possible confounders may be selected as a result of exploratory analysis. This should be:
   • restricted to variables that are associated with *both* the outcome and exposure, and are not on the causal pathway between them;
   • based on both the data being analysed and external knowledge, and after careful consideration of the direction of associations.

4 Note, however, that for **multiple linear regression**, *all* exposure variables that are clearly associated with the outcome should be included when estimating the effect of a particular exposure, *whether or not they are confounders* (with the exception that variables on the causal pathway between the exposure of interest and the outcome should *not* be included; see Section 29.8).

5 Note also that automated 'stepwise' regression procedures are unlikely to be appropriate in analyses whose aim is to estimate the effect of particular exposures (see Section 29.8).

38.6 ANALYSING FOR INTERACTIONS

Three sorts of interaction may be distinguished:

1 *Interaction between confounders.* The main difference between regression models and classical methods is that classical methods always allow for all interactions between confounders. This is in fact usually unnecessary.

2 *Interaction between a confounder and an exposure of interest.* Strictly speaking, the calculation of exposure effect estimates controlled for confounding variables is appropriate only if the exposure effect is the same for all levels of the confounder. In practice, of course, the effect will vary to at least some extent between strata; in other words there is likely to be some interaction between the exposure and the confounders controlled for in the analysis. In the presence of substantial interaction, the stratum-specific effects of the exposure should be reported.

3 *Interaction between exposures of interest.* If present, this may be of importance both for the scientific interpretation of an analysis and for its implications for preventive intervention.

An exhaustive search for interactions with all possible variables, however, is unlikely to be useful. Formal tests for interaction lack power, and statistically significant interactions identified by a systematic sweep of all variables may well be chance effects, while real interactions may go undetected. Sample sizes are typically inadequate to have high power of detecting any but the strongest interactions (see Section 35.4). Combining groups in the interaction parameter may increase the power of tests for interaction (see Section 29.5).

The purpose of a statistical analysis is to provide a simplified but useful picture of reality. If weak interactions are present, this is probably of little intrinsic interest, and the calculation of an overall pooled estimate of effect for an individual exposure is a reasonable approximation to the truth.

For these reasons, we suggest delaying analysis for interactions to the final analysis. Exposure–exposure and exposure–confounder interactions should then be examined, paying particular attention to those thought *a priori* to be worth investigation. These should be examined one at a time, to avoid a model with too many additional parameters. In assessing the evidence for interactions, as much attention should be paid to the presence of meaningful trends in effect estimates over the strata, as to the results of formal tests for interaction.

38.7 MAKING ANALYSES REPRODUCIBLE

In the early stages of a statistical analysis it is useful to work *interactively* with the computer, by trying a command, looking at the output, then correcting or refining the command before proceeding to the next command. However, we recommend that all analyses should eventually be done using files (programs) containing lists of commands.

It is usually the case that, after analyses are first thought to be complete, changes are found to be necessary. For example, more data may arrive, or corrections may be made, or it may be discovered that an important confounder has been omitted. This often means that the whole analysis must be performed again. If analyses were performed interactively, this can be a daunting task. The solution is to ensure that the whole analysis can be performed by running a series of programs.

A typical series of programs is illustrated in Table 38.2. We strongly recommend that you add frequent comment statements to your programs, which explain what is being done in each section; especially in complicated or long programs. This is useful for other members of the project team, and also invaluable when returning to your own program some time later to rerun it or to modify it for a new analysis. It is also important to *document* the analysis by recording the function of each program file, and the order in which they should be run.

Following this strategy has two important consequences. Firstly, it will now be straightforward to reproduce the entire analysis after corrections are made to the raw data. Secondly, you will always be able to check exactly how a derived variable was coded, which confounders were included in a particular analysis,

Table 38.2 Typical sequence of programs to perform the analyses needed to analyse a particular exposure–outcome association.

Program 1:	Read the raw data file into the statistical package, label variables so that it is easy to identify them, check that they have the correct value ranges, check consistency between variables, create derived variables by recoding and combining variables, save the resulting dataset
Program 2:	Use the new dataset to examine associations between the outcome variable and the exposures and confounders of interest, by producing appropriate graphs and tables and performing univariable analyses
Program 3:	Use Mantel–Haenszel and regression analyses to estimate exposure effects controlled for potential confounders
Program 4:	Examine interactions between exposures and between exposures and confounders
Program 5:	Produce final tables for the research report

and so on. Remember that reviewers' comments on a draft manuscript that was submitted for publication tend to be received many months after the paper was submitted (and even longer after the analysis was done). Minor modifications to the analysis will be straightforward if the analysis is reproducible, but can waste huge amounts of time if it is not.

38.8 COMMON PITFALLS IN ANALYSIS AND INTERPRETATION

Even when the analyses of primary interest are specified at the start of the study, a typical analysis will involve choices of variable groupings and modelling strategies that can make important differences to the conclusions. Further, it is common to investigate possible associations that were not specified in advance, for example if they were only recently reported. Three important reasons for caution in interpreting the results of analyses are:

1 **Multiple comparisons**. Even if there is no association between the exposure and outcome variables, we would expect one in twenty comparisons to be statistically significant at the 5 % level. Thus the interpretation of associations in a study in which the effect of many exposures was measured should be much more cautious than that for a study in which a specific a priori hypothesis was specified. Searching for all possible associations with an outcome variable is known as 'data-dredging' and may lead to dramatic but spurious findings.

2 **Subgroup analyses**. We should be particularly cautious about the interpretation of apparent associations in subgroups of the data, particularly where there is no convincing evidence of an overall association (see Section 34.2). It is extremely tempting to emphasize an 'interesting' finding in an otherwise negative study.

3 **Data-driven comparisons**. A related problem is that we should not group an exposure variable in order to produce the biggest possible association with the outcome, and then interpret the P-value as if this had always been the intended comparison. For example, when rearranging ten age groups into two larger

groups, we could compare 1 with 2–10 or 1 and 2 with 3–10 and so on. If we choose a particular grouping out of these nine possible ones because it shows the largest difference between 'younger' and 'older' individuals, then we have chosen the smallest P-value from nine possible ones. It is sensible to decide how variables will be grouped as far as possible before seeing how different groupings affect the conclusions of your study.

These problems *do not* mean that all studies must have hypotheses and methods of analysis that are specified at the outset. However, the interpretation of a finding will be affected by its context. If a reported association is one of fifty which were examined, this should be clearly stated when the research is reported. We would probably view such an association (even with a small P-value) as generating a hypothesis that might be tested in future studies, rather than as a definitive result.

38.9 CONCLUSIONS

In all but the simplest studies, there is no single 'correct' analysis or answer. Fast computers and excellent statistical software mean that it is easy to produce statistical analyses. The challenge to medical statisticians is to produce analyses that answer the research question as clearly and honestly as possible.

APPENDIX

STATISTICAL TABLES

Table A1 Areas in tail of the standard normal distribution.

Adapted from Table 3 of White et al. (1979) with permission of the authors and publishers.

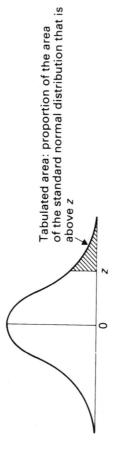

Tabulated area: proportion of the area of the standard normal distribution that is above z

Second decimal place of z

z	0.00	0.01	0.02	0.03	0.04	0.05	0.06	0.07	0.08	0.09
0.0	0.5000	0.4960	0.4920	0.4880	0.4840	0.4801	0.4761	0.4721	0.4681	0.4641
0.1	0.4602	0.4562	0.4522	0.4483	0.4443	0.4404	0.4364	0.4325	0.4286	0.4247
0.2	0.4207	0.4168	0.4129	0.4090	0.4052	0.4013	0.3974	0.3936	0.3897	0.3859
0.3	0.3821	0.3783	0.3745	0.3707	0.3669	0.3632	0.3594	0.3557	0.3520	0.3483
0.4	0.3446	0.3409	0.3372	0.3336	0.3300	0.3264	0.3228	0.3192	0.3156	0.3121
0.5	0.3085	0.3050	0.3015	0.2981	0.2946	0.2912	0.2877	0.2843	0.2810	0.2776
0.6	0.2743	0.2709	0.2676	0.2643	0.2611	0.2578	0.2546	0.2514	0.2483	0.2451
0.7	0.2420	0.2389	0.2358	0.2327	0.2296	0.2266	0.2236	0.2206	0.2177	0.2148
0.8	0.2119	0.2090	0.2061	0.2033	0.2005	0.1977	0.1949	0.1922	0.1894	0.1867
0.9	0.1841	0.1814	0.1788	0.1762	0.1736	0.1711	0.1685	0.1660	0.1635	0.1611
1.0	0.1587	0.1562	0.1539	0.1515	0.1492	0.1469	0.1446	0.1423	0.1401	0.1379
1.1	0.1357	0.1335	0.1314	0.1292	0.1271	0.1251	0.1230	0.1210	0.1190	0.1170
1.2	0.1151	0.1131	0.1112	0.1093	0.1075	0.1056	0.1038	0.1020	0.1003	0.0985
1.3	0.0968	0.0951	0.0934	0.0918	0.0901	0.0885	0.0869	0.0853	0.0838	0.0823
1.4	0.0808	0.0793	0.0778	0.0764	0.0749	0.0735	0.0721	0.0708	0.0694	0.0681

1.5	0.0668	0.0655	0.0643	0.0630	0.0618	0.0606	0.0594	0.0582	0.0571	0.0559
1.6	0.0548	0.0537	0.0526	0.0516	0.0505	0.0495	0.0485	0.0475	0.0465	0.0455
1.7	0.0446	0.0436	0.0427	0.0418	0.0409	0.0401	0.0392	0.0384	0.0375	0.0367
1.8	0.0359	0.0351	0.0344	0.0336	0.0329	0.0322	0.0314	0.0307	0.0301	0.0294
1.9	0.0287	0.0281	0.0274	0.0268	0.0262	0.0256	0.0250	0.0244	0.0239	0.0233
2.0	0.02275	0.02222	0.02169	0.02118	0.02068	0.02018	0.01970	0.01923	0.01876	0.01831
2.1	0.01786	0.01743	0.01700	0.01659	0.01618	0.01578	0.01539	0.01500	0.01463	0.01426
2.2	0.01390	0.01355	0.01321	0.01287	0.01255	0.01222	0.01191	0.01160	0.01130	0.01101
2.3	0.01072	0.01044	0.01017	0.00990	0.00964	0.00939	0.00914	0.00889	0.00866	0.00842
2.4	0.00820	0.00798	0.00776	0.00755	0.00734	0.00714	0.00695	0.00676	0.00657	0.00639
2.5	0.00621	0.00604	0.00587	0.00570	0.00554	0.00539	0.00523	0.00508	0.00494	0.00480
2.6	0.00466	0.00453	0.00440	0.00427	0.00415	0.00402	0.00391	0.00379	0.00368	0.00357
2.7	0.00347	0.00336	0.00326	0.00317	0.00307	0.00298	0.00289	0.00280	0.00272	0.00264
2.8	0.00256	0.00248	0.00240	0.00233	0.00226	0.00219	0.00212	0.00205	0.00199	0.00193
2.9	0.00187	0.00181	0.00175	0.00169	0.00164	0.00159	0.00154	0.00149	0.00144	0.00139
3.0	0.00135	0.00131	0.00126	0.00122	0.00118	0.00114	0.00111	0.00107	0.00104	0.00100
3.1	0.00097	0.00094	0.00090	0.00087	0.00084	0.00082	0.00079	0.00076	0.00074	0.00071
3.2	0.00069	0.00066	0.00064	0.00062	0.00060	0.00058	0.00056	0.00054	0.00052	0.00050
3.3	0.00048	0.00047	0.00045	0.00043	0.00042	0.00040	0.00039	0.00038	0.00036	0.00035
3.4	0.00034	0.00032	0.00031	0.00030	0.00029	0.00028	0.00027	0.00026	0.00025	0.00024
3.5	0.00023	0.00022	0.00022	0.00021	0.00020	0.00019	0.00019	0.00018	0.00017	0.00017
3.6	0.00016	0.00015	0.00015	0.00014	0.00014	0.00013	0.00013	0.00012	0.00012	0.00011
3.7	0.00011	0.00010	0.00010	0.00010	0.00009	0.00009	0.00008	0.00008	0.00008	0.00008
3.8	0.00007	0.00007	0.00007	0.00006	0.00006	0.00006	0.00006	0.00005	0.00005	0.00005
3.9	0.00005	0.00005	0.00004	0.00004	0.00004	0.00004	0.00004	0.00004	0.00003	0.00003

Table A2 Percentage points of the standard normal distribution.

	Percentage points	
P-value	One-sided	Two-sided
0.5	0.00	0.67
0.4	0.25	0.84
0.3	0.52	1.04
0.2	0.84	1.28
0.1	1.28	1.64
0.05	1.64	1.96
0.02	2.05	2.33
0.01	2.33	2.58
0.005	2.58	2.81
0.002	2.88	3.09
0.001	3.09	3.29
0.0001	3.72	3.89

Table A3 Percentage points of the *t* distribution.

Adapted from Table 7 of White *et al.* (1979) with permission of the authors and publishers.

	One-sided *P*-value								
	0.25	0.1	0.05	0.025	0.01	0.005	0.0025	0.001	0.0005
	Two-sided *P*-value								
d.f.	0.5	0.2	0.1	0.05	0.02	0.01	0.005	0.002	0.001
1	1.00	3.08	6.31	12.71	31.82	63.66	127.32	318.31	636.62
2	0.82	1.89	2.92	4.30	6.96	9.92	14.09	22.33	31.60
3	0.76	1.64	2.35	3.18	4.54	5.84	7.45	10.21	12.92
4	0.74	1.53	2.13	2.78	3.75	4.60	5.60	7.17	8.61
5	0.73	1.48	2.02	2.57	3.36	4.03	4.77	5.89	6.87
6	0.72	1.44	1.94	2.45	3.14	3.71	4.32	5.21	5.96
7	0.71	1.42	1.90	2.36	3.00	3.50	4.03	4.78	5.41
8	0.71	1.40	1.86	2.31	2.90	3.36	3.83	4.50	5.04
9	0.70	1.38	1.83	2.26	2.82	3.25	3.69	4.30	4.78
10	0.70	1.37	1.81	2.23	2.76	3.17	3.58	4.14	4.59
11	0.70	1.36	1.80	2.20	2.72	3.11	3.50	4.02	4.44
12	0.70	1.36	1.78	2.18	2.68	3.06	3.43	3.93	4.32
13	0.69	1.35	1.77	2.16	2.65	3.01	3.37	3.85	4.22
14	0.69	1.34	1.76	2.14	2.62	2.98	3.33	3.79	4.14
15	0.69	1.34	1.75	2.13	2.60	2.95	3.29	3.73	4.07
16	0.69	1.34	1.75	2.12	2.58	2.92	3.25	3.69	4.02
17	0.69	1.33	1.74	2.11	2.57	2.90	3.22	3.65	3.96
18	0.69	1.33	1.73	2.10	2.55	2.88	3.20	3.61	3.92
19	0.69	1.33	1.73	2.09	2.54	2.86	3.17	3.58	3.88
20	0.69	1.32	1.72	2.09	2.53	2.84	3.15	3.55	3.85
21	0.69	1.32	1.72	2.08	2.52	2.83	3.14	3.53	3.82
22	0.69	1.32	1.72	2.07	2.51	2.82	3.12	3.50	3.79
23	0.68	1.32	1.71	2.07	2.50	2.81	3.10	3.48	3.77
24	0.68	1.32	1.71	2.06	2.49	2.80	3.09	3.47	3.74
25	0.68	1.32	1.71	2.06	2.48	2.79	3.08	3.45	3.72
26	0.68	1.32	1.71	2.06	2.48	2.78	3.07	3.44	3.71
27	0.68	1.31	1.70	2.05	2.47	2.77	3.06	3.42	3.69
28	0.68	1.31	1.70	2.05	2.47	2.76	3.05	3.41	3.67
29	0.68	1.31	1.70	2.04	2.46	2.76	3.04	3.40	3.66
30	0.68	1.31	1.70	2.04	2.46	2.75	3.03	3.38	3.65
40	0.68	1.30	1.68	2.02	2.42	2.70	2.97	3.31	3.55
60	0.68	1.30	1.67	2.00	2.39	2.66	2.92	3.23	3.46
120	0.68	1.29	1.66	1.98	2.36	2.62	2.86	3.16	3.37
∞	0.67	1.28	1.65	1.96	2.33	2.58	2.81	3.09	3.29

Table A4 Two-sided *P*-values for the *t* distribution, according to the value of the test statistic.

The final column shows *P*-values for infinite degrees of freedom, equivalent to *P*-values from the normal distribution.

Value of test statistic (*t*)	Degrees of freedom for *t*							
	5	6	7	8	9	10	12	14
1.5	0.194	0.184	0.177	0.172	0.168	0.165	0.159	0.156
1.6	0.170	0.161	0.154	0.148	0.144	0.141	0.136	0.132
1.7	0.150	0.140	0.133	0.128	0.123	0.120	0.115	0.111
1.8	0.132	0.122	0.115	0.110	0.105	0.102	0.097	0.093
1.9	0.116	0.106	0.099	0.094	0.090	0.087	0.082	0.078
2.0	0.102	0.092	0.086	0.081	0.077	0.073	0.069	0.065
2.1	0.090	0.080	0.074	0.069	0.065	0.062	0.058	0.054
2.2	0.079	0.070	0.064	0.059	0.055	0.052	0.048	0.045
2.3	0.070	0.061	0.055	0.050	0.047	0.044	0.040	0.037
2.4	0.062	0.053	0.047	0.043	0.040	0.037	0.034	0.031
2.5	0.054	0.047	0.041	0.037	0.034	0.031	0.028	0.025
2.6	0.048	0.041	0.035	0.032	0.029	0.026	0.023	0.021
2.7	0.043	0.036	0.031	0.027	0.024	0.022	0.019	0.017
2.8	0.038	0.031	0.027	0.023	0.021	0.019	0.016	0.014
2.9	0.034	0.027	0.023	0.020	0.018	0.016	0.013	0.012
3.0	0.030	0.024	0.020	0.017	0.015	0.013	0.011	0.010
3.1	0.027	0.021	0.017	0.015	0.013	0.011	0.009	0.008
3.2	0.024	0.019	0.015	0.013	0.011	0.009	0.008	0.006
3.3	0.021	0.016	0.013	0.011	0.009	0.008	0.006	0.005
3.4	0.019	0.014	0.011	0.009	0.008	0.007	0.005	0.004
3.5	0.017	0.013	0.010	0.008	0.007	0.006	0.004	0.004
3.6	0.016	0.011	0.009	0.007	0.006	0.005	0.004	0.003
3.7	0.014	0.010	0.008	0.006	0.005	0.004	0.003	0.002
3.8	0.013	0.009	0.007	0.005	0.004	0.003	0.003	0.002
3.9	0.011	0.008	0.006	0.005	0.004	0.003	0.002	0.002
4.0	0.010	0.007	0.005	0.004	0.003	0.003	0.002	0.001
4.1	0.009	0.006	0.005	0.003	0.003	0.002	0.001	0.001
4.2	0.008	0.006	0.004	0.003	0.002	0.002	0.001	0.001
4.3	0.008	0.005	0.004	0.003	0.002	0.002	0.001	0.001
4.4	0.007	0.005	0.003	0.002	0.002	0.001	0.001	0.001
4.5	0.006	0.004	0.003	0.002	0.001	0.001	0.001	<0.001
4.6	0.006	0.004	0.002	0.002	0.001	0.001	0.001	<0.001
4.7	0.005	0.003	0.002	0.002	0.001	0.001	0.001	<0.001
4.8	0.005	0.003	0.002	0.001	0.001	0.001	<0.001	<0.001
4.9	0.004	0.003	0.002	0.001	0.001	0.001	<0.001	<0.001
5.0	0.004	0.002	0.002	0.001	0.001	0.001	<0.001	<0.001

			Degrees of freedom for t					∞ (same
16	18	20	25	30	40	50	60	as normal)
0.153	0.151	0.149	0.146	0.144	0.141	0.140	0.139	0.134
0.129	0.127	0.125	0.122	0.120	0.117	0.116	0.115	0.110
0.108	0.106	0.105	0.102	0.099	0.097	0.095	0.094	0.089
0.091	0.089	0.087	0.084	0.082	0.079	0.078	0.077	0.072
0.076	0.074	0.072	0.069	0.067	0.065	0.063	0.062	0.057
0.063	0.061	0.059	0.056	0.055	0.052	0.051	0.050	0.046
0.052	0.050	0.049	0.046	0.044	0.042	0.041	0.040	0.036
0.043	0.041	0.040	0.037	0.036	0.034	0.032	0.032	0.028
0.035	0.034	0.032	0.030	0.029	0.027	0.026	0.025	0.021
0.029	0.027	0.026	0.024	0.023	0.021	0.020	0.020	0.016
0.024	0.022	0.021	0.019	0.018	0.017	0.016	0.015	0.012
0.019	0.018	0.017	0.015	0.014	0.013	0.012	0.012	0.009
0.016	0.015	0.014	0.012	0.011	0.010	0.009	0.009	0.007
0.013	0.012	0.011	0.010	0.009	0.008	0.007	0.007	0.005
0.010	0.010	0.009	0.008	0.007	0.006	0.006	0.005	0.004
0.008	0.008	0.007	0.006	0.005	0.005	0.004	0.004	0.003
0.007	0.006	0.006	0.005	0.004	0.004	0.003	0.003	0.002
0.006	0.005	0.004	0.004	0.003	0.003	0.002	0.002	0.001
0.005	0.004	0.004	0.003	0.002	0.002	0.002	0.002	0.001
0.004	0.003	0.003	0.002	0.002	0.002	0.001	0.001	0.001
0.003	0.003	0.002	0.002	0.001	0.001	0.001	0.001	<0.001
0.002	0.002	0.002	0.001	0.001	0.001	0.001	0.001	<0.001
0.002	0.002	0.001	0.001	0.001	0.001	0.001	<0.001	<0.001
0.002	0.001	0.001	0.001	0.001	<0.001	<0.001	<0.001	<0.001
0.001	0.001	0.001	0.001	0.001	<0.001	<0.001	<0.001	<0.001
0.001	0.001	0.001	<0.001	<0.001	<0.001	<0.001	<0.001	<0.001
0.001	0.001	0.001	<0.001	<0.001	<0.001	<0.001	<0.001	<0.001
0.001	0.001	<0.001	<0.001	<0.001	<0.001	<0.001	<0.001	<0.001
0.001	<0.001	<0.001	<0.001	<0.001	<0.001	<0.001	<0.001	<0.001
<0.001	<0.001	<0.001	<0.001	<0.001	<0.001	<0.001	<0.001	<0.001
<0.001	<0.001	<0.001	<0.001	<0.001	<0.001	<0.001	<0.001	<0.001
<0.001	<0.001	<0.001	<0.001	<0.001	<0.001	<0.001	<0.001	<0.001
<0.001	<0.001	<0.001	<0.001	<0.001	<0.001	<0.001	<0.001	<0.001
<0.001	<0.001	<0.001	<0.001	<0.001	<0.001	<0.001	<0.001	<0.001
<0.001	<0.001	<0.001	<0.001	<0.001	<0.001	<0.001	<0.001	<0.001
<0.001	<0.001	<0.001	<0.001	<0.001	<0.001	<0.001	<0.001	<0.001

Table A5 Percentage points of the χ^2 distribution.

Adapted from Table 8 of White *et al*. (1979) with permission of the authors and publishers.

d.f. = 1. In the comparison of two proportions ($2 \times 2 \; \chi^2$ or Mantel–Haenszel χ^2 test) or in the assessment of a trend, the percentage points give a two-sided test. A one-sided test may be obtained by halving the *P*-values. (Concepts of one- and two-sidedness do not apply to larger degrees of freedom, as these relate to tests of multiple comparisons.)

d.f.	0.5	0.25	0.1	0.05	0.025	0.01	0.005	0.001
1	0.45	1.32	2.71	3.84	5.02	6.63	7.88	10.83
2	1.39	2.77	4.61	5.99	7.38	9.21	10.60	13.82
3	2.37	4.11	6.25	7.81	9.35	11.34	12.84	16.27
4	3.36	5.39	7.78	9.49	11.14	13.28	14.86	18.47
5	4.35	6.63	9.24	11.07	12.83	15.09	16.75	20.52
6	5.35	7.84	10.64	12.59	14.45	16.81	18.55	22.46
7	6.35	9.04	12.02	14.07	16.01	18.48	20.28	24.32
8	7.34	10.22	13.36	15.51	17.53	20.09	21.96	26.13
9	8.34	11.39	14.68	16.92	19.02	21.67	23.59	27.88
10	9.34	12.55	15.99	18.31	20.48	23.21	25.19	29.59
11	10.34	13.70	17.28	19.68	21.92	24.73	26.76	31.26
12	11.34	14.85	18.55	21.03	23.34	26.22	28.30	32.91
13	12.34	15.98	19.81	22.36	24.74	27.69	29.82	34.53
14	13.34	17.12	21.06	23.68	26.12	29.14	31.32	36.12
15	14.34	18.25	22.31	25.00	27.49	30.58	32.80	37.70
16	15.34	19.37	23.54	26.30	28.85	32.00	34.27	39.25
17	16.34	20.49	24.77	27.59	30.19	33.41	35.72	40.79
18	17.34	21.60	25.99	28.87	31.53	34.81	37.16	42.31
19	18.34	22.72	27.20	30.14	32.85	36.19	38.58	43.82
20	19.34	23.83	28.41	31.41	34.17	37.57	40.00	45.32
21	20.34	24.93	29.62	32.67	35.48	38.93	41.40	46.80
22	21.34	26.04	30.81	33.92	36.78	40.29	42.80	48.27
23	22.34	27.14	32.01	35.17	38.08	41.64	44.18	49.73
24	23.34	28.24	33.20	36.42	39.36	42.98	45.56	51.18
25	24.34	29.34	34.38	37.65	40.65	44.31	46.93	52.62
26	25.34	30.43	35.56	38.89	41.92	45.64	48.29	54.05
27	26.34	31.53	36.74	40.11	43.19	46.96	49.64	55.48
28	27.34	32.62	37.92	41.34	44.46	48.28	50.99	56.89
29	28.34	33.71	39.09	42.56	45.72	49.59	52.34	58.30
30	29.34	34.80	40.26	43.77	46.98	50.89	53.67	59.70
40	39.34	45.62	51.81	55.76	59.34	63.69	66.77	73.40
50	49.33	56.33	63.17	67.50	71.42	76.15	79.49	86.66
60	59.33	66.98	74.40	79.08	83.30	88.38	91.95	99.61
70	69.33	77.58	85.53	90.53	95.02	100.43	104.22	112.32
80	79.33	88.13	96.58	101.88	106.63	112.33	116.32	124.84
90	89.33	98.65	107.57	113.15	118.14	124.12	128.30	137.21
100	99.33	109.14	118.50	124.34	129.56	135.81	140.17	149.45

Table A6 Probits.

Adapted from Table 4 of Pearson & Hartley (1966) with permission of the Biometrika Trustees.

Probit = value of standard normal distribution corresponding to cumulative percentage | +5, optional: not included in this table

%	0.0	0.1	0.2	0.3	0.4	0.5	0.6	0.7	0.8	0.9
					Decimal place of %					
0	−∞	−3.09	−2.88	−2.75	−2.65	−2.58	−2.51	−2.46	−2.41	−2.37
1	−2.33	−2.29	−2.26	−2.23	−2.20	−2.17	−2.14	−2.12	−2.10	−2.07
2	−2.05	−2.03	−2.01	−2.00	−1.98	−1.96	−1.94	−1.93	−1.91	−1.90
3	−1.88	−1.87	−1.85	−1.84	−1.83	−1.81	−1.80	−1.79	−1.77	−1.76
4	−1.75	−1.74	−1.73	−1.72	−1.71	−1.70	−1.68	−1.67	−1.66	−1.65
5	−1.64	−1.64	−1.63	−1.62	−1.61	−1.60	−1.59	−1.58	−1.57	−1.56
6	−1.55	−1.55	−1.54	−1.53	−1.52	−1.51	−1.51	−1.50	−1.49	−1.48
7	−1.48	−1.47	−1.46	−1.45	−1.45	−1.44	−1.43	−1.43	−1.42	−1.41
8	−1.41	−1.40	−1.39	−1.39	−1.38	−1.37	−1.37	−1.36	−1.35	−1.35
9	−1.34	−1.33	−1.33	−1.32	−1.32	−1.31	−1.30	−1.30	−1.29	−1.29
10	−1.28	−1.28	−1.27	−1.26	−1.26	−1.25	−1.25	−1.24	−1.24	−1.23
11	−1.23	−1.22	−1.22	−1.21	−1.21	−1.20	−1.20	−1.19	−1.19	−1.18
12	−1.18	−1.17	−1.17	−1.16	−1.16	−1.15	−1.15	−1.14	−1.14	−1.13
13	−1.13	−1.12	−1.12	−1.11	−1.11	−1.10	−1.10	−1.09	−1.09	−1.08
14	−1.08	−1.08	−1.07	−1.07	−1.06	−1.06	−1.05	−1.05	−1.05	−1.04
15	−1.04	−1.03	−1.03	−1.02	−1.02	−1.02	−1.01	−1.01	−1.00	−1.00
16	−0.99	−0.99	−0.99	−0.98	−0.98	−0.97	−0.97	−0.97	−0.96	−0.96
17	−0.95	−0.95	−0.95	−0.94	−0.94	−0.93	−0.93	−0.93	−0.92	−0.92
18	−0.92	−0.91	−0.91	−0.90	−0.90	−0.90	−0.89	−0.89	−0.89	−0.88
19	−0.88	−0.87	−0.87	−0.87	−0.86	−0.86	−0.86	−0.85	−0.85	−0.85
20	−0.84	−0.84	−0.83	−0.83	−0.83	−0.82	−0.82	−0.82	−0.81	−0.81
21	−0.81	−0.80	−0.80	−0.80	−0.79	−0.79	−0.79	−0.78	−0.78	−0.78
22	−0.77	−0.77	−0.77	−0.76	−0.76	−0.76	−0.75	−0.75	−0.75	−0.74
23	−0.74	−0.74	−0.73	−0.73	−0.73	−0.72	−0.72	−0.72	−0.71	−0.71
24	−0.71	−0.70	−0.70	−0.70	−0.69	−0.69	−0.69	−0.68	−0.68	−0.68
25	−0.67	−0.67	−0.67	−0.67	−0.66	−0.66	−0.66	−0.65	−0.65	−0.65
26	−0.64	−0.64	−0.64	−0.63	−0.63	−0.63	−0.63	−0.62	−0.62	−0.62
27	−0.61	−0.61	−0.61	−0.60	−0.60	−0.60	−0.59	−0.59	−0.59	−0.59
28	−0.58	−0.58	−0.58	−0.57	−0.57	−0.57	−0.57	−0.56	−0.56	−0.56
29	−0.55	−0.55	−0.55	−0.54	−0.54	−0.54	−0.54	−0.53	−0.53	−0.53
30	−0.52	−0.52	−0.52	−0.52	−0.51	−0.51	−0.51	−0.50	−0.50	−0.50
31	−0.50	−0.49	−0.49	−0.49	−0.48	−0.48	−0.48	−0.48	−0.47	−0.47
32	−0.47	−0.46	−0.46	−0.46	−0.46	−0.45	−0.45	−0.45	−0.45	−0.44
33	−0.44	−0.44	−0.43	−0.43	−0.43	−0.43	−0.42	−0.42	−0.42	−0.42
34	−0.41	−0.41	−0.41	−0.40	−0.40	−0.40	−0.40	−0.39	−0.39	−0.39
35	−0.39	−0.38	−0.38	−0.38	−0.37	−0.37	−0.37	−0.37	−0.36	−0.36
36	−0.36	−0.36	−0.35	−0.35	−0.35	−0.35	−0.34	−0.34	−0.34	−0.33
37	−0.33	−0.33	−0.33	−0.32	−0.32	−0.32	−0.32	−0.31	−0.31	−0.31
38	−0.31	−0.30	−0.30	−0.30	−0.30	−0.29	−0.29	−0.29	−0.28	−0.28
39	−0.28	−0.28	−0.27	−0.27	−0.27	−0.27	−0.26	−0.26	−0.26	−0.26
40	−0.25	−0.25	−0.25	−0.25	−0.24	−0.24	−0.24	−0.24	−0.23	−0.23
41	−0.23	−0.23	−0.22	−0.22	−0.22	−0.21	−0.21	−0.21	−0.21	−0.20
42	−0.20	−0.20	−0.20	−0.19	−0.19	−0.19	−0.19	−0.18	−0.18	−0.18
43	−0.18	−0.17	−0.17	−0.17	−0.17	−0.16	−0.16	−0.16	−0.16	−0.15
44	−0.15	−0.15	−0.15	−0.14	−0.14	−0.14	−0.14	−0.13	−0.13	−0.13
45	−0.13	−0.12	−0.12	−0.12	−0.12	−0.11	−0.11	−0.11	−0.11	−0.10
46	−0.10	−0.10	−0.10	−0.09	−0.09	−0.09	−0.09	−0.08	−0.08	−0.08
47	−0.08	−0.07	−0.07	−0.07	−0.07	−0.06	−0.06	−0.06	−0.06	−0.05
48	−0.05	−0.05	−0.05	−0.04	−0.04	−0.04	−0.04	−0.03	−0.03	−0.03
49	−0.03	−0.02	−0.02	−0.02	−0.02	−0.01	−0.01	−0.01	−0.01	0.00

(continued)

Table A6 Probits (continued)

%	0.0	0.1	0.2	0.3	0.4	0.5	0.6	0.7	0.8	0.9
					Decimal place of %					
50	0.00	0.00	0.01	0.01	0.01	0.01	0.02	0.02	0.02	0.02
51	0.03	0.03	0.03	0.03	0.04	0.04	0.04	0.04	0.05	0.05
52	0.05	0.05	0.06	0.06	0.06	0.06	0.07	0.07	0.07	0.07
53	0.08	0.08	0.08	0.08	0.09	0.09	0.09	0.09	0.10	0.10
54	0.10	0.10	0.11	0.11	0.11	0.11	0.12	0.12	0.12	0.12
55	0.13	0.13	0.13	0.13	0.14	0.14	0.14	0.14	0.15	0.15
56	0.15	0.15	0.16	0.16	0.16	0.16	0.17	0.17	0.17	0.17
57	0.18	0.18	0.18	0.18	0.19	0.19	0.19	0.19	0.20	0.20
58	0.20	0.20	0.21	0.21	0.21	0.21	0.22	0.22	0.22	0.23
59	0.23	0.23	0.23	0.24	0.24	0.24	0.24	0.25	0.25	0.25
60	0.25	0.26	0.26	0.26	0.26	0.27	0.27	0.27	0.27	0.28
61	0.28	0.28	0.28	0.29	0.29	0.29	0.30	0.30	0.30	0.30
62	0.31	0.31	0.31	0.31	0.32	0.32	0.32	0.32	0.33	0.33
63	0.33	0.33	0.34	0.34	0.34	0.35	0.35	0.35	0.35	0.36
64	0.36	0.36	0.36	0.37	0.37	0.37	0.37	0.38	0.38	0.38
65	0.39	0.39	0.39	0.39	0.40	0.40	0.40	0.40	0.41	0.41
66	0.41	0.42	0.42	0.42	0.42	0.43	0.43	0.43	0.43	0.44
67	0.44	0.44	0.45	0.45	0.45	0.45	0.46	0.46	0.46	0.46
68	0.47	0.47	0.47	0.48	0.48	0.48	0.48	0.49	0.49	0.49
69	0.50	0.50	0.50	0.50	0.51	0.51	0.51	0.52	0.52	0.52
70	0.52	0.53	0.53	0.53	0.54	0.54	0.54	0.54	0.55	0.55
71	0.55	0.56	0.56	0.56	0.57	0.57	0.57	0.57	0.58	0.58
72	0.58	0.59	0.59	0.59	0.59	0.60	0.60	0.60	0.61	0.61
73	0.61	0.62	0.62	0.62	0.63	0.63	0.63	0.63	0.64	0.64
74	0.64	0.65	0.65	0.65	0.66	0.66	0.66	0.67	0.67	0.67
75	0.67	0.68	0.68	0.68	0.69	0.69	0.69	0.70	0.70	0.70
76	0.71	0.71	0.71	0.72	0.72	0.72	0.73	0.73	0.73	0.74
77	0.74	0.74	0.75	0.75	0.75	0.76	0.76	0.76	0.77	0.77
78	0.77	0.78	0.78	0.78	0.79	0.79	0.79	0.80	0.80	0.80
79	0.81	0.81	0.81	0.82	0.82	0.82	0.83	0.83	0.83	0.84
80	0.84	0.85	0.85	0.85	0.86	0.86	0.86	0.87	0.87	0.87
81	0.88	0.88	0.89	0.89	0.89	0.90	0.90	0.90	0.91	0.91
82	0.92	0.92	0.92	0.93	0.93	0.93	0.94	0.94	0.95	0.95
83	0.95	0.96	0.96	0.97	0.97	0.97	0.98	0.98	0.99	0.99
84	0.99	1.00	1.00	1.01	1.01	1.02	1.02	1.02	1.03	1.03
85	1.04	1.04	1.05	1.05	1.05	1.06	1.06	1.07	1.07	1.08
86	1.08	1.08	1.09	1.09	1.10	1.10	1.11	1.11	1.12	1.12
87	1.13	1.13	1.14	1.14	1.15	1.15	1.16	1.16	1.17	1.17
88	1.18	1.18	1.19	1.19	1.20	1.20	1.21	1.21	1.22	1.22
89	1.23	1.23	1.24	1.24	1.25	1.25	1.26	1.26	1.27	1.28
90	1.28	1.29	1.29	1.30	1.30	1.31	1.32	1.32	1.33	1.33
91	1.34	1.35	1.35	1.36	1.37	1.37	1.38	1.39	1.39	1.40
92	1.41	1.41	1.42	1.43	1.43	1.44	1.45	1.45	1.46	1.47
93	1.48	1.48	1.49	1.50	1.51	1.51	1.52	1.53	1.54	1.55
94	1.55	1.56	1.57	1.58	1.59	1.60	1.61	1.62	1.63	1.64
95	1.64	1.65	1.66	1.67	1.68	1.70	1.71	1.72	1.73	1.74
96	1.75	1.76	1.77	1.79	1.80	1.81	1.83	1.84	1.85	1.87
97	1.88	1.90	1.91	1.93	1.94	1.96	1.98	2.00	2.01	2.03
98	2.05	2.07	2.10	2.12	2.14	2.17	2.20	2.23	2.26	2.29
99	2.33	2.37	2.41	2.46	2.51	2.58	2.65	2.75	2.88	3.09

Table A7 Critical values for the Wilcoxon matched pairs signed rank test.

Reproduced from Table 21 of White *et al*. (1979) with permission of the authors and publishers.

N = number of non-zero differences; T = smaller of T_+ and T_-; Significant if $T <$ critical value.

	One-sided *P*-value						One-sided *P*-value			
	0.05	0.025	0.01	0.005			0.05	0.025	0.01	0.005
	Two-sided *P*-value						Two-sided *P*-value			
N	0.1	0.05	0.02	0.01		*N*	0.1	0.05	0.02	0.01
5	1					30	152	137	120	109
6	2	1				31	163	148	130	118
7	4	2	0			32	175	159	141	128
8	6	4	2	0		33	188	171	151	138
9	8	6	3	2		34	201	183	162	149
10	11	8	5	3		35	214	195	174	160
11	14	11	7	5		36	228	208	186	171
12	17	14	10	7		37	242	222	198	183
13	21	17	13	10		38	256	235	211	195
14	26	21	16	13		39	271	250	224	208
15	30	25	20	16		40	287	264	238	221
16	36	30	24	19		41	303	279	252	234
17	41	35	28	23		42	319	295	267	248
18	47	40	33	28		43	336	311	281	262
19	54	46	38	32		44	353	327	297	277
20	60	52	43	37		45	371	344	313	292
21	68	59	49	43		46	389	361	329	307
22	75	66	56	49		47	408	397	345	323
23	83	73	62	55		48	427	397	362	339
24	92	81	69	61		49	446	415	380	356
25	101	90	77	68		50	466	434	398	373
26	110	98	85	76						
27	120	107	93	84						
28	130	117	102	92						
29	141	127	111	100						

Table A8 Critical ranges for the Wilcoxon rank sum test.

Reproduced from Table A7 of Cotton (1974) with permission of the author and publishers.

n_1, n_2 = sample sizes of two groups; T = sum of ranks in group with smaller sample size; significant if T on boundaries or outside critical range.

	One-sided P-value					One-sided P-value		
	0.025	0.005	0.0005			0.025	0.005	0.0005
	Two-sided P-value					Two-sided P-value		
n_1, n_2	0.05	0.01	0.001		n_1, n_2	0.05	0.01	0.001
2, 8	3, 19				4, 13	18, 54	14, 58	10, 62
2, 9	3, 21				4, 14	19, 57	14, 62	10, 66
2, 10	3, 23				4, 15	20, 60	15, 65	10, 70
2, 11	4, 24				4, 16	21, 63	15, 69	11, 73
2, 12	4, 26				4, 17	21, 67	16, 72	11, 77
2, 13	4, 28				4, 18	22, 70	16, 76	11, 81
2, 14	4, 30				4, 19	23, 73	17, 79	12, 84
2, 15	4, 32				4, 20	24, 76	18, 82	12, 88
2, 16	4, 34				4, 21	25, 79	18, 86	12, 92
2, 17	5, 35				4, 22	26, 82	19, 89	13, 95
2, 18	5, 37				4, 23	27, 85	19, 93	13, 99
2, 19	5, 39	3, 41			4, 24	28, 88	20, 96	13, 103
2, 20	5, 41	3, 43			4, 25	28, 92	20, 100	14, 106
2, 21	6, 42	3, 45						
2, 22	6, 44	3, 47			5, 5	17, 38	15, 40	
2, 23	6, 46	3, 49			5, 6	18, 42	16, 44	
2, 24	6, 48	3, 51			5, 7	20, 45	17, 48	
2, 25	6, 50	3, 53			5, 8	21, 49	17, 53	
					5, 9	22, 53	18, 57	15, 60
3, 5	6, 21				5, 10	23, 57	19, 61	15, 65
3, 6	7, 23				5, 11	24, 61	20, 65	16, 69
3, 7	7, 26				5, 12	26, 64	21, 69	16, 74
3, 8	8, 28				5, 13	27, 68	22, 73	17, 78
3, 9	8, 31	6, 33			5, 14	28, 72	22, 78	17, 83
3, 10	9, 33	6, 36			5, 15	29, 76	23, 82	18, 87
3, 11	9, 36	6, 39			5, 16	31, 79	24, 86	18, 92
3, 12	10, 38	7, 41			5, 17	32, 83	25, 90	19, 96
3, 13	10, 41	7, 44			5, 18	33, 87	26, 94	19, 101
3, 14	11, 43	7, 47			5, 19	34, 91	27, 98	20, 105
3, 15	11, 46	8, 49			5, 20	35, 95	28, 102	20, 110
3, 16	12, 48	8, 52			5, 21	37, 98	29, 106	21, 114
3, 17	12, 51	8, 55			5, 22	38, 102	29, 111	21, 119
3, 18	13, 53	8, 58			5, 23	39, 106	30, 115	22, 123
3, 19	13, 56	9, 60			5, 24	40, 110	31, 119	23, 127
3, 20	14, 58	9, 63			5, 25	42, 113	32, 123	23, 132
3, 21	14, 61	9, 66	6, 69					
3, 22	15, 63	10, 68	6, 72					
3, 23	15, 66	10, 71	6, 75		6, 6	26, 52	23, 55	
3, 24	16, 68	10, 74	6, 78		6, 7	27, 57	24, 60	
3, 25	19, 71	11, 76	6, 81		6, 8	29, 61	25, 65	21, 69
					6, 9	31, 65	26, 70	22, 74
4, 4	10, 26				6, 10	32, 70	27, 75	23, 79
4, 5	11, 29				6, 11	34, 74	28, 80	23, 85
4, 6	12, 32	10, 34			6, 12	35, 79	30, 84	24, 90
4, 7	13, 35	10, 38			6, 13	37, 83	31, 89	25, 95
4, 8	14, 38	11, 41			6, 14	38, 88	32, 94	26, 100
4, 9	15, 41	11, 45			6, 15	40, 92	33, 99	26, 106
4, 10	15, 45	12, 48			6, 16	42, 96	34, 104	27, 111
4, 11	16, 48	12, 52			6, 17	43, 101	36, 108	28, 116
4, 12	17, 51	13, 55			6, 18	45, 105	37, 113	29, 121

Table A8 Critical ranges for the Wilcoxon rank sum test (continued)

	One-sided P-value					One-sided P-value		
	0.025	0.005	0.0005			0.025	0.005	0.0005
	Two-sided P-value					Two-sided P-value		
n_1, n_2	0.05	0.01	0.001		n_1, n_2	0.05	0.01	0.001
6, 19	46, 110	38, 118	29, 127		9, 15	79, 146	70, 155	60, 165
6, 20	48, 114	39, 123	30, 132		9, 16	82, 152	72, 162	61, 173
6, 21	50, 118	40, 128	31, 137		9, 17	84, 159	74, 169	63, 180
6, 22	51, 123	42, 132	32, 142		9, 18	87, 165	76, 176	65, 187
6, 23	53, 127	43, 137	33, 147		9, 19	90, 171	78, 183	66, 195
6, 24	55, 131	44, 142	34, 152		9, 20	93, 177	81, 189	68, 202
					9, 21	95, 184	83, 196	70, 209
7, 7	36, 69	32, 73	28, 77					
7, 8	38, 74	34, 78	29, 83		10, 10	78, 132	71, 139	63, 147
7, 9	40, 79	35, 84	30, 89		10, 11	81, 139	74, 146	65, 155
7, 10	42, 84	37, 89	31, 95		10, 12	85, 145	76, 154	67, 163
7, 11	44, 89	38, 95	32, 101		10, 13	88, 152	79, 161	69, 171
7, 12	46, 94	40, 100	33, 107		10, 14	91, 159	81, 169	71, 179
7, 13	48, 99	41, 106	34, 113		10, 15	94, 166	84, 176	73, 187
7, 14	50, 104	43, 111	35, 119		10, 16	97, 173	86, 184	75, 195
7, 15	52, 109	44, 117	36, 125		10, 17	100, 180	89, 191	77, 203
7, 16	54, 114	46, 122	37, 131		10, 18	103, 187	92, 198	79, 211
7, 17	56, 119	47, 128	38, 137		10, 19	107, 193	94, 206	81, 219
7, 18	58, 124	49, 133	39, 143		10, 20	110, 200	97, 213	83, 227
7, 19	60, 129	50, 139	41, 148					
7, 20	62, 134	52, 144	42, 154		11, 11	96, 157	87, 166	78, 175
7, 21	64, 139	53, 150	43, 160		11, 12	99, 165	90, 174	81, 183
7, 22	66, 144	55, 155	44, 166		11, 13	103, 172	93, 182	83, 192
7, 23	68, 149	57, 160	45, 172		11, 14	106, 180	96, 190	85, 201
					11, 15	110, 187	99, 198	87, 210
8, 8	49, 87	43, 93	38, 98		11, 16	114, 194	102, 206	90, 218
8, 9	51, 93	45, 99	40, 104		11, 17	117, 202	105, 214	92, 227
8, 10	53, 99	47, 105	41, 111		11, 18	121, 209	108, 222	94, 236
8, 11	55, 105	49, 111	42, 118		11, 19	124, 217	111, 230	97, 244
8, 12	58, 110	51, 117	43, 125					
8, 13	60, 116	53, 123	45, 131		12, 12	115, 185	106, 194	95, 205
8, 14	63, 121	54, 130	46, 138		12, 13	119, 193	109, 203	98, 214
8, 15	65, 127	56, 136	47, 145		12, 14	123, 201	112, 212	100, 224
8, 16	67, 133	58, 142	49, 151		12, 15	127, 209	115, 221	103, 233
8, 17	70, 138	60, 148	50, 158		12, 16	131, 217	119, 229	105, 243
8, 18	72, 144	62, 154	51, 165		12, 17	135, 225	122, 238	108, 252
8, 19	74, 150	64, 160	53, 171		12, 18	139, 233	125, 247	111, 261
8, 20	77, 155	66, 166	54, 178					
8, 21	79, 161	68, 172	56, 184		13, 13	137, 214	125, 226	114, 237
8, 22	82, 166	70, 178	57, 191		13, 14	141, 223	129, 235	116, 248
					13, 15	145, 232	133, 244	119, 258
9, 9	63, 108	56, 115	50, 121		13, 16	150, 240	137, 253	122, 268
9, 10	65, 115	58, 122	52, 128		13, 17	154, 249	140, 263	125, 278
9, 11	68, 121	61, 128	53, 136					
9, 12	71, 127	63, 135	55, 143		14, 14	160, 246	147, 259	134, 272
9, 13	73, 134	65, 142	56, 151		14, 15	164, 256	151, 269	137, 283
9, 14	76, 140	67, 149	58, 158		14, 16	169, 265	155, 279	140, 294
					15, 15	185, 280	171, 294	156, 309

Table A9 Random numbers.

Reproduced from Table XXXIII of Fisher and Yates (1963) following Armitage (1971) by permission of the authors and publishers.

03	47	43	73	86	36	96	47	36	61	46	98	63	71	62	33	26	16	80	45	60	11	14	10	95
97	74	24	67	62	42	81	14	57	20	42	53	32	37	32	27	07	36	07	51	24	51	79	89	73
16	76	62	27	66	56	50	26	71	07	32	90	79	78	53	13	55	38	58	59	88	97	54	14	10
12	56	85	99	26	96	96	68	27	31	05	03	72	93	15	57	12	10	14	21	88	26	49	81	76
55	59	56	35	64	38	54	82	46	22	31	62	43	09	90	06	18	44	32	53	23	83	01	30	30
16	22	77	94	39	49	54	43	54	82	17	37	93	23	78	87	35	20	96	43	84	26	34	91	64
84	42	17	53	31	57	24	55	06	88	77	04	74	47	67	21	76	33	50	25	83	92	12	06	76
63	01	63	78	59	16	95	55	67	19	98	10	50	71	75	12	86	73	58	07	44	39	52	38	79
33	21	12	34	29	78	64	56	07	82	52	42	07	44	38	15	51	00	13	42	99	66	02	79	54
57	60	86	32	44	09	47	27	96	54	49	17	46	09	62	90	52	84	77	27	08	02	73	43	28
18	18	07	92	46	44	17	16	58	09	79	83	86	19	62	06	76	50	03	10	55	23	64	05	05
26	62	38	97	75	84	16	07	44	99	83	11	46	32	24	20	14	85	88	45	10	93	72	88	71
23	42	40	64	74	82	97	77	77	81	07	45	32	14	08	32	98	94	07	72	93	85	79	10	75
52	36	28	19	95	50	92	26	11	97	00	56	76	31	38	80	22	02	53	53	86	60	42	04	53
37	85	94	35	12	83	39	50	08	30	42	34	07	96	88	54	42	06	87	98	35	85	29	48	39
70	29	17	12	13	40	33	20	38	26	13	89	51	03	74	17	76	37	13	04	07	74	21	19	30
56	62	18	37	35	96	83	50	87	75	97	12	25	93	47	70	33	24	03	54	97	77	46	44	80
99	49	57	22	77	88	42	95	45	72	16	64	36	16	00	04	43	18	66	79	94	77	24	21	90
16	08	15	04	72	33	27	14	34	09	45	59	34	68	49	12	72	07	34	45	99	27	72	95	14
31	16	93	32	43	50	27	89	87	19	20	15	37	00	49	52	85	66	60	44	38	68	88	11	80
68	34	30	13	70	55	74	30	77	40	44	22	78	84	26	04	33	46	09	52	68	07	97	06	57
74	57	25	65	76	59	29	97	68	60	71	91	38	67	54	13	58	18	24	76	15	54	55	95	52
27	42	37	86	53	48	55	90	65	72	96	57	69	36	10	96	46	92	42	45	97	60	49	04	91
00	39	68	29	61	66	37	32	20	30	77	84	57	03	29	10	45	65	04	26	11	04	96	67	24
29	94	98	94	24	68	49	69	10	82	53	75	91	93	30	34	25	20	57	27	40	48	73	51	92

31 03 37 02 02 68 29 21 47 60 74 71 00 19 67 12 11 64 62 83 59 66 82 90 16
38 30 94 45 38 86 30 90 70 76 02 34 37 94 02 66 74 19 09 06 06 75 94 27 11
98 95 50 75 02 16 56 53 92 16 91 04 45 78 79 38 26 51 32 33 20 16 10 24 35
32 08 84 51 48 62 91 74 01 40 41 81 66 75 87 50 01 97 38 42 38 86 16 23 38
62 89 26 55 27 85 48 43 52 00 91 53 82 86 34 13 49 33 44 96 47 91 25 96 31

66 11 00 16 57 90 37 20 83 76 68 09 65 05 11 86 95 71 05 64 14 67 40 67 66
80 95 74 52 07 08 22 12 98 22 86 14 41 27 52 90 05 88 73 75 11 45 84 90 14
59 44 38 37 49 90 43 82 33 59 55 93 62 60 07 19 75 02 96 33 00 18 51 05 68
30 13 93 95 47 36 49 16 54 39 08 31 33 02 04 02 14 40 51 97 90 73 78 46 26
33 17 74 67 02 62 89 78 78 40 06 75 10 90 01 20 93 15 06 15 79 97 58 19 14

74 05 77 91 52 83 06 78 56 59 77 59 51 03 92 13 15 85 35 22 60 70 93 26 05
51 09 77 05 58 93 16 29 51 06 15 99 62 71 61 64 99 42 98 09 23 88 10 97 07
48 29 24 56 29 16 63 92 95 44 12 11 08 32 73 54 47 66 87 54 85 85 86 71 68
94 16 67 44 94 74 85 55 17 32 42 67 50 10 42 70 80 78 37 58 53 65 61 99 26
43 39 39 29 15 50 01 27 08 13 55 06 63 78 26 41 22 36 59 87 75 68 52 65 14

83 30 74 96 02 99 36 27 95 44 26 96 94 41 12 72 50 61 41 71 71 58 77 53 17
23 70 32 99 25 07 36 18 02 07 39 18 02 93 96 12 33 23 52 23 19 21 59 26 90
17 49 14 17 97 20 89 43 41 13 88 45 48 47 10 96 69 49 04 31 99 55 52 23 41
34 72 10 99 18 60 48 12 30 24 76 03 33 81 35 68 68 73 99 31 69 81 50 20 60
60 65 54 62 82 12 29 57 35 90 09 03 59 37 45 36 41 28 58 94 90 05 38 25 91

49 66 31 07 45 04 04 80 94 74 82 19 93 77 09 91 00 33 80 98 37 74 57 50 34
47 38 13 94 53 31 46 54 31 08 28 86 46 62 33 79 94 53 81 73 43 39 04 22 85
88 94 39 80 35 60 05 44 89 72 83 24 27 03 05 21 22 97 82 73 48 77 13 79 09
87 67 61 04 16 37 70 07 48 02 49 22 82 32 39 49 42 75 95 22 14 18 80 75 88
33 76 00 89 90 32 69 30 37 94 36 38 78 85 55 90 06 03 00 39 00 70 23 96 90

(continued)

Table A9 Random numbers (continued).

53	74	23	99	67	61	32	28	69	84	94	62	67	86	24	98	33	41	19	95	47	53	53	38	09
63	38	06	86	54	99	00	65	26	94	02	82	90	23	07	79	62	67	80	60	75	91	12	81	19
35	30	58	21	46	06	72	17	10	94	25	21	31	75	96	49	28	24	00	49	55	65	79	78	07
63	43	36	82	69	65	51	18	37	88	61	38	44	12	45	32	92	85	88	65	54	34	81	85	35
98	25	37	55	26	01	91	82	81	46	74	71	12	94	97	24	02	71	37	07	03	92	18	66	75
02	63	21	17	69	71	50	80	89	56	38	15	70	11	48	43	40	45	86	98	00	83	26	91	03
64	55	22	21	82	48	22	28	06	00	61	54	13	43	91	82	78	12	23	29	06	66	24	12	27
85	07	26	13	89	01	10	07	82	04	59	63	69	36	03	69	11	15	83	80	13	29	54	19	28
58	54	16	24	15	51	54	44	82	00	62	61	65	04	69	38	18	65	18	97	85	72	13	49	21
34	85	27	84	87	61	48	64	56	26	90	18	48	13	26	37	70	15	42	57	65	65	80	39	07
03	92	18	27	46	57	99	16	96	56	30	33	72	85	22	84	64	38	56	98	99	01	30	98	64
62	95	30	27	59	37	75	41	66	48	86	97	80	61	45	23	53	04	01	63	45	76	08	64	27
08	45	93	15	22	60	21	75	46	91	98	77	27	85	42	28	88	61	08	84	69	62	03	42	73
07	08	55	18	40	45	44	75	13	90	24	94	96	61	02	57	55	66	83	15	73	42	37	11	61
01	85	89	95	66	51	10	19	34	88	15	84	97	19	75	12	76	39	43	78	64	63	91	08	25
72	84	71	14	35	19	11	58	49	26	50	11	17	17	76	86	31	57	20	18	95	60	78	46	75
88	78	28	16	84	13	52	53	94	53	75	45	69	30	96	73	89	65	70	31	99	17	43	48	76
45	17	75	65	57	28	40	19	72	12	25	12	74	75	67	60	40	60	81	19	24	62	01	61	16
96	76	28	12	54	22	01	11	94	25	71	96	16	75	88	68	64	36	74	45	19	59	50	88	92
43	31	67	72	30	24	02	94	08	63	38	32	36	66	02	69	36	38	25	39	48	03	45	15	22
50	44	66	44	21	66	06	58	05	62	68	15	54	35	02	42	35	48	96	32	14	52	41	52	48
22	66	22	15	86	26	63	75	41	99	58	42	36	72	24	58	37	52	18	51	03	37	18	39	11
96	24	40	14	51	23	22	30	88	57	95	67	47	29	83	94	69	40	06	07	18	16	36	78	86
31	73	91	61	19	60	20	72	93	48	98	57	07	23	69	65	95	39	69	58	56	80	30	19	44
78	60	73	99	84	43	89	94	36	45	56	69	47	07	41	90	22	91	07	12	78	35	34	08	72

```
96 52 02 00 34   93 07 54 41 30   44 97 77 98 31   94 09 09 36 06   39 35 79 30 60
39 32 80 38 83   56 81 62 60 89   27 95 21 24 99   26 08 77 54 11   25 07 42 21 98
18 52 59 59 88   29 99 55 74 93   56 08 57 93 71   13 92 63 14 09   84 90 16 30 67
64 14 63 47 13   54 44 80 89 07   48 11 12 82 11   54 32 55 47 96   80 98 72 49 39
01 63 86 01 22   56 14 13 53 56   19 82 88 99 43   74 04 18 70 54   82 05 67 63 66

60 93 27 49 87   03 81 33 14 94   77 60 30 89 25   86 67 44 76 45   92 18 80 97 94
34 58 56 05 38   09 38 74 76 98   09 18 71 47 75   63 93 49 94 42   26 79 50 18 26
45 91 78 94 29   19 19 52 90 52   57 15 35 20 01   68 08 48 90 23   80 23 70 47 59
48 34 14 98 42   73 94 95 32 14   45 45 15 34 54   42 29 15 83 55   76 35 46 60 96
76 33 30 91 33   53 45 50 01 48   21 47 25 56 92   96 61 76 52 16   81 96 16 80 82

60 81 89 93 27   14 58 66 72 84   59 76 38 15 40   65 63 77 33 92   32 35 32 70 49
76 29 27 06 90   82 94 32 05 53   72 19 05 63 58   90 84 74 10 20   69 89 08 99 20
34 76 62 24 55   74 71 78 04 96   54 04 23 30 22   97 06 02 16 14   58 53 80 82 93
11 29 85 48 53   33 14 94 85 54   07 36 39 23 00   21 25 97 24 10   79 07 74 14 01
85 99 83 21 00   62 40 96 64 28   93 72 34 89 87   74 62 51 73 42   38 82 15 32 91

05 86 75 56 56   34 99 27 94 72   84 96 37 47 62   11 38 80 74 67   18 38 95 72 77
98 08 89 66 16   71 66 07 95 64   41 69 30 88 95   82 39 95 53 37   00 87 56 68 71
23 35 58 31 52   20 74 54 44 64   00 33 81 14 76   14 81 75 81 39   72 59 20 82 23
10 93 64 24 73   01 98 03 02 79   05 88 80 91 32   20 28 57 79 02   74 36 97 46 22
70 98 89 79 03   35 33 80 20 92   13 82 40 44 71   56 06 31 37 58   18 24 54 38 08

56 23 48 60 65   39 92 13 13 27   65 35 46 71 78   83 03 34 24 88   00 80 82 43 50
61 08 07 87 97   13 68 29 95 83   45 48 62 88 61   57 29 10 86 87   22 79 98 03 05
90 10 59 83 68   29 32 70 67 13   08 43 71 30 10   36 92 50 38 23   95 60 62 89 73
37 67 28 15 19   81 86 91 71 66   96 83 60 17 69   93 30 29 31 01   33 84 40 31 59
84 36 07 10 55   53 51 35 37 93   02 49 84 18 79   75 38 51 21 29   95 90 46 20 71
```

Bibliography

Agresti A. (1996) *An introduction to categorical data analysis*. Wiley, New York.

Altman D.G., Machin D., Bryant T.N. & Gardner M.J. (2000) *Statistics with confidence*, 2nd edition. BMJ Books, London.

Ananth C.V. & Kleinbaum D.G. (2000) Regression models for ordinal responses: a review of methods and applications. *International Journal of Epidemiology* **26**: 1323–1333.

Antman E.M., Lau J., Kupelnick B., Mosteller F. & Chalmers T.C. (1992) A comparison of results of meta-analyses of randomized control trials and recommendations of clinical experts. Treatments for myocardial infarction. *JAMA* **268**: 240–248.

Armitage P. & Berry G. (2002) *Statistical methods in medical research*, 4th edition. Blackwell Science, Oxford.

Armstrong B.G. & Sloan M. (1989) Ordinal regression models for epidemiologic data. *American Journal of Epidemiology* **129**: 191–204.

Assmann S.F., Pocock S.J., Enos L.E. & Kasten L.E. (2001) Subgroup analysis and other (mis)uses of baseline data in clinical trials. *Lancet* **355**: 1064–1069.

Begg C., Cho M., Eastwood S., Horton R., Moher D., Olkin I. *et al.* (1996) Improving the quality of reporting of randomized controlled trials. The CONSORT statement. *JAMA* **276**: 637–639.

Begg C.B. & Mazumdar M. (1994) Operating characteristics of a rank correlation test for publication bias. *Biometrics* **50**: 1088–1101.

Bland J.M. & Altman D.G. (1986) Statistical methods for assessing agreement between two methods of clinical measurement. *Lancet* **i**: 307–310.

Bland J.M. & Altman D.G. (1995) Comparing methods of measurement: why plotting difference against standard method is misleading. *Lancet* **346**: 1085–1087.

Blomqvist N. (1977) On the relation between change and initial value. *Journal of The American Statistical Association* **72**: 746–749.

Breslow N.E. & Day N.E. (1980) *Statistical methods in cancer research. Volume 1 – The analysis of case–control studies*. International Agency for Research on Cancer, Lyon.

Breslow N.E. & Day N.E. (1987) *Statistical methods in cancer research. Volume II – The design and analysis of cohort studies*. International Agency for Research on Cancer, Lyon.

Bryk A.S. & Raudenbush S.W. (2001). *Hierarchical linear models*, 2nd edition. Sage Publications, Thousand Oaks.

Carpenter J. & Bithell J. (2000) Bootstrap confidence intervals: when, which, what? A practical guide for medical statisticians. *Statistics in Medicine* **19**: 1141–1164.

Christensen E., Neuberger J., Crowe J., Altman D.G., Popper H., Portmann B. et al. (1985) Beneficial effect of azathioprine and prediction of prognosis in primary biliary cirrhosis. Final results of an international trial. *Gastroenterology* **89**: 1084–1091.

Clarke M., Oxman A.D. (eds) *Cochrane Reviewers Handbook 4.1.5* [updated April 2002]. In: The Cochrane Library, Issue 2, 2002. Update Software, Oxford. Updated quarterly: available at http://www.cochrane.org/cochrane/hbook.htm.

Clarke R. & Croft P. (1998) *Critical reading for the reflective practitioner: a guide for primary care.* Butterworth Heinemann, Oxford.

Clayton D. & Hills M. (1993) *Statistical models in epidemiology.* Oxford University Press, Oxford.

Cochran W.G. (1954) Some methods for strengthening the common χ^2 tests. *Biometrics* **10**: 417–451.

Colditz G.A., Brewer T.F., Berkey C.S. et al. (1994) Efficacy of BCG vaccine in the prevention of tuberculosis. Meta-analysis of the published literature. *JAMA* **271**: 698–702.

Collett D. (2002) *Modelling binary data*, 2nd edition. Chapman & Hall, London.

Collett D. (2003) *Modelling survival data in medical research*, 2nd edition. Chapman & Hall, London.

Collins R., Yusuf S. & Peto R. (1985) Overview of randomised trials of diuretics in pregnancy. *British Medical Journal* **290**: 17–23.

Conover W.J. (1999) *Practical nonparametric statistics*, 3rd edition. Wiley, New York.

Cook D.J., Sackett D.L. & Spitzer W.O. (1995) Methodologic guidelines for systematic reviews of randomized control trials in health care from the Potsdam consultation on meta-analysis. *Journal of Clinical Epidemiology* **48**: 167–171.

Cox D.R. & Oakes D. (1984) *Analysis of survival data.* Chapman & Hall, London.

Crombie I.K. (1996) *The pocket guide to critical appraisal.* BMJ Books, London.

Davison A.V. & Hinkley D.V. (1997) *Bootstrap methods and their applications.* Cambridge University Press, Cambridge.

Donner A. & Klar N. (2000) *Design and analysis of cluster randomization trials in health research.* Arnold, London.

Draper N.R. & Smith H. (1998) *Applied regression analysis*, 3rd edition. Wiley, New York.

Dunn G. (1989) *Design and analysis of reliability studies.* Arnold, London.

DerSimonian R. & Laird N. (1986) Meta-analysis in clinical trials. *Controlled Clinical Trials* **7**: 177–188.

Efron B. & Tibshirani. R.J. (1993) *An introduction to the bootstrap.* Chapman & Hall, New York.

Egger M., Davey Smith G. & Altman D. (eds) (2001) *Systematic reviews in practice: meta-analysis in context.* BMJ Books, London.

Egger M., Davey Smith G., Schneider M. & Minder C. (1997a) Bias in meta-analysis detected by a simple, graphical test. *British Medical Journal* **315**: 629–634.

Egger M., Schneider M. & Davey Smith G. (1997b) Spurious precision? Meta-analysis of observational studies. *British Medical Journal* **316**: 140–144.

Elliott P., Wakefield J., Best N. & Briggs D. (eds.) (2000) *Spatial epidemiology.* Oxford University Press, Oxford.

Engels E.A., Schmid C.H., Terrin N.T., Olkin I. & Lau J. (2000) Heterogeneity and statistical significance in meta-analysis: an empirical study of 125 meta-analyses. *Statistics in Medicine* **19**: 1707–1828.

Everitt B. & Dunn G. (2001) *Applied multivariate data analysis*, 2nd edition. Arnold, London.

Fine P.E.M. (1995) Variation in protection by BCG: implications of and for heterologous immunity. *Lancet* **346**: 1339–1345.

Fisher R.A. & Yates F. (1963) *Statistical tables for biological, agricultural and medical research*, 6th edition. Oliver & Boyd, Edinburgh.

Fleiss J. (1981) *Statistical methods for rates and proportions*, 2nd edition. Wiley, New York.

Friedman L.M., Furberg C. & Demets D.L. (1998) *Fundamentals of clinical trials*. Springer-Verlag, New York.

Frost C. & Thompson S.G. (2000) Correcting for regression dilution bias: comparison of methods for a single predictor variable. *Journal of the Royal Statistical Society A* **163**: 173–189.

Goldstein H. (1995) *Multilevel statistical models*, 2nd edition. Arnold, London. Also available for downloading from http://www.arnoldpublishers.com/support/goldstein.htm.

Gordis L. (2000) *Epidemiology*, 2nd edition. W.B. Saunders, Philadelphia.

Greenhalgh T. (2000) *How to read a paper: the basics of evidence based medicine*. BMJ Books, London.

Gulliford M.C., Ukoumunne O.C. & Chinn S. (1999) Components of variance and intraclass correlations for the design of community-based surveys and intervention studies: data from the Health Survey for England 1994. *American Journal of Epidemiology* **149**: 876–883.

Hayes R.J. (1988) Methods for assessing whether change depends on initial value. *Statistics in Medicine* **7**: 915–927.

Hayes R.J. & Bennet S. (1999) Simple sample size calculation for cluster-randomized trials. *International Journal of Epidemiology* **28**: 319–326.

Hernán M.A., Hernández-Diaz S., Werler M.M. & Mitchell A.A. (2002) Causal knowledge as a prerequisite for confounding evaluation: an application to birth defects epidemiology. *American Journal of Epidemiology* **155**: 176–184.

Hosmer D.W. & Lemeshow S. (2000) *Applied logistic regression*. Wiley, New York.

Huber P.J. (1967) The behaviour of maximum likelihood estimates under nonstandard conditions. In: *Proceedings of the fifth Berkeley symposium on mathematical statistics and probability*, 221–233. University of California, Berkeley.

Huxley R., Neil A. & Collins R. (2002) Unravelling the fetal origins hypothesis: is there really an association between birthweight and subsequent blood pressure? *Lancet* **360**: 659–665.

Kalbfleisch J.D. & Prentice R.L. (1980) *The statistical analysis of failure time data*. Wiley, New York.

Kirkwood B.R., Cousens S.N., Victora C.G. & de Zoysa I. (1997) Issues in the design and interpretation of studies to evaluate the impact of community-based interventions. *Tropical Medicine and International Health* **2**: 1022–1029.

Kleinbaum D.G. (1996) *Survival analysis*. Springer-Verlag, New York.

Liang K.Y. & Zeger S.L. (1986) Longitudinal data analysis using generalized linear models. *Biometrika* **72**: 13–22.

Magder L.S. & Hughes J.P. (1997) Logistic regression when the outcome is measured with uncertainty. *American Journal of Epidemiology* **146**: 195–203.

Moher D., Cook D.J., Eastwood S., Olkin I., Rennie D. & Stroup D.F. (1999) Improving the quality of reports of meta-analyses of randomised controlled trials: the QUOROM statement. Quality of Reporting of Meta-analyses. *Lancet* **354**: 1896–1900.

Moher D., Dulberg C.S. & Wells G.A. (1994) Statistical power, sample size, and their reporting in randomized controlled trials. *JAMA* **272**: 122–124.

Moher D., Schulz K.F. & Altman D. (2001) The CONSORT statement: revised recommendations for improving the quality of reports of parallel-group randomized trials. *JAMA* **285**: 1987–1991.

Murray C.J.L. & Lopez A.D. (eds) (1996) *The global burden of disease.* Harvard University Press, Cambridge, MA.

Oakes M. (1986) *Statistical inference.* Wiley, Chichester.

Oldham P.D. (1962) A note on the analysis of repeated measurements of the same subjects. *Journal of Chronic Diseases* **15**: 969.

Pearson E.S. & Hartley H.O. (1966) *Biometrika tables for statisticians*, Volume 1, 3rd edition. Cambridge University Press, Cambridge.

Phillips A.N. & Davey Smith G. (1991) How independent are "independent" effects? Relative risk estimation when correlated exposures are measured imprecisely. *Journal of Clinical Epidemiology* **44**: 1223–1231.

Phillips A.N. & Davey Smith G. (1993) The design of prospective epidemiological studies: more subjects or better measurements? *Journal of Clinical Epidemiology* **46**: 1203–1211.

Pocock S.J. (1983) *Clinical trials: a practical approach.* Wiley, Chichester.

Robins J.M., Breslow N. & Greenland S. (1986). Estimators of the Mantel–Haenszel variance consistent in both sparse data and large-strata limiting models. *Biometrics* **42**: 311–323.

Robins J.M. & Tsiatis A.A. (1991) Correcting for non-compliance in randomized trials using rank preserving structural failure time models. *Communications in Statistics Theory and Methods* **20**: 2609–2631.

Rodrigues L. & Kirkwood B.R. (1990) Case–control designs in the study of common diseases: updates on the demise of the rare disease assumption and the choice of sampling scheme for controls. *International Journal of Epidemiology* **19**: 205–213.

Rothman K.J. (2002) *Epidemiology: an introduction.* Oxford University Press, New York.

Rothman K.J. & Greenland S. (1998) *Modern epidemiology*, 2nd edition. Lippincott Williams & Wilkins, Philadelphia.

Royall R.M. (1997) *Statistical evidence – a likelihood paradigm.* Chapman & Hall, London.

Royston P. (1993) A toolkit for testing for non-normality in complete and censored samples. *The Statistician* **42**: 37–43.

Sackett D.L., Straus S., Richardson W.S., Rosenberg W. & Haynes R.B. (2000) *Evidence-based medicine: how to practice and teach EBM*, 2nd edition. Churchill Livingstone, Edinburgh.

Schlesselman J.J. & Stolley P.D. (1982) *Case–control studies: design, conduct, analysis.* Oxford University Press, New York.

Schulz K.F., Chalmers I., Hayes R.J. & Altman D.G. (1995) Empirical evidence of bias. Dimensions of methodological quality associated with estimates of treatment effects in controlled trials. *JAMA* **273**: 408–412.

Shapiro S.S. & Wilk M.B. (1965) An analysis of variance test for normality (complete samples). *Biometrika* **52**: 591–611.

Siegel S. & Castellan, N.J. (1988) *Nonparametric statistics for the behavioral sciences.* McGraw-Hill, New York.

Silagy C. & Haines A. (2001) *Evidence based practice in primary health care.* BMJ Books, London.

Smith P.G. & Day N.E. (1984) The design of case-control studies: the influence of confounding and interaction effects. *International Journal of Epidemiology*, **13**: 356–365.

Smith P.G. & Morrow R. (1996) *Field trials of health interventions in developing countries.* Macmillan, London.

Smith P.G., Rodrigues L.C. & Fine P.E.M. (1984) Assessment of the protective efficacy of vaccines against common diseases using case-control and cohort studies. *International Journal of Epidemiology* **13**: 87–93.

Snedecor G.W. & Cochran W.G. (1989) *Statistical methods*, 8th edition. Iowa State University Press, Iowa.

Sprent P. & Smeeton N.C. (2000) *Applied nonparametric statistical methods*, 3rd edition. Chapman & Hall, London.

Sterne J.A.C. & Davey Smith G. (2001) Sifting the evidence – what's wrong with significance tests? *British Medical Journal* **322**: 226–231.

Sterne J.A.C. & Egger M. (2001) Funnel plots for detecting bias in meta-analysis: guidelines on choice of axis. *Journal of Clinical Epidemiology* **54**: 1046–1055.

Sterne J.A.C., Gavaghan D. & Egger M. (2000) Publication and related bias in meta-analysis: power of statistical tests and prevalence in the literature. *Journal of Clinical Epidemiology* **53**: 1119–1129.

Szklo M. & Nieto F.J. (2000) *Epidemiology: beyond the basics.* Aspen, Maryland.

Thompson S.G. & Barber J.A. (2000) How should cost data in pragmatic randomised trials be analysed? *British Medical Journal* **320**: 1197–1200.

Ukoumunne O.C., Gulliford M.C., Chinn S., Sterne J.A.C. & Burney P.G. (1999) Methods for evaluating area-wide and organisation-based interventions in health and health care: a systematic review. *Health Technology Assessment* **3**: 1–92. Available at http://www.hta.nhsweb.nhs.uk.

Victora C.G., Huttly S.R., Fuchs S.C. & Olinto T.A. (1997) The role of conceptual frameworks in epidemiological analysis: a hierarchical approach. *International Journal of Epidemiology* **26**: 224–227.

Weisberg S. (1985) *Applied linear regression.* Wiley, New York.

White H. (1980) A heteroskedasticity-consistent covariance matrix estimator and a direct test for heteroskedasticity. *Econometrica* **48**: 817–830.

White I., Frost C. & Tokanuga S. (2001) Correcting for measurement error in binary and continuous variables using replicates. *Statistics in Medicine* **20**: 3441–3457.

White I.R., Walker S. & Babiker A. (2002). strbee: randomization-based efficacy estimator. *Stata Journal* **2**: 140–150.

White J., Yeats A. & Skipworth G. (1979) *Tables for statisticians*, 3rd edition. Stanley Thornes, Cheltenham.

WHO Expert Committee on physical status. (1995) *The use and interpretation of anthropometry*. WHO Technical Report Series, no. 854, Geneva.

Zeger S.L. & Liang KY. (1986) Longitudinal data analysis for discrete and continuous outcomes. *Biometrics* 1986; **42**: 121–130.

Index

SUMMARY GUIDE TO METHODS OF ANALYSIS: II

BINARY OUTCOME VARIABLE	Section
Single exposure group	
Proportion, with confidence interval	15.5
Test that the proportion has a particular value	15.6
Odds, with confidence interval	16.7
Two exposure groups	
Measures of exposure effect:	
Difference between proportions (risk difference)	16.3
Risk ratio	16.4, 16.5
Odds ratio	16.6, 16.7
χ^2 test for 2×2 tables	17.2
Exact test for small samples	17.3
Logistic regression	19.2
More than two exposure groups	
χ^2 test for $r \times 2$ tables	17.4
Logistic regression with indicator variables	19.4
Ordered or numerical exposure variable	
χ^2 test for trend	17.5
Logistic regression	19.5
Multiple exposure variables (control of confounding)	
Mantel–Haenszel method	18.4
Logistic regression	20.2
Regression analysis of risk ratios	20.4
Direct standardization of proportions	25.2
Paired or matched measurements	
Comparison of two proportions	21.2
Odds ratios and McNemar's χ^2 test	21.3
Conditional logistic regression	21.5

CATEGORICAL OUTCOME VARIABLE WITH MORE THAN TWO LEVELS

χ^2 test for larger tables	17.4
Multinomial logistic regression	20.5
Ordinal logistic regression	20.5

(Continued from inside front cover)